Biopharmaceutics of Ocular Drug Delivery

Edited by
Peter Edman, Ph.D.

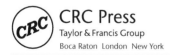

CRC Press
Taylor & Francis Group
Boca Raton London New York

CRC Press is an imprint of the
Taylor & Francis Group, an **informa** business

CRC Press
Taylor & Francis Group
6000 Broken Sound Parkway NW, Suite 300
Boca Raton, FL 33487-2742

Reissued 2019 by CRC Press

© 1993 by Taylor & Francis Group, LLC
CRC Press is an imprint of Taylor & Francis Group, an Informa business

No claim to original U.S. Government works

A Library of Congress record exists under LC control number:

Publisher's Note
The publisher has gone to great lengths to ensure the quality of this reprint but points out that some imperfections in the original copies may be apparent.

Disclaimer
The publisher has made every effort to trace copyright holders and welcomes correspondence from those they have been unable to contact.

ISBN 13: 978-0-367-24859-8 (hbk)
ISBN 13: 978-0-367-24865-9 (pbk)
ISBN 13: 978-0-429-28475-5 (ebk)

Visit the Taylor & Francis Web site at http://www.taylorandfrancis.com and the CRC Press Web site at http://www.crcpress.com

DEDICATED TO DINNE, ELIN, AND OSCAR

PHARMACOLOGY AND TOXICOLOGY: BASIC AND CLINICAL ASPECTS

Mannfred A. Hollinger, Series Editor
University of California, Davis

Published Titles
Inflammatory Cells and Mediators in Bronchial Asthma,
  Devendra K. Agrawal and Robert G. Townley
Pharmacology of the Skin, Hasan Mukhtar
The Basis of Toxicity Testing, Donald H. Ecobichon
In Vitro *Methods of Toxicology,* Ronald R. Watson

Forthcoming Titles
Alcohol Consumption, Cancer, and Birth Defects, Anthony J. Garro
Beneficial and Toxic Effects of Aspirin, Susan E. Feinman
Classical Receptor Theory, Terry P. Kenakin
Human Drug Metabolism from Molecular Biology to Man, Elizabeth Jeffreys
Neural Control of Airways, Peter J. Barnes
PAF Receptor Signal Mechanisms, Shivendra D. Shukla
Placental Pharmacology, B. B. Rama Sastry
Placental Toxicology, B. B. Rama Sastry
Preclinical and Clinical Modulation of Anticancer Drug Toxicity, Kennth D. Tew,
  Peter Houghton, and Janet Houghton
Rational Drug Design, Davis B. Weiner and William V. Williams

CONTENTS

Series Preface   vi
Preface   vii
The Editor   ix
Contributors   x

1. Anatomy and Physiology of the Eye. Physiological Aspects of Ocular
      Drug Therapy   1
    Johan Stjernschantz and Maria Astin

2. Formulation of Ophthalmic Solutions and Suspensions.
      Problems and Advantages   27
    Marc M. M. Van Ooteghem

3. The Effects of Preservatives on Corneal Permeability of Drugs   43
    Keith Green

4. Solid Polymeric Inserts/Disks as Drug Delivery Devices   61
    Marco Fabrizio Saettone

5. The Development and Use of *In Situ* Formed Gels, Triggered by pH   81
    Robert Gurny, Houssam Ibrahim, and Pierre Buri

6. Liposomes and Nanoparticles as Ocular Drug Delivery Systems   91
    Michael Mezei and Dale Meisner

7. Use of Hyaluronic Acid in Ocular Therapy   105
    Stéphanie F. Bernatchez, Ola Camber, Cyrus Tabatabay,
      and Robert Gurny

8. Improved Ocular Drug Delivery by Use of Chemical
      Modification (Prodrugs)   121
    Vincent H. L. Lee

9. Bioadhesives in Ocular Drug Delivery   145
    Eliot M. Slovin and Joseph R. Robinson

10. Pharmacokinetics in Ocular Drug Delivery   159
    Ronald D. Schoenwald

Index   193

SERIES PREFACE

The series, *Pharmacology and Toxicology: Basic and Clinical Aspects,* has been created in recognition of the fact that, from time to time, a new area of interest within a discipline matures to a critical mass that merits organization and integration of the respective observations into a free-standing monograph. In order for such an undertaking to be successful, each editor and/or author must be qualified to identify and select sources best suited to communicate essential aspects of that subject. Such is the case with this volume of the series, *Biopharmaceutics of Ocular Drug Delivery.* Dr. Edman has assembled a list of international contributors whose expertise in their respective areas is well known. They have succeeded in organizing the relevant subject matter in such a way that the monograph will be of extreme value to anyone interested in ocular drug delivery.

Mannfred A. Hollinger, Ph.D.
Series Editor
Professor and Chair
Department of Medical Pharmacology and Toxicology
University of California, Davis
Davis, California

PREFACE

Administration of drugs to the eye is a difficult topic. There are several factors which have to be considered before an optimal ocular pharmaceutical formulation can be done. A good understanding of anatomy and physiology is necessary. Knowledge about tear flow dynamics and pharmacokinetical behavior of drugs in the eye is also necessary. The purpose of this book is to give the reader a good understanding of the problems associated with ocular drug delivery and also to highlight the promising research on new delivery systems for improved drug therapy. The contributing authors are all leading scientists in the ophthalmic area and in their chapters they have summarized and reviewed the current state-of-the-art in each research area.

The book starts with a brief overview and updating of the main knowledge involved in formulation and usage of ophthalmic solutions and suspensions. Influence of surfactants and preservatives on ocular drug absorption is also deeply discussed. A large part of the book is devoted to new drug delivery systems, e.g., new pharmaceutical vehicles, inserts, liposomes, nanoparticles, and prodrugs. Ocular drug delivery is a difficult field that changes rapidly, but it is my hope that this book can be a starting point for biopharmaceutical scientists interested in expanding the knowledge within this area.

Peter Edman

THE EDITOR

Peter Edman, Ph.D., is Director of the Pharmaceutical Department at Astra Draco AB at Lund, Sweden. Dr. Edman obtained his training at the University of Uppsala, Sweden, receiving the M.S.Pharm. degree in 1977 and the Ph.D. degree in Pharmaceutical Biochemistry in 1981. He became an Associate Professor of Pharmaceutical Biochemistry in 1986 and Professor in Pharmaceutics/Drug Formulation in 1988.

While working as an academician Dr. Edman has had positions as Section Leader in the Pharmaceutical Division of the Swedish Medical Products Agency (1983 to 1985) and Director of Pharmaceutical Research and Development at Pharmacia AB in Uppsala (1985 to 1991). His current research interests are in new drug delivery systems, especially those intended for nasal and ocular use. Parenteral administration of microspheres as a targeting system for drugs is another topic where he has published several research articles.

Dr. Edman has authored a number of scientific publications, reviews, and book chapters and directed several M.S. and Ph.D. students. He is a member of the Board of the Pharmaceutical and Biopharmaceutical Section of the Swedish Academy of Pharmaceutical Sciences. He is also a member of the Controlled Release Society and the International Association for Pharmaceutical Technology (APV).

CONTRIBUTORS

Maria Astin, M.Sc.
Research Associate
Glaucoma Research Laboratories
Kabi Pharmacia Ophthalmics
Uppsala, Sweden

Stéphanie F. Bernatchez, M.Sc.
Doctoral Student
School of Pharmacy
University of Geneva
Geneva, Switzerland

Pierre Buri, Ph.D.
Professor
School of Pharmacy
University of Geneva
Geneva, Switzerland

Ola Camber, Ph.D.
Director
Pharmaceutical Research and
  Development
Kabi Pharmacia Therapeutics
Uppsala, Sweden

Keith Green, Ph.D., D.Sc.
Regents' Professor
Department of Ophthalmology
Medical College of Georgia
Augusta, Georgia

Robert Gurny, Ph.D.
Professor
School of Pharmacy
University of Geneva
Geneva, Switzerland

Houssam Ibrahim, Ph.D.
Manager
Debiopharm S.A.
Lausanne, Switzerland

Vincent H. L. Lee, Ph.D.
Professor and Chairman
Department of Pharmaceutical Sciences
School of Pharmacy
University of Southern California
Los Angeles, California

Dale Meisner, Ph.D.
Senior Research Scientist
Department of Pharmaceutical Research
  and Development
Merck Frosst Canada, Inc.
Pointe Claire-Dorval, Quebec, Canada

Michael Mezei, Ph.D.
Professor
College of Pharmacy
Dalhousie University
Halifax, Nova Scotia, Canada

Marc M. M. Van Ooteghem, Ph.D.
Professor
Department of Pharmaceutics
College of Pharmaceutical Sciences
University of Antwerp
Antwerp, Belgium

Joseph R. Robinson, Ph.D.
Professor
School of Pharmacy
University of Wisconsin
Madison, Wisconsin

Marco Fabrizio Saettone, Ph.D.
Professor
Department of Pharmaceutical
  Technology/Biopharmaceutics
Institute of Pharmaceutical Chemistry
University of Pisa
Pisa, Italy

Ronald D. Schoenwald, Ph.D.
Professor
Division of Pharmaceutics
College of Pharmacy
University of Iowa
Iowa City, Iowa

Eliot M. Slovin, M.S.
Research Assistant
School of Pharmacy
University of Wisconsin
Madison, Wisconsin

Johan Stjernschantz, M.D., Ph.D.
Director
Glaucoma Research Laboratories
Kabi Pharmacia Ophthalmics
Uppsala, Sweden

Cyrus Tabatabay, M.D.
Privat Docent
School of Pharmacy
University of Geneva
Geneva, Switzerland

Chapter 1

ANATOMY AND PHYSIOLOGY OF THE EYE. PHYSIOLOGICAL ASPECTS OF OCULAR DRUG THERAPY

Johan Stjernschantz and Maria Astin

TABLE OF CONTENTS

I.   General Introduction 2

II. A Practical Approach to the Anatomy and Physiology of the Eye 3
    A.   The Anterior Segment of the Eye 3
        1.   The Cornea 3
        2.   The Conjunctiva and the Eyelids.................................. 5
        3.   The Lacrimal Apparatus 7
        4.   The Anterior Uvea, the Chamber System, and the
            Chamber Angle 9
            a.   The Ciliary Body....................................... 10
            b.   The Iris.. 12
            c.   The Trabecular Meshwork and Schlemm's Canal 13
            d.   The Intraocular Pressure................................ 13
        5.   The Lens... 14
    B.   The Posterior Segment of the Eye..................................... 15
        1.   The Retina and the Optic Nerve 15
        2.   The Vitreous... 17
        3.   The Choroid and the Sclera..................................... 17
        4.   Extraocular Orbital Structures................................... 18

III. Physiological Aspects of Ocular Drug Therapy 19
    A.   Eye Tissues as Barriers in Ocular Drug Delivery....................... 19
    B.   Importance of Aqueous Humor Drainage and Ciliary
        Epithelium Organic Anion Pump System............................. 19
    C.   Inaccessibility of Drugs to the Vitreous 20
    D.   The Cornea and the Vitreous as Drug Reservoirs....................... 20
    E.   Consensual Eye Responses 21
    F.   Importance of Autacoids and Neuropeptides in Drug Responses
        of the Eye 22

Acknowledgments.. 22

References.. 22

I. GENERAL INTRODUCTION

The eye is a unique organ, from an anatomical and physiological point of view, in that it contains several highly different structures with specific physiological functions. For instance, the cornea and the crystalline lens are the only tissues in the body in addition to cartilage which have no blood supply, whereas the choroid and the ciliary processes are highly vascularized and exhibit very high blood flows. The retina with the optic nerve, an extension of the diencephalon of the central nervous system, has a very specific function in the visual perception and transduction phenomena. The high demand of absence of light scattering in the various media of the optical pathway to achieve good visual acuity has resulted in a particular symmetrical organization of collagen fibrils in the cornea and of lens fibers in the crystalline lens. Furthermore, the aqueous humor normally contains no cells and the protein content of it is very low. Finally, the vitreous is a semisolid hydrogel with few cells scattered in it.

The embryologic development of the eye starts by outpocketings from the forebrain, the so-called optic vesicles which get in contact with the surface ectoderm (Figure 1). The contact between the optic vesicle and the ectoderm induces the formation of a lens placode which subsequently develops into the crystalline lens. At a very early stage the invagination of the optic vesicle also starts (Figure 1). The invagination leads to two membranes opposing each other and extending all around the globe from the edge of the iris at the pupil. The inner layer develops into the neural part of the retina and the outer layer develops into the pigment epithelium. These two layers can also be found in the ciliary body, the inner layer corresponding to the neural part of the retina being the nonpigmented epithelial cell layer and the outer layer corresponding to the retinal pigment epithelium being the pigment epithelium of the ciliary processes.

The epithelium of the posterior part of the iris contains both cell layers which are deeply pigmented. Curiously enough, the sphincter muscle and the dilator muscle of the iris develop from the epithelium and thus are of neuroectodermal origin. In contrast to this, the ciliary muscle and practically all of the muscles in the body are of mesodermal origin. The cornea and the conjunctiva derive from the surface ectoderm. Generally, the sclera surrounding the eye is regarded as equivalent to the dura mater of the brain, whereas the choroid has been compared with pia mater of the brain. Both the sclera and the choroid originate from the mesenchyme surrounding the developing eye.

A great problem in ophthalmic research is constituted by the fact that marked species differences exist even between higher vertebrates such as mammals. Thus, the rabbit eye, which is often used as a model in anterior segment pharmacology and pharmaceutic delivery research, differs in many respects from the human eye. In the rabbit, for example, the ciliary muscle is poorly developed, almost rudimentary, and consequently cholinergic agonists as a rule have very little effect on the intraocular pressure in this species. The rabbit retina is virtually avascular with only a small wing shaped area being vascularized. The rabbit blinks only about 5 times per hour which is in sharp contrast to the human eye. Therefore, the kinetics of drugs applied on the surface of the rabbit eye may be quite different from that of drugs applied on the human eye. The outflow system of aqueous humor in the eyes of rabbits, cats, and dogs is also somewhat different from that in primates, including humans, in that in the former species no canal of Schlemm exists.

In many animal species (e.g., the rabbit and the cat) there is a nictitating membrane which is missing from the human and other primate eyes. The nictitating membrane may affect drug kinetics because it will absorb many substances and may serve as a depot. The lacrimal gland also differs between species. Animals with a nictitating membrane have an accessory lacrimal gland called Harder's gland at the inner corner of the eye. In most monkeys

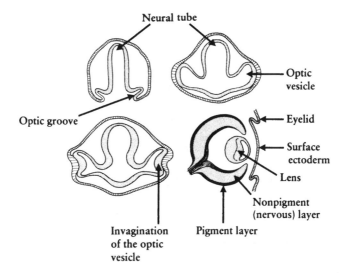

FIGURE 1.   Embryologic development of the eye.

the bulbar conjunctiva is pigmented, a fact that may affect drug kinetics. Finally, in lower animal species, such as rats and mice, the eye may not be ideal as a model since the crystalline lens occupies most of the globe. Thus, even if many of the animal models for studying anterior segment pharmacology from a technical point of view are quite satisfactory, extrapolation of results from these models to the human eye may in fact be very difficult. An example of this is the variety of responses that can be obtained with neuropeptides and autacoids in the mammalian eye, differing markedly between species.

II. A PRACTICAL APPROACH TO THE ANATOMY AND PHYSIOLOGY OF THE EYE

The intention of this chapter is to give a condensed general view of the anatomy and physiology of the eye much from the perspective of ocular drug delivery. Consequently, most of the attention is focused on the anterior segment of the eye. Even so, the approach has to be very practical and therefore only the most essential facts have been included. Entire books have been published on the cornea, the anatomy of the eye, the physiology of the eye, etc.; the reader is kindly referred to these for more comprehensive information.

A. THE ANTERIOR SEGMENT OF THE EYE
Generally, the anterior segment of the eye comprises the cornea, conjunctiva, iris, ciliary body, the anterior and posterior chambers, and the lens. In addition, the lacrimal apparatus and the eyelids will be included in this concept. The posterior segment of the eye refers to the parts of the eye which are situated behind the lens.

1. The Cornea
The cornea is the anteriormost transparent membrane of the eye continuing posteriorly as the sclera. The border between the nontransparent sclera and the cornea is called the limbus. In the human eye the cornea has a refractive power of approximately 43 diopters and accounts for about 70% of the refractive power of the eye. The thickness of the human cornea is about 0.57 mm in the central part. In the periphery the cornea is somewhat thicker. Normally there are no blood vessels in the cornea. The peripheral parts of the cornea get

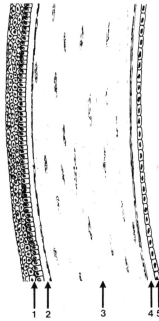

1. Epithelium

2. Bowman's membrane

3. Stroma

4. Descemet's membrane

5. Endothelium

FIGURE 2.   Section through the cornea. Basement membrane of the epithelium is not shown.

oxygen and nutrition from the capillaries of the limbal area. The rest of the cornea is probably nourished primarily by the aqueous humor, but most of the oxygen originates from the lacrimal film. In certain diseases the cornea may become vascularized.

The cornea consists of five layers, the epithelium, Bowman's membrane, the stroma, Descemet's membrane, and the endothelium (Figure 2). In addition to these layers there is a basement membrane of the epithelium, which is situated between the epithelial cell layer and Bowman's membrane. The epithelial cell layer consists of five or six layers of cells. The most superficial of these layers consists of squamous cells similar to those of the skin except for not being keratinized. There are numerous microvilli protruding into the lacrimal film from these cells. It is believed that these microvilli together with the glycocalix attached to the cells retard the tear fluid, thus preventing the cells from drying. The innermost epithelial cell layer, the germinal layer, is columnar in shape. An important feature of the superficial cell layers is the junctional complexes between adjacent cells. Tight junctions surround the entire cell.[1] Water soluble molecules with low lipophilicity which do not to any greater extent traverse cell membranes are markedly hindered by these junctional complexes and therefore pass poorly into the epithelium. Typically, sodium fluorescein, a very water soluble substance, is used as a diagnostic tool to study the integrity of the superficial epithelial cell layers. Staining indicates that the tight junctions have broken up and that there is direct access of this hydrophilic molecule to the cornea.

The corneal epithelium contains large amounts of acetylcholine and choline esterases.[2] The acetylcholine resides in the epithelial cells primarily; these cells also exhibit choline acetyltransferase and acetylcholine esterase. The physiological function of acetylcholine in the corneal epithelium is not known.[2] An interesting consequence of the presence of esterases in the corneal epithelium is that these enzymes can be utilized in the delivery of esterified prodrugs to the eye. Such prodrugs comprise, e.g., dipivalyl epinephrine and prostaglandin esters which are efficiently hydrolyzed in the corneal epithelium.[3]

Bowman's membrane is a thin structure consisting of a fibrillar material, probably mainly collagen. It contains no cells and the membrane is found only in the eyes of human and other primates. The stroma of the cornea consists of many parallel lamellae containing primarily collagen fibrils, organized in such a way that the collagen fibrils in two adjacent lamellae are perpendicular to each other. This high degree of geometrical symmetry is very important because in such a lattice system of collagen fibrils, light scattering is eliminated by interference between the adjacent fibrils.[4] The corneal stroma contains about 75 to 80% water based on wet weight. Glycosaminoglycans can be found between the collagen fibrils. The glycosaminoglycans are mainly keratan sulfate, chondroitin, and chondroitin sulfate A. The glycosaminoglycans, being negatively charged, play a certain role in corneal hydration since they interact with water and electrolytes. The corneal stroma also contains some albumin, which probably originates from the blood vessels at the limbus. Keratocytes, cells reminiscent of fibrocytes, are important in the turnover of collagen and in the metabolism of the stroma. While lipophilicity promotes penetration through the epithelial cell layer, water soluble drugs penetrate the corneal stroma more effectively.

Descemet's membrane is the basement membrane of the endothelial cells. The corneal endothelium is a single cell layer facing the anterior chamber. The cells cover entirely Descemet's membrane, and if cells are lost the adjacent cells enlarge to compensate for the cells lost. The posterior cell membrane of the endothelial cells seems to be covered by a viscous substance, probably hyaluronic acid,[5] which increases wettability of the lipid membrane. In the newborn there are about 4000 cells per square millimeter, but in the endothelium of adult persons the cell density is only 1400 to 2500 per square millimeter. It is generally accepted that the endothelial cells do not divide in primates, and although this may be a misconception there is certainly very little mitotic activity, which is not enough to compensate for the loss due to aging and, e.g., trauma. In some animal species, such as the rabbit, the endothelial cells of the cornea divide. The endothelial cells have a very important function because they transfer bicarbonate and sodium ions into the aqueous humor, thus being the most important factor in the regulation of corneal hydration. There is also a chloride transport into the tear fluid from the epithelium that contributes to the regulation of corneal hydration.[6] If the endothelial cell density falls below a critical range of 400 to 700 per square millimeter decompensation follows, leading to edema in the stroma. Although there are tight junctions between the endothelial cells, this layer is more leaky than the superficial epithelial cell layers.[6] Most drugs readily penetrate the endothelial cell layer from the stroma.

The cornea is one of the most densely innervated tissues with respect to nociceptive sensory input. These nerves derive via the ophthalmic branch from the trigeminal ganglion. The nerves form a subepithelial plexus from which nerve fibers penetrate Bowman's membrane and directly supply the epithelial cell layer. Neuropeptides, such as substance P,[7] have been found in the sensory nerves of the cornea. Adrenergic nerves have also been demonstrated in the cornea subepithelially, but the exact function of these nerves, if any, is obscure. Trophic factors or neuropeptides released from the sensory nerves in the cornea, on the other hand, may have an important function because in situations with interference of the ophthalmic branch of the fifth cranial nerve a neurotrophic keratitis may develop.

2. The Conjunctiva and the Eyelids

The conjunctiva can be regarded as a mucous membrane covering the inner surface of the eyelids and the visible part of the sclera. The conjunctiva is usually divided into three parts: the palpebral conjunctiva, the forniceal conjunctiva, and the bulbar conjunctiva (see Figure 3). In addition, there are two special parts of the conjunctiva: the plica semilunaris and the caruncle in the nasal corner of the eye. The plica semilunaris is a rudiment of the nictitating membrane that is found in many animals, e.g., rabbits and cats.

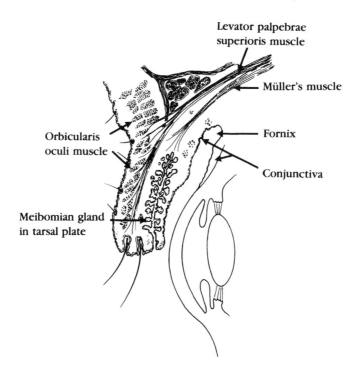

FIGURE 3. Schematic picture of the conjunctiva and the upper eyelid; only major structures are indicated, proportions distorted.

The conjunctival epithelium consists of a stratified columnar epithelium, which is not keratinized. At the limbus and the mucocutaneous junction on the eyelid margin the cells are squamous instead of columnar in shape. The cells of the superficial layer have numerous microvilli which are covered by a glycocalix and mucin. The mucin originates from goblet cells, which are dispersed in great quantity in the conjunctiva. In the basal cell layer melanocytes and Langerhans' cells can be found. Keratinization of the epithelium is pathological and is found in certain diseases, such as severe dry eye syndrome and ocular pemphigoid, and after chemical injuries. The thickness of the epithelium varies in different parts of the conjunctiva. In addition to blood vessels the conjunctiva also contains lymph vessels. The conjunctiva is innervated mainly by sensory nerves originating in the trigeminal ganglion and by sympathetic nerves originating in the superior cervical sympathetic ganglion.

The eyelids consist of four main layers: the skin, the muscle layer, a layer of fibrous tissue or the tarsus, and the conjunctiva (Figure 3). The skin of the eyelids is very thin. Some sweat glands can be found in the skin. The eyelid margin contains cilia (eyelashes). Special glands are situated close to the follicles of the cilia and empty their secretion into the follicles. These are called the glands of Zeis and are modified sebaceous glands that lubricate the eyelashes. The glands of Moll, a type of sweat glands, frequently also empty into the eyelash follicles. The exact function of the glands of Moll is not known.

There are three main muscles in the upper eyelid: the orbicularis oculi muscle, the levator palpebrae superioris muscle, and Müller's muscle. In the lower eyelid the levator palpebrae superioris muscle is missing. Except for Müller's muscle these muscles are of the striated type. The levator palpebrae muscle is innervated by the oculomotor nerve, and the orbicularis oculi muscle by the facial nerve. Müller's muscle is a smooth muscle innervated by the sympathetic nervous system. The striated muscles are used for closing and opening of the

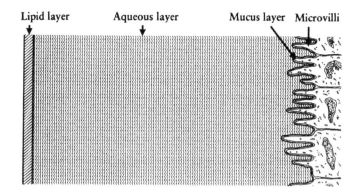

Lipid layer   Aqueous layer   Mucus layer Microvilli

FIGURE 4. The tear film.

eye; the exact function of Müller's muscle is not known, but loss of sympathetic tone causes ptosis, a decrease in palpebral fissure, whereas stimulation of Müller's muscle (e.g., by certain sympathomimetics) causes an increase in the palpebral fissure.

The fibrous layer forms the tarsus of the eyelids. The tarsus contains collagen and some elastic fibers. The meibomian glands are located in the tarsus (Figure 3) and are large sebaceous glands. They are the largest glands in the eyelids. They empty through orifices in the lid margin. The secretions of the meibomian glands form the superficial lipid layer of the tear film.

Normally a human being blinks about 15 times per minute. However, there is a large variation between individuals in blinking frequency. The blinking frequency also varies in different situations in the same individual. Some animals may blink only a few times per hour (e.g., the rabbit), while others (e.g., some monkeys) blink up to 45 times per minute. Various stimuli (e.g., tactile, optic, and auditory stimuli) cause reflex blinking.

3. The Lacrimal Apparatus

Good visual function requires the surface of the eye to be covered by fluid to maintain a uniform surface. In addition, the tear fluid has a nutritional function as well as an anti-bacterial function. The tear fluid also lubricates the eye and washes away debris.

The tear film consists of three main layers, as depicted in Figure 4. The outermost layer is a thin lipid layer, which is derived from the Meibomian glands and possibly the glands of Zeis. The middle layer, which constitutes the tear fluid, is about 7 μm thick and is mainly secreted by the lacrimal gland but also by the accessory glands of Krause and Wolfring. Finally, the innermost layer is a mucoid layer mainly secreted by the goblet cells in the conjunctiva. Some mucin is also secreted by the lacrimal gland. It is generally considered that the mucin layer is important for wetting of the corneal and conjunctival epithelium. When the mucin is spread over the surface it makes the hydrophobic surface of the epithelium more hydrophilic and thus increases wettability.[8] The lipid layer reduces evaporation and also prevents overflow of the tear fluid onto the skin during blinking.

Up to 25% of the tear fluid is lost due to evaporation. The composition of human tears is shown in Table 1. It is particularly interesting that the tear fluid contains proteins with marked antibacterial activity (e.g., lysozyme and lactoferrin). Of the immunoglobulins, mainly IgG and IgA are found in the tear fluid. The pH of tears is usually between 7.3 and 7.7, normally around 7.4 (i.e., close to that of plasma). The osmotic pressure of tears equals about 0.9% saline (i.e., about the same as for plasma).

The lacrimal gland, which is responsible for most of the tear fluid secretion, is situated in the superior temporal angle of the orbit. The levator palpebrae superioris muscle divides

TABLE 1
Physical Properties and Chemical Composition of Human Tears

Physical Properties

Osmotic pressure	0.9% NaCl (300 mOsm/l)
pH	7.4 (7.3 to 7.7)
Refractive index	1.357
Volume	0.50 to 0.67 g/16 h (waking)

Electrolytes

Bicarbonate	26 mEq/l[a]
Chloride	120 to 135 mEq/l
Potassium	15 to 29 mEq/l
Sodium	142 mEq/l
Calcium	2.29 mg/100ml

Nitrogenous Substances

Total protein	0.669 to 0.800 g/100 ml
Albumin	0.394 g/100 ml
Globulin	0.275 g/100 ml
Ammonia	0.005 g/100 ml
Urea	0.04 mg/100 ml
Nitrogen	
Total nitrogen	158 mg/100 ml
Nonprotein nitrogen	51 mg/100 ml

Carbohydrates

Glucose	2.5 (0 to 5.0) mg/100 ml

Sterols

Cholesterol and cholesterol esters	8 to 32 mg/100 ml

Miscellaneous Organic Acids, Vitamins, Enzymes

Citric acid	0.6 mg/100 ml
Ascorbic acid	0.14 mg/100 ml
Lysozyme	1438 (viscosimetric) (800 to 2500) units/ml
Lactoferrin[b]	1.6 to 2.1 mg/ml

[a]   mEq/l = milliequivalents per liter.
[b]   Values obtained from References 77–79.

Partly adapted from Milder, B., *Adler's Physiology of the Eye*, C. V. Mosby, St. Louis, 1987. With permission.

the lacrimal gland into two parts: an orbital part and a palpebral part. The ducts from the gland empty into the upper temporal fornix of the conjunctiva. Some tear fluid is also secreted by the accessory lacrimal glands of Krause and the glands of Wolfring. These are situated at the upper fornix of the conjunctiva. Lacrimal secretion is regulated by motor nerves of facial nerve origin synapsing in the pterygopalatine ganglion, by sensory nerves originating in the trigeminal ganglion, and by sympathetic nerves originating in the superior cervical ganglion.

The tear fluid is spread over the surface of the eye during blinking. When the upper lid approaches the lower lid the tear fluid is forced nasally to end up at the eyelid lacrimal puncta, which are situated on the nasal part of the lid margins. The lacrimal puncta are connected to the lacrimal sac via the canaliculi. The lacrimal sac is drained through the nasolacrimal duct, which empties laterally to the inferior nasal choncha.

The normal tear flow in human beings varies widely, but an average figure is around 1 μl/min.[9] Tear secretion is divided into two categories: basal secretion and reflex secretion. The latter may be due to peripheral sensory stimulation, such as irritation of the cornea, or to central sensory stimulation, such as occurs, e.g., during crying. Emotional lacrimation seems to be unique to the human being and is not found in animals. The continuous flow of tear fluid propagated by blinking is very important from a drug delivery point of view. Drugs that sting or irritate upon instillation tend to be washed away quickly and thus the contact time with the corneal and conjunctival epithelium is reduced. This will affect negatively the bioavailability of the drug. Usually it is considered that in 5 min essentially all drug has been washed away from the surface of the eye.

4. The Anterior Uvea, the Chamber System, and the Chamber Angle

The anterior uvea comprises the ciliary body and the iris. Between the lens, ciliary processes, and the iris there is a small cavity called the posterior chamber (Figure 5). Between the iris, the chamber angle, and the cornea there is another cavity called the anterior chamber. The posterior and anterior chambers communicate through the pupil (Figure 5). This chamber system is filled with aqueous humor, a fluid somewhat reminiscent of the cerebrospinal fluid. The aqueous humor normally contains no cells and very little protein. This is necessary to avoid light scattering which would interfere with light transmittance. The ion composition is almost identical with that of plasma. In some species, such as the rabbit, the aqueous humor contains large amounts of ascorbic acid, and this substance is pumped into the posterior chamber against a concentration gradient. The exact function of ascorbic acid in the aqueous humor is not known.

There is a continuous flow of aqueous humor; the aqueous has an important role in bringing nutrients and oxygen to the avascular structures of the eye, such as the lens and the corneal endothelium, and the trabecular meshwork. At the same time it carries away metabolites (e.g., lactate) from surrounding structures. In addition to these functions the continuous flow of aqueous humor is important because it creates a certain pressure in the eye above the atmospheric pressure. The total volume of the chamber system in the human eye is 200 to 300 μl. In the rabbit the volume is also around 200 to 300 μl, but in the cynomolgus monkey it is only around 100 to 150 μl. In the cat the volume of the chamber system may be as large as 1 ml. The rate of aqueous humor flow is approximately 1 to 1.5% of the chamber volume per minute. In the human eye it is around 2 to 3 μl/min.

Aqueous humor is secreted by the ciliary processes into the posterior chamber. It enters the anterior chamber through the pupil and leaves the eye through the trabecular meshwork and Schlemm's canal (Figure 5). Schlemm's canal is directly connected with the episcleral veins outside the eye. Part of the aqueous humor leaves the eye through another route, the so-called uveoscleral outflow pathway. This outflow pathway was first described in 1966.[10] When aqueous humor leaves the eye via the uveoscleral route it bypasses most of the trabecular meshwork and percolates through the ciliary muscle to enter into the supraciliary and suprachoroidal space. This is the space between the choroid/ciliary body and the sclera. From here the fluid relatively easily can leave the eye through porosities in the sclera (e.g., where blood vessels and nerves penetrate the sclera). Certain drugs, such as prostaglandins and possibly epinephrine, enhance the uveoscleral outflow of aqueous humor.

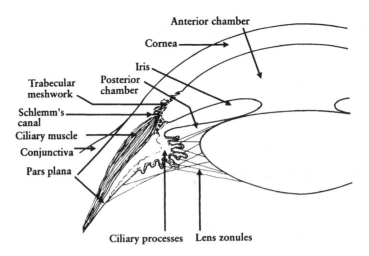

FIGURE 5.   Anterior segment of the eye.

a. The Ciliary Body

The ciliary body comprises the ciliary muscle and the ciliary processes. The ciliary muscle (see Figure 5) is a smooth muscle which consists of longitudinal bundles, circular bundles, and oblique bundles. In man and other primates the longitudinal muscle fibers insert partly into the scleral spure and partly into the trabecular meshwork. Contraction of the muscle will distend the trabecular meshwork. The ciliary muscle is cholinergically innervated with nerve fibers originating in the ciliary ganglion. Cholinergic muscarinic agonists such as acetylcholine and pilocarpine contract the muscle. The main function of the ciliary muscle is to enable accommodation. When the ciliary muscle contracts the lens zonules relax and, due to its elasticity, the lens changes its shape to become more convex. Thus the refractive power increases, which enables focusing on nearby objects.

The ciliary processes are highly vascularized foldings of the ciliary body which protrude into the posterior chamber. In the human eye there are about 70 processes. The processes are covered by a double layer epithelium (Figure 6). The inner of these epithelial cell layers (the one facing the posterior chamber) is not pigmented and is therefore called the non-pigmented epithelial cell layer. Embryologically, due to the invagination of the optic cup it corresponds to the neural part of the retina. The outer epithelial cell layer facing the stroma of the processes is markedly pigmented and is called the pigmented epithelial cell layer. Embryologically it corresponds to the pigment epithelium of the retina. Due to the invagination during the embryologic development the apical sides of these two epithelial cell layers are facing each other.

The nonpigmented epithelial cells are attached to each other by junctional complexes and the tight junctions between the cells constitute an obstacle for larger molecules such as proteins to diffuse into the aqueous humor of the posterior chamber (Figure 6). This barrier, ultimately formed by the nonpigmented epithelial cells and the tight junctions between them, is called the blood-aqueous barrier, and because of it the aqueous humor normally contains very small amounts of proteins and colloids. The nonpigmented epithelial cells are typical secreting cells, exhibiting a large number of mitochondria and a well-developed endoplasmatic reticulum. Furthermore, high activity of Na/K ATPase has been detected in the cell membranes, particularly in the basal and lateral infoldings of the cells.[11] The nonpigmented epithelial cells actively transfer sodium ions and chloride or bicarbonate ions into the infoldings at the basal side and the lateral side between the cells. This creates an osmotic

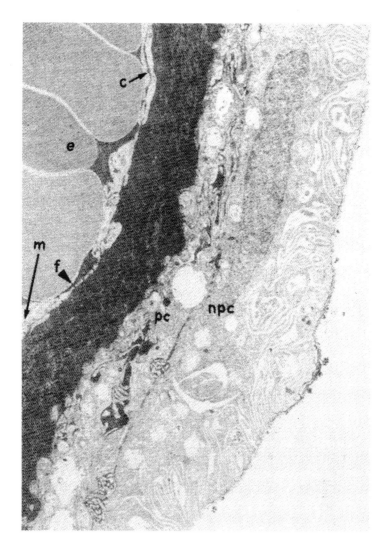

FIGURE 6. Electron micrograph of the ciliary epithelium of the albino rabbit eye. Horseradish peroxidase has been injected intravenously, and its location is demonstrated by the electron-dense material. c = intracellular cleft of vascular endothelium, e = erythrocyte, f = fenestrae, m = micropinocytotic vesicles, npc = nonpigmented cell, pc = pigmented cell. Note the absence of staining between nonpigmented epithelial cells due to the blood-aqueous barrier. Melanin is absent from the pigmented cells (albino). (From Uusitalo, R., Palkama, A., and Stjernschantz, J., *Exp. Eye Res.*, 17, 49, 1973. With permission.)

gradient attracting water. Although the exact mechanism of aqueous humor production is not known it is generally accepted that practically all aqueous humor is formed by an active pump mechanism.[12] Ultrafiltration, however, has to take place from the capillaries into the stroma of the ciliary processes.

The stroma of the ciliary processes is highly vascularized and the capillaries are fenestrated. Consequently, the extravascular plasma protein content in the stroma is very high, approximately 75% of the intravascular plasma protein content in rabbits, for example.[13,14] The plasmacolloidal (oncotic) pressure that follows exerts a negative pressure on aqueous humor formation and would in fact tend to reabsorb fluid from the posterior chamber. Therefore, it is necessary to use an effective pump mechanism to produce aqueous humor;

pure ultrafiltration would not suffice. There are no lymph vessels inside the eye. Thus plasma proteins in the stroma of the ciliary processes have to leave the eye either by reabsorption into blood vessels, through the iris root into the chamber angle, or through the uveoscleral outflow pathways. The blood flow in the ciliary body does not seem to be autoregulated to any greater extent. Sympathetic stimulation causes marked vasoconstriction, and an increase in intraocular pressure also reduces the blood flow in the ciliary body.[15,16] Quite surprisingly, parasympathetic stimulation (by stimulating the oculomotor nerve with which the cholinergic nerves to the ciliary ganglion run) also causes vasoconstriction in the ciliary body of rabbits but not of cats or monkeys.[17]

The ciliary body is innervated by sympathetic nerves, most of which innervate the blood vessels, and by cholinergic nerves, most of which innervate the ciliary muscle. There are also some sensory nerves. Some cholinergic and adrenergic nerves have been shown to exist in the vicinity of the ciliary epithelium and it may be that there is a direct innervation of the ciliary epithelium,[18] although final evidence for this is still lacking. β-Adrenergic agonists (e.g., isoprenaline in monkeys[19] and epinephrine in human beings[20]) tend to increase aqueous humor production. β-Adrenergic receptors have been localized to the ciliary epithelium and are positively coupled via a G-protein to adenylate cyclase, converting ATP into cAMP. Since β-adrenergic antagonists effectively reduce the intraocular pressure by reducing the aqueous humor formation it would seem that there is a physiologic adrenergic tone promoting aqueous humor formation. This adrenergic tone is probably based on circulating catecholamines rather than the sympathetic innervation of the ciliary body. During sleep aqueous humor production falls, and no inhibiting effect on this parameter can be achieved with β-blockers.[21] Thus, it would seem that catecholamines can stimulate aqueous humor production but that there is a basal level of production which is not dependent on catecholamines.

b. The Iris

The iris consists of the pigmented epithelial cell layer, the iridial sphincter and dilator muscles, and the stroma. As mentioned in the introduction, the epithelial cell layer is actually a fusion of both the pigmented and the nonpigmented cell layers. It is heavily pigmented. In the stroma, anterior to the muscle layer, melanocytes containing melanin are scattered. Persons with few melanocytes in the stroma exhibit a blue, grey, or green color of the iris. This is due to the fact that the pigmentation in the epithelial layer is shining through the muscle layer and the stroma. Persons with many melanocytes in the stroma exhibit brown irides.

The sphincter muscle is mainly innervated by cholinergic nerves originating in the ciliary ganglion. Contraction of the muscle causes miosis, a decrease in the pupil size. The dilator muscle, being situated further to the periphery with muscle fibers organized radially, causes mydriasis, a dilatation of the pupil. The dilatator muscle of the iris is innervated mainly by adrenergic nerves originating in the superior cervical ganglion. Some adrenergic nerves also pass to the sphincter muscle and some cholinergic nerves pass to the dilatator muscle, but their exact function is not known. In addition to the autonomic innervation there is also abundant sensory innervation of the iris. Several neuropeptides have been localized to sensory nerves in the iris [e.g., substance P and calcitonin gene-related peptide (CGRP)][22,23] and both substance P and CGRP can be released, upon nerve stimulation, from the iris.[24,25] Substance P causes miosis in rabbits[24,26] but has very little effect in the cat, monkey, and man[27] whereas CGRP has marked vascular effects in rabbits, causing increased blood flow and a breakdown of the blood-aqueous barrier.[23] Interestingly enough, in cats CGRP has quite different effects from those in rabbits. In cats CGRP causes a decrease in intraocular pressure[28] which probably is due to an increase in the facility of outflow of aqueous humor.[29]

In man and other primates cholecystokinin and fragments of this peptide appear to be potent miotics.[30,31] The physiologic significance of the neuropeptides in the iris is not fully understood but it appears that they may be important in trauma and irritation by being released rapidly through axon reflex mechanisms.

On the anterior surface of the iris there is no covering epithelial cell layer. Consequently the trabeculae of the stroma can be directly visualized in slit lamp microscopy. Opposite to the situation in the ciliary processes, the capillaries of the iris are very tight, and there is practically no leakage of plasma proteins from these vessels.[32,33] The iris is not as vascularized as the ciliary processes and the blood flow seems to be poorly autoregulated.[15]

Sympathetic stimulation causes a marked decrease in blood flow. Interestingly, the same is also true for parasympathetic stimulation[17] both in rabbits and cats as well as in primates. The mechanism of this cholinergic vasoconstriction in the iris has not yet been fully worked out.[34]

c. The Trabecular Meshwork and Schlemm's Canal

The trabecular meshwork is the structure between the cornea, the sclera, and the iris in the chamber angle (see Figure 5). It consists of a large number of collagen beams covered by endothelial cells. The collagen beams crisscross each other forming a three-dimensional network that somewhat has the shape of a sponge. The part of the meshwork situated close to the cornea and the sclera is called the corneoscleral meshwork; the part situated further medially is called the uveal meshwork. Aqueous humor is drained through the meshwork into a small vessel in the sclera called Schlemm's canal. The juxtacanalicular tissue is the tissue between the inner wall of Schlemm's canal and the corneoscleral meshwork. Most of the resistance to outflow of aqueous humor is believed to reside in this tissue of the outflow pathway. Vacuoles traversing the entire inner wall of Schlemm's canal have been described and, for instance, erythrocytes and other cellular elements can pass into Schlemm's canal through such vacuoles.[35-37] Schlemm's canal is directly connected to the episcleral veins through collecting channels. Some of these collecting channels can be seen in the microscope and are called aqueous veins.

The main cause of the increased intraocular pressure in open angle glaucoma is increased resistance to outflow of aqueous humor in the trabecular meshwork and juxtacanalicular tissue.[38] Cholinergic drugs such as pilocarpine reduce the intraocular pressure primarily by contracting the longitudinal muscle fibers of the ciliary muscle thus stretching the trabecular meshwork, which enhances outflow of aqueous humor.[39]

d. The Intraocular Pressure

The intraocular pressure is dependent on the flow of aqueous humor and the resistance in the outflow pathways; and to these should be added the pressure in the episcleral veins into which aqueous humor is drained. The intraocular pressure can thus be expressed according to the formula:

$$IOP = Pe + F \cdot R \qquad (1)$$

where IOP is the intraocular pressure, Pe the episcleral venous pressure, F the flow of aqueous humor, and R the resistance to outflow. Usually, the outflow facility, the reciprocal of outflow resistance, is measured; and Equation 1 can therefore be expressed:

$$IOP = Pe + F/C \qquad (2)$$

where C is the outflow facility of aqueous humor. However, it was earlier mentioned that part of the aqueous humor may actually leave the eye through the uveoscleral pathway.

Since the pressure gradient between the anterior chamber and the suprachoroidal space is very small, almost negligible, uveoscleral outflow can be regarded as pressure insensitive, and experiments have indeed demonstrated that increasing the intraocular pressure does not increase the outflow of aqueous humor through the uveoscleral pathways. Thus, a more accurate expression of the intraocular pressure is

$$IOP = Pe + (F_{tot} - F_u)/C \tag{3}$$

where F_{tot} is total aqueous flow and F_u the part of aqueous leaving the eye through the uveoscleral pathway. Thus, any drug which substantially increases uveoscleral outflow is going to have a marked reducing effect on the intraocular pressure. The prostaglandins constitute a new group of intraocular pressure-lowering drugs which seem to exert their effect by increasing uveoscleral outflow.[40,41]

Several prostaglandins have been shown to be very effective intraocular pressure-reducing agents in animals[42] and $PGF_{2\alpha}$ and its isopropyl ester reduce the intraocular pressure in man.[43]

5. The Lens

The crystalline lens is situated behind the iris in front of the vitreous. The lens is completely surrounded by the lens capsule. The lens capsule consists of a collagen-like material that is quite elastic. The lens capsule does not contain any cells and is embryologically formed from the lens epithelium. The lens is important for the visual function because it has a refractive power of about 20 diopters. It enables, together with the ciliary muscle, accommodation and protects the retina from the harmful ultraviolet radiation.

A schematic picture of the lens is shown in Figure 7. The lens is suspended by small filaments called the zonules of Zinn. The zonules attach to the ciliary processes and pars plana. On the anterior surface of the lens there is an epithelial cell layer. The cells are cuboidal and form a single layer. At the equator of the lens (Figure 7) the cells elongate to form lens fibers. In the pre-equatorial zone the epithelial cells undergo mitosis. Typically the lens fibers lose the nucleus and many cell organelles and become fibers packed with protein. The fibers have a hexagonal shape and new fibers are formed continuously throughout the life. In the middle of the lens the fibers coalesce and form the nucleus of the lens. The transparency of the lens depends on the regular geometry of the lens fibers.

The lens contains slightly more than 30% proteins of the total weight. It has the highest protein content of all tissues in the body. About 85% of the proteins in the lens are water soluble. These proteins are called the crystallines. The crystallines are subdivided into alpha crystallines (about 15%), beta crystallines (about 55%), and gamma crystallines (about 15%). The alpha crystallines are the largest of these proteins with a molecular weight of about 1,000,000. The beta crystallines have a molecular weight of about 50,000 to 200,000, and the gamma crystallines have a molecular weight of about 20,000.

With age, the lens gets more rigid and the accommodative function is lost. This is called presbyopia. Clinically significant presbyopia starts at about age 45 and is usually completed around the age of 60 when an accommodative capacity of approximately 3 diopters has been lost. Only persons with myopia (nearsightedness) can thereafter manage without reading glasses.

In spite of the fact that the lens, with age, gains in convexity, the refractive power of the lens is reduced in presbyopia. This so-called lens paradox is probably due to the fact that the refractive index of the lens decreases, which causes a net decrease in refractive power of the lens in the presbyopic age. When the crystallines and other proteins start to aggregate, light is scattered in the lens, which can be seen as an opacification. Opacification

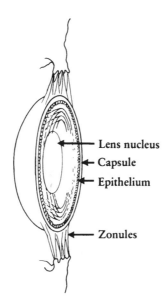

FIGURE 7.   Schematic picture of the crystalline lens.

of the lens is called cataract. There are several types of cataract as well as etiologies of cataract. A widening of the spaces between the lens fibers, with destruction of cell membranes and accumulation of water, is commonly seen in cataract.

The lens receives glucose, amino acids, oxygen, and other nutrients mainly from the aqueous humor. The aqueous humor also has an important role in removing metabolites from the lens. During the embryologic development the hyaloid artery enters the lens from the posterior segment. However, this artery regresses after the embryologic development and can be found frequently in the vitreous as a vestigial fibrous stalk.

The lens is a rather effectively sequestered organ from the blood and immune system. First, the lens is suspended in the posterior chamber; the blood-aqueous barrier normally prevents cells and immunoglobulins from entering the aqueous humor. Second, the lens is protected by its capsule, and third, the proteins in the lens fibers are protected by the plasma membrane. Therefore, the lens proteins may be recognized by the immune system (e.g., in mature cataracts with lysis of lens fibers or after a cataract operation with remnants of the lens left in the eye), which may cause inflammation.

B. THE POSTERIOR SEGMENT OF THE EYE

The posterior segment of the eye comprises the retina with the optic nerve, the vitreous, the choroid, and the sclera. The anteriormost part of the sclera close to the limbus belongs to the anterior segment.

1. The Retina and the Optic Nerve

The retina and the optic nerve are embryologically an extension of the diencephalon. The optic nerve enters the eye in the posterior pole through a porous collagen membrane structure called lamina cribrosa. The optic nerve in a human being contains approximately one million separate neurons, and it has been estimated that up to 30% of these can be lost without detectable loss in visual function.[44,45] A prerequisite is, of course, that the neurons are lost somewhat uniformly. The optic nerve is surrounded by cerebrospinal fluid and dura

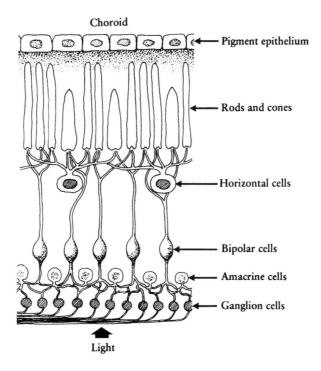

FIGURE 8.   Schematic picture of the retina.

mater of the brain. Increased pressure in the brain is transmitted to the optic nerve head causing it to become edematous, which can be easily detected by ophthalmoscopy. The reason for the swelling is probably an interference with axoplasmatic flow in the optic nerve.[49] The retina extends anteriorly to the pars plana of the ciliary body. The border between the ciliary body and the retina is called ora serrata. Since there are no photoreceptors in the optic nerve head it is a blind spot in the visual field.

The retina consists of two major functional parts: the neural layer and the pigment epithelium. The photoreceptors face the pigment epithelium, which is the outermost layer of the retina (Figure 8). Thus, with respect to the light entering the eye, the retina is situated upside down because the photoreceptors are facing away from the light. There are two kinds of photoreceptors: rods and cones. The cones transmit color signals. In primates three types of cones have been demonstrated, those absorbing the yellow-red, blue, and green. The macula is situated somewhat laterally to the optic nerve head. The center of the macula is called the fovea and contains only cones. There are no blood vessels in the fovea.

The photoreceptors are coupled to bipolar neurons which are coupled to the ganglion cells of the retina. The axons of the ganglion cells extend into the optic nerve. There are at least two complex horizontal networks in the retina. The one closer to the photoreceptor layer is based on horizontal neurons, and these cells seem to connect photoreceptor cells. The inner horizontal network is based on amacrine cells. The amacrine neurons seem to connect the vertical neural pathways at the level of bipolar and ganglion cells. In addition to the neural elements of the retina there are glial cells called Müller cells. The visual pigment in rods is rhodopsin, whereas the pigments in cones are less well defined as yet. Rhodopsin consists of opsin and a chromophore, which is 11-cis-retinal. Rhodopsin is widely distributed and is found both in the vertebrate eye and in the invertebrate compound eye. When rhodopsin is bleached by light it dissociates into opsin and all-trans-retinal. This event triggers an electrophysiological signal possibly involving guanylate cyclase and formation of cGMP.[46,47] All-trans-retinal has to be isomerized to 11-cis-retinal, which then together with opsin can regenerate rhodopsin.

The pigment epithelium of the retina forms a barrier between the choroid and the retina. This barrier is very tight and the pigmented epithelial cells are connected with tight junctions. The pigment epithelium selectively transfers nutrients to the retina from the choroid, and there is also a pump mechanism of fluid in the direction of the choroid through the pigment epithelium. Furthermore, the pigment epithelium has a very important function in that it, by means of phagocytosis, removes the tips of the outer segments of the photoreceptors, which are continuously shed.[48]

The inner two thirds of the retina in primates receives the blood supply from the retinal artery. The outermost one third receives oxygen and nutrients from the choriocapillaries in the choroid. The blood flow of the retina is effectively autoregulated as in the brain.[15] Unfortunately, there is very little collateral circulation in the retina. Consequently, various obstructions of blood flow, such as arterial emboli, as a rule cause rapid and irreversible damage in the retina. However, retina can survive during detachment from the choroid for a relatively long period of time. In glaucoma the increased intraocular pressure causes damage in the optic nerve head and the retina. Clinically this is manifested by defects in the visual field. There is usually a simultaneous excavation of the optic nerve head (cupping). The cupping is believed to be due to degenerative processes in the neural and glial tissue as well as to a thinning and posterior displacement of the lamina cribrosa, secondary to increased intraocular pressure and possibly other factors.[49]

2. The Vitreous

The vitreous is a hydrogel which fills the cavity between the retina and the lens. It is separated from the lens capsule and the posterior chamber by the anterior vitreous membrane (anterior hyaloid membrane) and it is anchored by ligaments to the retina. There are three main zones of the vitreous in the human eye: the cortical layer, the intermediate zone, and the central channel. The cortical vitreous, which is closest to the retina, is a gel-like mass consisting of collagen fibrils and hyaluronic acid. Hyalocytes, special cells of the vitreous, are dispersed in the outer parts of the cortical vitreous particularly in the vicinity of pars plana.[50] The rest of the vitreous may be in liquid state or in a gel state containing collagen and hyaluronic acid. In some animals most of the vitreous is in a liquid state (e.g., in the owl monkey). In the rabbit there is a small flow of fluid through the vitreous, backwards from the posterior chamber,[51] but this has not been shown in primates.[51,52]

The water content of the vitreous is very high at 98 to 99.7%. The turnover of water in the vitreous has been reported to be about 10 to 15 min. The pH of the vitreous is approximately 7.5. There is no flow through the vitreous, only diffusion. In the human eye the vitreous can to a large extent be replaced by water, and with age the vitreous usually liquefies at least partly. The vitreous is an excellent culture media for bacteria and, unfortunately, antibiotics normally penetrate very poorly into the vitreous. In the inflamed eye, however, penetration of antibiotics into the vitreous is somewhat improved.

3. The Choroid and the Sclera

The choroid is a highly vascularized tissue between the retina and the sclera. It is the posterior part of the uvea, the anterior part comprising the iris and the ciliary body. The choroid consists of three main parts: the vessel layer, the choriocapillary layer, and Bruch's membrane, which is in direct contact with the retinal pigment epithelium. The vessel layer contains veins and arteries of large and medium size. Melanocytes can be found dispersed between the blood vessels in the stroma. The choriocapillary layer consists of a very fine and dense network of capillaries. The capillaries are of the fenestrated type and consequently very permeable to plasma proteins and colloids.[13,14] The capillary network underlying the fovea is particularly well developed. As mentioned previously, in the fovea there are no blood vessels, and consequently most of the nutrition is derived from the underlying choriocapillaries. Interestingly enough, in contrast to the very well autoregulated blood flow of the retina, autoregulation of choroidal blood flow seems to be lacking almost entirely.[15] For instance, sympathetic stimulation dramatically reduces the choroidal blood flow, as does an increase in the intraocular pressure.[15,53]

Bruch's membrane is a few micron thick structure situated between the choriocapillaries and the pigment epithelium of the retina. Bruch's membrane consists of the basal laminae of the pigment epithelium and endothelial cells of the choriocapillaries and, in addition, of collagen and elastic fibers.

Between the choroid and the sclera there is the suprachoroidal or perichoroidal space. This is a very thin, almost potential space consisting of various connective tissue lamellae with melanocytes and macrophages scattered in the loose tissue. It can be characterized as a sponge tissue. In the suprachoroidal space there are numerous nerves that run forward to the anterior segment of the eye. The suprachoroidal space is also important with respect to aqueous humor dynamics, because a substantial part of the aqueous humor that leaves the eye via the uveoscleral route ends up in the suprachorodial space and is finally drained out from the eye through porosites in the sclera.

The sclera is the outermost tunic of the eye, protecting the sensitive inner parts of the eye together with the cornea. The sclera is about 0.5 to 1 mm thick, being thicker at the posterior pole. The sclera is a relatively resistant structure consisting mainly of collagen bundles and some elastic fibers. Fibroblasts and melanocytes are scattered in the network of the bundles. Porosites in the sclera exist at the entry of blood vessels and nerves into the eye. There are very few blood vessels in the sclera. The extraocular muscles insert with their tendons into the sclera and Tenon's capsule, a loose collagenous structure covering the sclera.

4. Extraocular Orbital Structures

The eyeball is embedded in orbital fat which facilitates movement and rotation. Six extraocular muscles insert into the sclera: the superior and inferior rectus muscles, the lateral and medial rectus muscles, and the superior and inferior oblique muscles. All these muscles are striated and are innervated by the third cranial nerve (n. oculomotorius), except for the superior oblique muscle, which is innervated by the fourth cranial nerve (n. trochlearis), and the lateral rectus muscle, which is innervated by the sixth cranial nerve (n. abducens). In the orbit of some species there are also large vein plexa (e.g., in the rabbit). The ciliary ganglion is situated posteriorly in the orbit. The ciliary ganglion is the main parasympathetic ganglion of the eye. Most of the preganglionic fibers originate in the Edinger-Westphal nucleus of the oculomotor nuclear complex in the brain and run to the ciliary ganglion along with the third cranial nerve. These fibers innervate the iridial sphincter muscle, the ciliary muscle, and, most likely to some extent, blood vessels in the anterior uvea.[36] The cholinergic input to the lacrimal gland and choroidal blood vessels originates from the facial-intermediate nerve and synapse in the pterygopalatine ganglion, which is not located in the orbit.[54] Stimulation of these nerves causes lacrimation and a marked vasodilation in the choroid.[55,56] The vasodilation is probably based on a release of vasoactive intestinal polypeptide (VIP).[57]

In retrobulbar anesthesia, the anesthetic is injected into the fat of the orbit in which it is spread around, thereby intefering with nerve conductance in the ciliary nerves conveying somatosensory and autonomic input. In some species, such as the rabbit, retrobulbar anesthesia may be difficult to perform due to the large retrobulbar orbital vein plexa.

III. PHYSIOLOGICAL ASPECTS OF OCULAR DRUG THERAPY

A. EYE TISSUES AS BARRIERS IN OCULAR DRUG DELIVERY

Most drugs are administered to the eye through the topical route. Consequently, the cornea, conjunctiva, and sclera form the most essential barriers to drug penetration into the eye. In some situations this is of no concern or is even an advantage (e.g., when anesthetizing the cornea or when treating superficial infections or inflammations of the eye). However, frequently it is desirable that the drug penetrates into the eye (e.g., for reducing the intraocular pressure in the treatment of glaucoma or for treating intraocular inflammations such as iritis). Generally, the cornea must be considered a very tight barrier to drug penetration. The tight junctions around the epithelial cells make it difficult for water soluble substances to pass into the corneal stroma. Essentially the only way of passing through the epithelium for water soluble substances is the paracellular one. Therefore, if the tight junctions are broken up (e.g., by benzalkonium chloride) penetration of water soluble substances can be increased substantially. Lipophilic substances, on the other hand, seem to penetrate well into the corneal epithelium, and for these substances the corneal stroma reduces penetration.

The corneal epithelium can be utilized elegantly in prodrug delivery due to the high content of esterases. Thus a hydrophilic substance can be made lipophilic by esterification, and the ester bond is hydrolyzed in the epithelium. The penetration into the eye of water soluble substances such as epinephrine and prostaglandin $F_{2\alpha}$ has been increased by more than ten times by esterification of the molecules.[3,58]

The conjunctival epithelium also constitutes a relatively tight barrier to drug penetration, although not as tight as the corneal epithelium.[59] However, the vasculature of the conjunctiva will absorb a substantial part of the drug that has passed the epithelium. The rest that enters the sclera seems to have rather good access into the eye, probably at the trabecular meshwork, the iris root, and also at the pars plana. The pars plana is not so heavily vascularized as the ciliary processes. Through the route of pars plana some drug may actually also have access to the anterior part of the vitreous. In general the sclera does not form a very tight barrier to penetration of solutes even of relatively large molecular weight.[59] However, substances entering the eyeball posteriorly will be effectively picked up by the choroidal circulation; thus, drugs cannot to any greater extent be administered (e.g., to the retina) by retrobulbar injection.

Drugs administered systemically (e.g., through the oral or intravenous route) also have poor access to the aqueous humor and the vitreous. This is because of the blood-aqueous barrier which prevents substances from entering into the aqueous humor, and because of the blood-retinal barrier, which consists of the pigment epithelium and the vascular endothelium in the retina, preventing drugs from entering into the extravascular space of the retina and into the vitreous.

B. IMPORTANCE OF AQUEOUS HUMOR DRAINAGE AND CILIARY EPITHELIUM ORGANIC ANION PUMP SYSTEM

The continuous flow of aqueous humor drains the drug from the anterior chamber rather effectively. Part of the drug diffuses into the iris; many drugs containing amine groups and generally drugs that are cations bind to melanin in the iris. Melanin is a polyanion; drugs which classically bind strongly to melanin are chloroquine and chlorpromazine, as well as β-adrenergic antagonists such as timolol. The melanin binding, as a rule, is reversible and thus the drug-melanin complex may in fact form a slow release system. Very little of the drug enters into the posterior chamber because of the continuous flow of aqueous humor through the pupil, and virtually no drug enters the vitreous in phakic eyes.

The aqueous humor drainage may also be beneficial (e.g., with respect to the delivery of antiglaucoma drugs) since the drug will reach the target tissue, the trabecular meshwork, and the ciliary muscle rapidly. With many antiglaucoma drugs a peak effect is noted 1 to 2 h after topical administration. Drugs that need access to the ciliary epithelium may also benefit from the aqueous flow because they get into the chamber angle and iris root quickly. The distance from the iris root to the ciliary processes is short and there is no epithelial barrier to cross.

The ciliary epithelium is rather unique in that it transports organic anions from the aqueous humor into the stroma of the ciliary processes.[60] This is based on a carrier-mediated transport system, which is sensitive to temperature and ouabain and can be prevented by probenicid. The transport system of the ciliary epithelium is in many respects reminiscent of that of the renal tubuli, the choroid plexus, and the liver.[61] For instance, penicillin is transported out of the eye by this system. Naturally occurring organic anions, such as prostaglandins, are also substrates of this transport system,[62-64] and it is highly questionable whether any prostaglandin at all can pass posteriorly between the crystalline lens and the ciliary epithelium, virtually all being transported into the ciliary processes. From the ciliary processes the organic anions are probably carried out from the eye with the blood.

C. INACCESSIBILITY OF DRUGS TO THE VITREOUS

There are several situations in which it would be desirable for a drug to have access to the vitreous. Such situations are, for example, infection of the vitreous in endophthalmitis and various vitreoretinopathies. Unfortunately, the access of drugs to the vitreous is usually poor because there is virtually no penetration through the crystalline lens or between the ciliary processes and the crystalline lens. Neither is there satisfactory access from the blood vessels in the retina or from the choroid due to the pigment epithelium. Retrobulbar injection of drugs may result in penetration through the sclera, but the highly vascularized choroid will be a physiological barrier, and finally, of course, the pigment epithelium will hinder the movement of the drug into the retina and the vitreous. Thus, the only remaining route will be through the pars plana of the ciliary body. Subconjunctival injection may to some extent deliver the drug to the vitreous through the pars plana. In aphakic and pseudophakic eyes penetration of drugs from the aqueous humor to the vitreous is somewhat improved, particularly if the lens capsule has been removed. During inflammation, however, many barriers such as the blood-aqueous barrier and the blood-retinal barrier become leaky and, therefore, as a rule the penetration of antibiotics and other drugs is enhanced during such pathological conditions.

Generally, from a practical clinical point of view it is not advisable to routinely perform intravitreal injections because of the danger of complications, but in certain sight-threatening conditions intravitreal injections are carried out. It should also be remembered that certain drugs (e.g., antibiotics) are neurotoxic and, therefore, should not be injected into the vitreous.

D. THE CORNEA AND THE VITREOUS AS DRUG RESERVOIRS

Both the cornea and the vitreous may act as drug reservoirs. Of these the cornea is more important. It is not exactly clear which part of the cornea harbors the drug, but probably in cases of lipophilic substances the epithelium may harbor it, whereas in cases of hydrophilic substances the stroma is more likely. The cornea may be a reservoir for fluorescein. By administering this very water soluble substance repeatedly on the cornea, concentrations high enough to be measured with fluorophotometry can be achieved. From the stroma the fluorescein will diffuse into the aqueous humor of the anterior chamber and, depending on the concentration of fluorescein in the cornea, a reflection coefficient, and the rate of aqueous humor flow, a certain concentration of fluorescein is obtained in the aqueous humor. By measuring the decay in corneal and aqueous humor fluorescein concentration it is thus possible to determine the rate of the aqueous humor flow in an intact eye.[65,66] It is not inconceivable that the cornea may act as a reservoir for many drugs, particularly prodrugs, which upon hydrolysis become water soluble thus preventing them from diffusing back into the tear film.

As a rule, substances even of high molecular weight diffuse freely in the vitreous.[64] Injection of fluorescein-marked dextran, with a molecular weight of about 200,000, into the vitreous of rabbits has been shown to give rise to a slow release system of dextran into the posterior chamber.[65] Since this is a very slow system (weeks to months), the diffusion of tracer into the aqueous humor of the posterior chamber during shorter periods of time (e.g., a day) is almost linear; thus it is possible to some extent to estimate the flow of aqueous humor simply by measuring the concentration of fluorescein-dextran in the anterior chamber by fluorophotometry.[65] Although this flow measuring method exhibits a certain inaccuracy, it nevertheless demonstrates that the vitreous can indeed act as a depot for certain large molecular compounds provided these are not actively picked up by the retina or the retinal pigment epithelium.

E. CONSENSUAL EYE RESPONSES

A very peculiar phenomenon is frequently encountered in physiological and pharmacological experiments, namely the existence of a consensual response in the contralateral control eye. This phenomenon is most often encountered in intraocular pressure studies. It occurs in both animals and man. Not uncommonly, the intraocular pressure of the untreated control eye also decreases upon treatment. Although this may be due partly to a systemic effect (e.g., the blood pressure), to an involuntary transfer of traces of the drug from one eye to the other, or to a carryover effect via the blood, there is ample data to suggest that some other mechanism must exist, possibly a neuronal reflex via the brain. Loading one eye with a certain weight has been shown, after the load is removed, to reduce the intraocular pressure and the episcleral venous pressure not only of the treated eye but also of the contralateral untreated eye.[68] This could conceivably not be mediated through a vascular pathway, but is most likely based on a reflex mechanism. Pressor receptors have been postulated to exist in the eye,[69,70] but this concept remains controversial. On the other hand, there are good reasons to believe that some of the consensual responses seen with β-blockers are carryover effects via the blood.

Consensual responses are also encountered in rabbits during ocular irritation. Sporadically, the blood-aqueous barrier of the untreated eye disrupts, a phenomenon that has been postulated to be based on a neuronal reflex mechanism, possibly through antidromic transmission of nerve signals in the fifth cranial nerve to the untreated eye. However, it should be remembered that the rabbit eye is very sensitive and easily reacts with a breakdown of the blood-aqueous barrier even to minimal trauma. If the manipulation of one eye somehow were to trigger the somatosensory system, it could be that careless handling of the animal causing subthreshold irritation of the contralateral control eye would be enough to induce a disruption of the blood-aqueous barrier also in the control eye. Thus, part of the consensual responses seen in the rabbit may be artifacts.

Sympathetic ophthalmitis is a condition characterized by inflammation of a nontraumatized eye usually a few weeks to years after a perforating trauma to the other eye. This consensual ocular response of the healthy eye is probably triggered by an immune mechanism upon the trauma to the other eye. The effect is carried with the immune system from the affected eye to the other eye. The reason for this phenomenon may be that during trauma some tissues normally sequestered in the eye are recognized by the immune system. Subsequently, a cross reaction of antigen recognition in the healthy eye takes place, leading to inflammation.

F. IMPORTANCE OF AUTACOIDS AND NEUROPEPTIDES IN DRUG RESPONSES OF THE EYE

In the anterior uvea of many species there is a relatively high capacity for eicosanoid synthesis, particularly prostaglandin.[71,72] Prostaglandins have been demonstrated in the aqueous humor; particularly PGE_2 may be released in inflammations of the anterior uvea, but it is likely that prostaglandins also have normal physiologic functions (e.g., in neuronal transmission phenomena), as shown in other organs.[73,74] Thus, it is not inconceivable that certain drugs may exert at least part of the effect through a release of prostaglandins. Some drugs that seem to involve prostaglandins are epinephrine, para-aminoclonidine, and verapamil.[75] The intraocular pressure-lowering effect of these substances in animal models can at least partly be blocked by prior treatment with cyclo-oxygenase inhibitors.

Since there is some indirect evidence that prostaglandins may release neuropeptides (e.g., substance P[24] in the eye), it is quite possible that the final effect of certain intraocular pressure-lowering agents is based on a very complex interaction with both eicosanoids and neuropeptides. It is relevant in this regard that at least calcitonin gene-related peptide has been shown potently to reduce the intraocular pressure in cats,[28] a phenomenon probably based on an increase in outflow facility of aqueous humor.[29] In monkeys too, this peptide causes increased outflow facility of aqueous humor, although the response is much more subtle.[76] One may conclude that it is likely that the mechanism behind many drug effects in the eye is much more complex than what has so far been believed.

ACKNOWLEDGMENTS

We would like to thank Ms. Iréne Aspman for invaluable help in typing the manuscript as well as Mr. Mats Linder for producing the figures.

REFERENCES

1. **McLaughlin, B. J., Caldwell, R. B., Sasaki, Y., and Wood, T. O.,** Freeze-fracture quantitative comparison of rabbit corneal epithelial and endothelial membranes, *Curr. Eye Res.,* 4, 951, 1985.
2. **Kaufman, P. L., Wiedman, T., and Robinson, J. R.,** Cholinergics, in *Pharmacology of the Eye,* Sears, M. L., Ed., Springer-Verlag, Berlin, 1984, 149.
3. **Camber, O., Edman, P., and Olsson, L.-I.,** Permeability of prostaglandin F_{2a} and prostaglandin F_{2a} esters across cornea *in vitro,* *Int. J. Pharmaceutics,* 29, 259, 1986.
4. **Maurice, D.,** The physics of corneal transparency, in *Transparency of the Cornea,* Duke-Elder, S., Ed., Charles C. Thomas, Springfield, IL, 1960.
5. **Madsen, K., Schenholm, M., Jahnke, G., and Tengblad, A.,** Hyaluronate binding to intact corneas and cultured endothelial cells, *Invest. Ophthalmol. Vis. Sci.,* 30, 2132, 1989.
6. **Klyce, S. D. and Beuerman, R. W.,** Structure and function of the cornea, in *The Cornea,* Kaufman, H. E., Barron, B. A., McDonald, M. B., and Waltman, S. R., Eds., Churchill Livingstone, New York, 1988, 3.
7. **Tervo, K., Tervo, T., Eränkö, L., Vannas, A., Cuello, C., and Eränkö, O.,** Substance P-immunoreactive nerves in the human cornea and iris, *Invest. Ophthalmol. Vis. Sci.,* 23, 671, 1982.
8. **Lemp, M. A., Holly, F. J., Iwata, S., and Dohlman, C. H.,** The precorneal tear film. I. Factors in spreading and maintaining a continuous tear film over the corneal surface, *Arch. Ophthalmol.,* 83, 89, 1970.
9. **Mishima, S., Gasset, A., Klyce, S., and Baum, J.,** Determination of tear volume and tear flow, *Invest. Ophthalmol.,* 5, 264, 1966.
10. **Bill, A.,** Conventional and uveoscleral drainage of aqueous humor in the cynomolgus monkeys (Macaca irus) at normal and high intraocular pressures, *Exp. Eye Res.,* 5, 45, 1966.

11. **Shiose, Y. and Sears, M. L.**, Fine structural localization of nucleoside phosphatase activity in the ciliary epithelium of albino rabbits, *Invest. Ophthalmol.*, 5, 152, 1966.
12. **Sears, M. L.**, The aqueous, in *Adler's Physiology of the Eye*, Moses, R. A., Ed., C. V. Mosby, St. Louis, 1981, 204.
13. **Bill, A.**, The albumin exchange in the rabbit eye, *Acta Physiol. Scand.*, 60, 18, 1964.
14. **Bill, A.**, Capillary permeability to and extravascular dynamics of myoglobin, albumin and gammaglobulin in the uvea, *Acta Physiol. Scand.*, 73, 204, 1968.
15. **Alm, A. and Bill, A.**, The oxygen supply to the retina. II. Effects of high intraocular pressure and of increased arterial carbon dioxide tension on uveal and retinal blood flow in cats. A study with labelled microspheres including flow determinations in the brain and some other tissues, *Acta Physiol. Scand.*, 84, 306, 1972.
16. **Alm, A. and Bill, A.**, The effect of stimulation of the sympathetic chain on retinal oxygen tension and uveal, retinal and cerebral blood flow in cats, *Acta Physiol. Scand.*, 88, 84, 1973.
17. **Stjernschantz, J. and Bill, A.**, Effect of intracranial stimulation of the oculomotor nerve on ocular blood flow in the monkey, cat and rabbit, *Invest. Ophthalmol.*, 18, 99, 1979.
18. **Uusitalo, R. and Palkama, A.**, Evidence for the nervous control of secretion in the ciliary processes, *Prog. Brain Res.*, 34, 513, 1971.
19. **Bill, A.**, Effects of norepinephrine, isoproterenol and sympathetic stimulation on aqueous humor dynamics in vervet monkeys, *Exp. Eye Res.*, 10, 31, 1970.
20. **Townsend, D. J. and Brubaker, R. F.**, Immediate effect of epinephrine on aqueous formation in the human eyes as measured by fluorophotometry, *Invest. Ophthalmol. Vis. Sci.*, 19, 256, 1980.
21. **Topper, J. E. and Brubaker, R. F.**, Effects of timolol, epinephrine and acetazolamide on aqueous flow during sleep, *Invest. Ophthalmol. Vis. Sci.*, 26, 1315, 1985.
22. **Tervo, K., Tervo, T., Eränkö, L., Eränkö, O., and Cuello, A. C.**, Immunoreactivity for substance P in the gasserian ganglion, ophthalmic nerve and the anterior segment of the rabbit eye, *Histochem. J.*, 13, 435, 1980.
23. **Unger, W. G., Terenghi, G., Ghatei, M. A., Ennis, K. K., Butler, J. M., Zhang, S. Q., Too, H. P., Polak, J. M., and Bloom, S. R.**, Calcitonin gene-related polypeptide as a mediator of the neurogenic ocular injury response, *J. Ocular Pharmacol.*, 1, 189, 1985.
24. **Bill, A., Stjernschantz, J., Mandahl, A., Brodin, E., and Nilsson, G.**, Substance P: Release on trigeminal nerve stimulation, effects in the eye, *Acta Physiol. Scand.*, 106, 371, 1979.
25. **Wahlestedt, C., Beding, B., Ekman, R., Oksala, O., Stjernschantz, J., and Håkanson, R.**, Calcitonin gene-related peptide in the eye: Release by sensory nerve stimulation and effects associated with neurogenic inflammation, *Regulatory Peptides*, 16, 107, 1986.
26. **Stjernschantz, J.**, Autacoids and neuropeptides, in *Pharmacology of the Eye*, Sears, M. L., Ed., Springer-Verlag, Berlin, 1984, 311.
27. **Unger, W. G. and Tighe, J.**, The response of the isolated iris sphincter muscle of various mammalian species to substance P, *Exp. Eye Res.*, 39, 677, 1984.
28. **Oksala, O. and Stjernschantz, J.**, Effects of calcitonin gene-related peptide in the eye: A study in rabbits and cats, *Invest. Ophthalmol. Vis. Sci.*, 29, 1006, 1988.
29. **Oksala, O. and Stjernschantz, J.**, Increase in outflow facility of aqueous humor in cats induced by calcitonin gene-related peptide, *Exp. Eye Res.*, 47, 787, 1988.
30. **Bill, A., Andersson, S. E., and Almegård, B.**, Cholecystokinin causes contraction of the pupillary sphincter in monkeys but not in cats, rabbits, rats and guinea pigs: Antagonism by Lorglumide, *Acta Phys. Scand.* 138, 479, 1990.
31. **Almegård, B., Stjernschantz, J., and Bill, A.**, CCK contracts isolated human and monkey iris sphincters: A study with CCK-antagonists, *Europ. J. Pharmacol.*, 211, 183, 1992.
32. **Vegge, T.**, An electron microscopic study of the permeability of iris capillaries to horseradish peroxidase in the vervet monkey (Cercopithecus ethiops), *Z. Zellforsch. Mikrosk. Anat.*, 121, 74, 1971.
33. **Uusitalo, R., Palkama, A., and Stjernschantz, J.**, Electron microscopical study of the blood-aqueous barrier in the ciliary body and iris of the rabbit, *Exp. Eye Res.*, 17, 49, 1973.
34. **Stjernschantz, J.** Cholinergic vasoconstriction in the eye, *J. Ocular Pharmacol.*, 6, 195, 1990.
35. **Holmberg, Å.**, The fine structure of the inner wall of Schlemm's canal, *Arch. Ophthalmol.*, 62, 956, 1959.
36. **Bill, A.**, Scanning electron microscopic studies of the canal of Schlemm, *Exp. Eye Res.*, 10, 214, 1970.
37. **Bill, A.**, Blood circulation and fluid dynamics in the eye, *Physiol. Rev.*, 55, 383, 1975.
38. **Hoskins, H. D., Jr. and Kass, M. A.**, *Becker-Schaffer's Diagnosis and Therapy of the Glaucomas*, 6th ed., C. V. Mosby, St. Louis, 1989, 277.
39. **Bárány, E. H.**, The mode of action of pilocarpine on outflow resistance in the eye of a primate (Cercopithecus ethiops), *Invest. Ophthalmol.*, 1, 712, 1962.

40. **Crawford, K. and Kaufman, P. L.,** Pilocarpine antagonizes PGF$_{2a}$-induced ocular hypotension: evidence for enhancement of uveoscleral outflow by PGF$_{2a}$, *Arch. Ophthalmol.,* 105, 1112, 1987.

41. **Nilsson, S. F. E., Samuelson, M., Bill, A., and Stjernschantz, J.,** Increased uveoscleral outflow as a possible mechanism of ocular hypotension caused by prostaglandin F$_{2a}$-1-isopropyl ester in the cynomolgus monkey, *Exp. Eye Res.,* 48, 707, 1989.

42. **Bito, L. Z., Camras, C. B., Gum, G. G., and Resul, B.,** The ocular hypotensive effects and side effects of prostaglandins on the eyes of experimental animals, in *The Ocular Effects of Prostaglandins and Other Eicosanoids,* Bito, L. Z. and Stjernschantz, J., Eds., Alan R. Liss, New York, 1989, 349.

43. **Alm, A. and Villumsen, J.,** Effects of topically applied PGF$_{2a}$ and its isopropyl ester, on normal and glucomatous human eyes, in *The Ocular Effects of Prostaglandins and Other Eicosanoids,* Bito, L. Z. and Stjernschantz, J., Eds., Alan R. Liss, New York, 1989, 447.

44. **Quigley, H. A. and Green, W. R.,** The histology of human glaucoma cupping and nerve damage: Clinicopathologic correlation in 21 eyes, *Ophthalmology,* 10, 1803, 1979.

45. **Quigley, H. A., Addicks, E. M., and Green, W. R.,** Optic nerve damage in human glaucoma. III. Quantitative correlation of nerve fiber loss and visual field defect in glaucoma, ischemic neuropathy, papilledema and toxic neuropathy, *Arch. Ophthalmol.,* 100, 135, 1982.

46. **Fesenko, E. E., Kolesnikov, S. S., and Lyubarski, A. L.,** Induction by cyclic GMP of cationic conductance in plasma membrane of retinal rod outer segment, *Nature, (London),* 313, 310, 1985.

47. **Nakatani, K. and Yau, K.-W.,** cGMP opens the light-sensitive conductance in retinal rods, *Biophys. J.,* 47, 356a, 1985.

48. **Young, R. W. and Bok, D.,** Participation of the retinal pigment epithelium in the rod outer segment process, *J. Cell Biol.,* 42, 392, 1969.

49. **Anderson, D. R.,** The optic nerve, in *Adler's Physiology of the Eye,* Moses, R. A., Ed., C. V. Mosby, St. Louis, 1987, 491.

50. **Szirmai, J. A. and Balazs, E. A.,** Studies on the structure of the vitreous body. III. Cells in the cortical layer, *Arch. Ophthalmol.,* 59, 34, 1958.

51. **Hayreh, S. S.,** Posterior drainage of the intraocular fluid from the vitreous, *Exp. Eye Res.,* 5, 123, 1966.

52. **Gärtner, J.,** Die Bedeutung des perivasculären Raums der Zentralgefässe für den vitreopapillären Stofftransport beim normalen Mäuseauge und beim menschlichen Auge unter patologischen Bedingungen, *V. Graefes Arch. Ophthalmol.,* 175, 13, 1968.

53. **Alm, A.,** The effect of sympathetic stimulation on blood flow through the uvea, retina and optic nerve in monkeys, *Exp. Eye Res.,* 25, 19, 1977.

54. **Ruskell, G. L.,** Facial parasympathetic innervation of the choroidal blood vessels in monkeys, *Exp. Eye Res.,* 12, 166, 1971.

55. **Stjernschantz, J. and Bill, A.,** Vasomotor effects of facial nerve stimulation: Noncholinergic vasodilation in the eye, *Acta Physiol. Scand.,* 109, 45, 1980.

56. **Nilsson, S. F. E., Linder, J., and Bill, A.,** Characteristics of uveal vasodilation produced by facial nerve stimulation in monkeys, cats and rabbits, *Exp. Eye Res.,* 40, 841, 1985.

57. **Nilsson, S. F. E. and Bill, A.,** Vasoactive intestinal polypeptide (VIP): Effects in the eye and on regional blood flows, *Acta Physiol. Scand.,* 121, 385, 1984.

58. **Wei, C.-P., Andersson, J. A., and Leopold, I.,** Ocular absorption and metabolism of topically applied epinephrine and a dipivalyl ester of epinephrine, *Invest. Ophthalmol.,* 17, 315, 1978.

59. **Maurice, D. M. and Mishima, S.,** Ocular pharmacokinetics, in *Pharmacology of the Eye,* Sears, M. L., Ed., Springer-Verlag, Berlin, 1984, 19.

60. **Forbes, M. and Becker, B.,** The transport of organic anions by the rabbit eye. II. *In vivo* transport of iodopyrocet (Diodrast), *Am. J. Ophthalmol.,* 50, 867, 1960.

61. **Bárány, E. H.,** Organic cation uptake *in vitro* by the rabbit iris-ciliary body, renal cortex and choroid plexus, *Invest. Ophthalmol.,* 15, 341, 1976.

62. **Bito, L. Z.,** Accumulation and apparent active transport of prostaglandins by some rabbit tissues *in vitro,* *J. Physiol. (London),* 221, 371, 1972.

63. **Bito, L. Z.,** Comparative study of concentrative prostaglandin accumulation by various tissues of mammals and marine vertebrates and invertebrates, *Comp. Biochem. Physiol.,* 42a, 65, 1972.

64. **Bito, L. Z. and Salvador, E. V.,** Intraocular fluid dynamics. III. The site and mechanism of prostaglandin transfer across the blood intraocular fluid barriers, *Exp. Eye Res.,* 14, 233, 1972.

65. **Jones, R. F. and Maurice, D. M.,** New methods of measuring the rate of aqueous flow in man with fluorescein, *Exp. Eye Res.,* 5, 208, 1966.

66. **Brubaker, R. F.,** The flow of aqueous humor in the human eye, *Trans. Am. Ophthalmol. Soc.,* 80, 391, 1982.

67. **Johnson, F. and Maurice, D.,** A simple method of measuring aqueous humor flow with intravitreal fluoresceinated dextrans, *Exp. Eye Res.,* 39, 791, 1984.

68. **Krakau, C. E. T. and Wilke, K.,** Effects of loading of the eye on the intraocular pressure and on the episcleral venous pressure, *Acta Ophthalmol.,* 52, 107, 1974.

69. **Belmonte, C., Simon, J., and Gallego, A.,** Effects of intraocular pressure changes on the afferent activity of ciliary nerves, *Exp. Eye Res.,* 12, 342, 1971.

70. **Gallego, R. and Belmonte, C.,** Nervous efferent activity in the ciliary nerves related to intraocular pressure changes, *Exp. Eye Res.,* 19, 331, 1974.

71. **Bhattacherjee, P., Kulkarni, P. S., and Eakins, K. E.,** Metabolism of arachidonic acid in rabbit ocular tissues, *Invest. Ophthalmol. Vis. Sci.,* 18, 172, 1979.

72. **Kulkarni, P. S. and Srinivasan, B. D.,** Cyclooxygenase and lipoxygenase pathways in anterior uvea and conjunctiva, in *The Ocular Effects of Prostaglandins and Other Eicosanoids,* Bito, L. Z. and Stjernschantz, J., Eds., Alan R. Liss, New York, 1989, 39.

73. **Hedquist, P.,** Modulating effect of prostaglandin E_2 on noradrenalin release from the isolated cat spleen, *Acta Physiol. Scand.,* 75, 511, 1969.

74. **Junstad, M. and Wennmalm, Å.,** Release of prostaglandin from the rabbit isolated heart following vagal nerve stimulation of acetylcholine infusion, *Br. J. Pharmacol.,* 52, 375, 1974.

75. **Camras, C. B. and Podos, S. M.,** The role of endogenous prostaglandins in clinically used and investigational glaucoma therapy, in *The Ocular Effects of Prostaglandins and Other Eicosanoids,* Bito, L. Z. and Stjernschantz, J., Eds., Alan R. Liss, New York, 1989, 459.

76. **Almegård, B. and Andersson, S. E.,** Outflow facility in the monkey eye: Effects of calcitonin gene-related peptide, cholecystokinin, galanin, substance P and capsaicin, *Exp. Eye Res.,* 51, 685, 1990.

77. **Ballow, M., Donshik, P. C., Rapacz, P., and Samartino, L.,** Tear lactoferrin in patients with external inflammatory ocular disease, *Invest. Ophthalmol. Vis. Sci.,* 28, 543, 1987.

78. **Fullard, R. J.,** Identification of proteins in small tear volumes with and without size exclusion HPLC fractionation, *Curr. Eye Res.,* 7, 163, 1988.

79. **Fullard, R. J. and Tucker, D. L.,** Changes in human tear protein levels with progressively increasing stimulus, *Invest. Ophthalmol. Vis. Sci.,* 32, 2290, 1991.

Chapter 2

FORMULATION OF OPHTHALMIC SOLUTIONS AND SUSPENSIONS. PROBLEMS AND ADVANTAGES

Marc M. M. Van Ooteghem

TABLE OF CONTENTS

I.   Introduction 28

II.   The Elimination Process 28

III.   Properties Influencing Drug Retention 29
        A.   Instilled Volume... 29
        B.   Drugs and Adjuvants 29
        C.   Surface Tension 30
        D.   Osmolality... 31
        E.   Hydrogen Ion Concentration or pH..................................... 31
        F.   Viscosity 32
        G.   Suspended Drugs 33

IV.   Methods to Prolong the Residence of the Solution............................. 34
        A.   Formulation of the Solution 34
                1.   Drugs 34
                2.   Adjuvants 34
        B.   Instilled Volume... 35
        C.   Administration of the Solution 36

References.. 36

0-8493-7296-8/93/$0.00 + $.50

27

I. INTRODUCTION

Solutions and aqueous suspensions are the pharmaceutical forms most widely used to administer drugs that must be active on the eye surface or in the eye after passage through the cornea or conjunctiva.

These forms have some advantages: they are easily administered by the nurse or by the patient himself, and the drug is in a solved state and may be immediately active (in the case of a suspension, the drug is suspended in a saturated solution). These forms also have disadvantages: the very short time the solution stays at the eye surface, its poor bioavailability, the instability of the dissolved drug, and the necessity of using preservatives.

A considerable disadvantage of using eye drops is the rapid elimination of the solution and their poor bioavailability. This rapid elimination is due to the solution state of the preparation and may be influenced by the composition of the solution.

In this chapter the elimination process will be discussed, and the parameters influencing the elimination and the possibilities to prolong the retention of the solution at the eye surface will be examined.

II. THE ELIMINATION PROCESS

Sørensen and Jensen[1] instilled a suspension containing a radioactive tracer (^{99m}Tc) on the eyes of human volunteers and registered the radioactivity decay. The radioactivity was reduced by two thirds within 2 min and the tracer was completely eliminated after 15 min. The decay occurred in 3 steps: a very fast elimination during the first 2 min, followed by a rapid one between 2 and 5 min, and finally a slow elimination 5 to 15 min after instillation.

The rapid elimination has different causes: the amount and the structure of the tear film present, the capacity of the lower eyelid sack, and the different defense mechanisms of the eye against foreign matter.

The cornea and the conjunctiva are protected by tears and by the eyelids, which are responsible for the cleaning of the eye surface and for the elimination of foreign matter such as ophthalmic solutions or ophthalmic suspensions. The eye surface is covered by a thin (± 5 to 9-μm thick) precorneal tear film. About 7 to 8 μl of tears are spread out on the visible eye surface while about 3 μl of tears are present in the inferior conjunctival sac. The tear film on the eye surface is composed of three layers: a mucin layer adhering to the epithelium of the cornea and the conjunctiva, an aqueous layer which represents 90% of the precorneal tear film, and a thin lipid layer at the outside of the film. The basal tears are continuously secreted by different lacrimal and accessory glands. The average secretion of basal tears is 1.2 μl·min^{-1}.[2] The tears flow continuously over the eye surface of the cornea and conjunctiva, where a part of the water evaporates, while the remaining tears are drained through the puncti to the lacrimal sac. A sensory stimulation of the nerve endings in the cornea (e.g., by foreign bodies or ophthalmic solution) elicits reflex tears after 30 s.[3] The volume of reflex tears, which is influenced by the irritating power of the solutions instilled, varies from 3 μl·min^{-1} to between 300 and 400 μl·min^{-1}.[4] Reflex tears eliminate the ophthalmic solution from the eye surface more rapidly than basal tears. The decay of radioactivity observed by Sørensen and Jensen,[1] which occurred 2 to 5 min after instillation, was due to the secretion of reflex tears.

The elimination rate of an instilled solution is also influenced by eyelid movements. The upper eyelid moves vertically over two thirds of the eye surface. This downward motion appears to act as a "scraper", causing the surface of the cornea to be cleaned and the ophthalmic solution to be pushed downward. The main motion of the lower eyelid is a horizontal translation in the nasal direction, sometimes as much as 4 or 6 mm. This action appears to move the tear fluid, foreign matter, and ophthalmic solutions to the nasal corner of the lid junction, where the liquid exits, via the puncti.[5] The velocity of the eyelids during a blink is not constant and varies from individual to individual. By closing, the eyelids move at velocities between 0 cm·s^{-1} and 10 to 30 cm·s^{-1}.[6] The thickness of the tear film being about 7 μm, the rate of shear during a blink fluctuates between 0 and 14,000 to 43,000 s^{-1}.[7] The force exercised by the eyelid during a blink varies between 0.2 and 0.8 N.[8] Involuntary, usually unconscious, quick eye closure that occurs throughout the day is called periodic blinking. In relaxed adults the average frequency of this blinking is 15 to 16 per min, the range being 3 to 28 per min.[9] Stimuli (e.g., ophthalmic solutions) may provoke an increase in the blinking frequency, eliciting reflex blinks. The reflex blink elicited by a stimulus occurs with a latency of about 100 msec.[10] The velocity of the eyelid movement is the same as in the case of periodic blinking. The reflex blink quickly eliminates the stimulus, such as an instilled solution, from the eye surface. In the experiments of Sørensen and Jensen[1] reflex blinking seems to be responsible for the fast decay of the radioactivity during the first 2 min immediately after the instillation of the suspension.

III. PROPERTIES INFLUENCING DRUG RETENTION

Drug retention on the eye surface may be influenced by the instilled volume and the irritation power of the solution, which elicit reflex tears and reflex blinks, and by some physical properties of the solution. The irritation may be due to the dissolved drugs and adjuvants, the surface tension, the osmolality and pH of the solution, and the particle size of the suspended drugs. The retention of the solution is also influenced by the viscosity of the vehicle.

A. INSTILLED VOLUME

Under normal conditions the human tear volume is about 7 μl, with 1 μl in the precorneal tear film and about 3 μl in each marginal tear meniscus.[2] The unperturbed tear volume is relatively constant; the average tear turnover rate is 16%/min.[2] Only 3 μl of a solution can be incorporated in the precorneal film without causing it to destabilize.[11] In the lower eyelid sack a maximum of 30 μl of solution can be added.[2] However, the capacity is different for each person.[12] The instillation of a greater volume causes reflex blinks, which increase the drainage rate to the nasolacrimal canal, spilling on the cheeks and splashing the excess of the solution on the eyelashes.[13-16] The instillation of 20 and 50 μl of a drug solution could give similar therapeutic responses.[17-19] The normal tear volume is restored 2 to 3 min after the instillation of an excess, mostly in the first 15 to 30 s after the instillation.[20]

The rate of drainage of the solution, which is incorporated in the lower eyelid sack, is related to the instilled volume; the smaller the volume the slower the drainage rate. The decrease in fluorescence after the instillation of 20 μl and smaller volumes of a solution containing fluorescein is slower when 1 μl is instilled than when 20 μl are used.[12] The solution is also mixed with the resident tears, reducing the concentration of the drug. Assuming a tear volume of 7 μl in the precorneal area, the dilution with 1, 5, 10, and 20 μl solution is, respectively, 8, 2.4, 1.7, and 1.35 times after the instillation.[12] This concentration decrease minimizes the efficiency of the drug. Ideally, a high concentration of the drug in a small volume is desirable. The instilled drop should have a volume of between 10 and 15 μl.

B. DRUGS AND ADJUVANTS

The eye is very sensitive to many substances. These substances may directly react as allergens with the antigens of the tissue cells (type I hypersensitivity).[21,22] They often irritate the sensory nerve ends in the cornea.[23]

No relation exists between the structure of the substance and its irritation power; this is different for each substance.[24] The ocular irritation of substances in rabbit eyes has been evaluated by the Draize method.[25] As the tear secretion and the blink frequency of rabbit eyes are one hundred times smaller compared to human eyes, the substance remains on the surface of rabbit eyes for a longer period. Therefore it is very difficult to extrapolate the irritancy of substances on human eyes from the results of the Draize test. The tolerance of a substance should be determined on the human eye; the eye is examined 5, 10, 30, and 55 min after the instillation of the solution of the substance.[26] From their use on human eyes it appears that 165 drugs and adjuvants elicit ocular irritation.[27] Most of the antibiotics (amoxycillin, bacitracin, several penicillins, cephalosporins, chloramphenicol, chlortracycline, clindamycin, colistin, neomycin, gentamicin, kanamycin, polymyxin B, streptomycin, tobramycin, amphotericin B), several sulfonamides, miotics (echothiophate, aceclidine, neostigmine, pilocarpine), mydriatics (atropine, homatropine, tropicamide), antiviral agents (acyclovir, idoxuridine), agents used to treat glaucoma (timolol, dipivefrin), antihistamines (antazoline), sympathomimetics (ephedrine, epinephrine, hydroxyamphetamine, phenylephrine, naphazoline), and several mercuric and silver compounds (mercuric oxide, organomercurials, colloidal silver, siliver nitrate, silver protein) have irritant properties.[23,27-31]

Local anesthetics immediately cause a temporary irritation and lacrimation after instillation. Several adjuvants, such as preservatives (benzalkonium chloride, 2-phenylethanol, chlorhexidine) and some viscolyzers, have irritative properties.[27,31-35]

Systemic administration of some drugs may influence the tear secretion. Atropine, scopolamine, antihistamines, β-adrenergic blocking agents, general anesthetics (nitrous oxide, halothan, enfluran), diuretics, and tranquilizers (tricyclic antidepressants, MAO-inhibitors, benzodiazepines, meprobamate) reduce the tear secretion. Systemic-administered pilocarpine, carbachol, neostigmine, sympathomimetics (ephedrine, epinephrine), cytostatics (fluorouracil), bromhexidine, and a chronic use of heroin, histamine, etc., increase the tear secretion.[37-41]

C. SURFACE TENSION

The epithelial surface of the cornea and conjunctiva is covered with a thin tear film. The innermost layer of the tear film in contact with the epithelium cells is composed of a mucus layer. When the mucus layer is completely removed and the cornea exposed to the air its critical surface tension equals 28 or 31 $mN \cdot m^{-1}$, according to Holly, Lemp, et al.[42,43] But Tiffany[44,45] estimated the critical surface tension of the eye surface to be 67.5 to 69.3 $mN \cdot m^{-1}$. The difference in the values is probably due to the incomplete removal of the mucus layer. The surface tension of tear fluid at the eye temperature is 43.6 to 46.6 $mN \cdot m^{-1}$ for normal eyes and 49.6 $mN \cdot m^{-1}$ for dry eyes.[46,47] The instillation of a solution containing drugs or adjuvants that lower the surface tension may disrupt the outermost lipid layer of the tear film into numerous oily droplets which are solubilized.[48,49] The protective effect of the oily film against evaporation of the tear film aqueous layer disappears and dry spots will be formed.[50,51] The dry spots are painful and irritant and elicit reflex blinks to eliminate the surfactant. The irritation will not always happen immediately after the instillation — in many cases it appears 30 min to 1 h after the application; it is dependent on the substance and on its concentration.[52,53] The tear film is destabilized when the surface tension of the instilled solution is much lower than the surface tension of the lacrimal fluid.[47,54] The irritation power of surfactants decreases in the following order: cationic, anionic, ampholytic, nonionic.[55,56] The surfactants may also remove the mucus layer and disrupt tight junctional complexes, increasing the permeability of the cornea.[57-59] This may explain the increased transcorneal penetration of drugs in the presence of surfactants.[60-63]

D. OSMOLALITY

The osmolality of the lacrimal fluid is mainly dependent on the number of dissolved ions and crystalloids. Proteins contribute very little (about 1 in 10,000) to the total osmotic pressure of tears because of their molecular weight and low concentration.[64]

The osmolality of the tears after prolonged eye closure or during sleep varies from 280 to 293 mOsm·kg^{-1}.[65] During the day when the eyes are open, and due to the evaporation process, the osmolality progresses at a rate of 1.43 mOsm·kg^{-1}·h^{-1} and varies between 302 and 318 mOsm·kg^{-1} (extreme values 231 to 446 mOsm·kg^{-1}) in normal eyes.[65-68] The osmolality differs across the ocular surface; the tear fluid in the conjunctival sac has a higher osmolality than the fluid of the tear strip.[69] The tear film osmolality is increased in the case of ocular surface diseases such as keratoconjunctivitis sicca (dry eye), thyroid eye disease in which the palperal fissures are widened, and in contact lens wearers after 40 years.[68,70,71]

When the eye surface is covered with a hypotonic solution the permeability of the epithelium is increased considerably and water flows into the cornea.[72] The corneal tissues swell, increasing the pressure on the nerves and causing an anesthetizing action up the cornea.[73]

In the case where the eye surface is covered with hypertonic solution, water flows from the aqueous layer through the cornea to the eye surface.[74] A desquamation of superficial cells is also observed after instillation of hypertonic solutions in rabbits.[75]

An ophthalmic solution instilled in the eye is mixed with the tears present. The osmotic pressure of the mixture depends upon the osmolality of the tears, and upon the osmolality and the volume of the amount instilled. The instillation of hypo- or hypertonic solutions could elicit reflex tears and reflex blinks due to discomfort and irritation. Depending on the drop size, solutions with an osmolality lower than 100 or 266 mOsm·kg^{-1} and higher than 480 or 640 mOsm·kg^{-1} are irritant.[76-80] The original osmolality will be restored 1 or 2 min after instillation of the nonisotonic solution depending on the drop size.[81] The instillation of a hypotonic drug solution creates an osmotic gradient between the tear film and the surrounding tissues. This induces a flux of water from the eye surface to the cornea, temporarily increasing the drug concentration on the eye surface.[82]

E. HYDROGEN ION CONCENTRATION OR pH

The pH of tears is determined by different substances dissolved in the aqueous layer of the tears: carbon dioxide, bicarbonate, and proteins such as the basic lysozyme and an acidic specific tear prealbumin.[83] The fatty acids secreted by the meibomian glands are mixed with the aqueous phase secreted by the lacrimal glands to give an acid solution with a pH of about 6.6.[84] After spreading of the tear film, carbon dioxide evaporates and the pH of the lacrimal fluid increases. When the eye remains open for 50 s the pH rises to pH 9.[85] However, due to frequent blinking and secretion of fresh tears, the pH increases slowly during the waking hours of the day and varies between 6.9 and 7.5[86-91] The tear fluid becomes more alkaline because the amount of carbon dioxide that evaporates is not always completely compensated by the carbon dioxide present in the freshly secreted tears.[89-92] Moreover, in contact-lens wearers the tears are more acid due to the impediment of the efflux of carbon dioxide.[93,94] The lacrimal fluid is more alkaline in the case of diseases such as keratoconjunctivitis sicca (dry eye), severe ocular rosacea, and lacrimal stenosis, after cataract extraction, and also in newborns.[83,95-98]

The tear fluid has a small buffer capacity. This is principally due to the carbon dioxide and the carbonate dissolved in the aqueous phase of the tears. The pH is not influenced by the addition of 0.05 μg of HCl or by the addition of 0.0125 μg NaOH to 10 μl of human tears (± volume of tears on the eye).[99] However, the pH of the tears decreases or increases rapidly with the addition of greater amounts of acids or alkali.[100]

The exposure of the eye surface to an acid fluid causes damage to the ocular tissues resulting from a reaction with cellular proteins, forming insoluble complexes. An alkalinization of the tear film tends to produce an interaction of the hydroxyl ions with the cell membranes. At a high pH the lipids in the cell membranes will be saponified causing disruption of the structural integrity of the cells.[101,102] The damage is dependent on the concentration of hydrogen and hydroxyl ions and on the exposure time.

When a drop of acid or alkaline solution is instilled, the solution will be mixed with the tears present. The tears are not able to neutralize this important volume, so reflex tears will be secreted to dilute the instilled drop and to eliminate the solution.[103,104] The time necessary to neutralize the solution and recover the original pH varies from a few to 20 min. The pH, volume, and buffer capacity of the instilled solution, as well as the age of the patient, will influence the recovery time.[83,103]

In some cases the instillation of a solution with a pH different from the tears will be irritant and will cause a painful sensation. This depends on the volume instilled, the buffer capacity and composition of the solution, and the contact time with the eye surface. Lake water of pH 6.3, isotonic buffer solution containing mono-, di-, and tri-sodium phosphate of pH 5.8 and 6.7, citrate buffer solution of pH 5.0, and borate solution of pH 6.5 and 9.0 are irritant.[76,79,103,105]

To prolong the retention of a drug at the eye surface, it is necessary that the ophthalmic solution have a pH between 7.0 and 7.7. If it is impossible to prepare a solution with these pH values (e.g., instability of the drug), the solution does not contain a strong buffer and only a low concentration of a weak buffer system.

F. VISCOSITY

The viscosity of ophthalmic solutions is often increased to prolong their retention on the eye surface and to increase the bioavailability of the drug.[106,117] The viscosity may also be increased to diminish the frictional resistance occurring between the cornea and the eyelid with each blink.[118] This friction has been assumed to be of the boundary type and decreases with the viscosity of the precorneal tear fluid and the velocity of the eyelid movement.[119]

After the instillation of a viscous ophthalmic solution, a part is incorporated in the precorneal tear film and in the marginal tear strip, increasing the available volume of the solution.[11] The other part of the solution remains in the eyelid sack and is able to restore a thick precorneal film at each blink. For most viscous solutions this phenomenon seems to persist for as long as 20 min. The thickness of the precorneal film formed principally depends on the viscosity of the solution instilled, but decreases as the surface tension of the solution increases.[11]

The values for tear viscosity given in the literature vary between 1.052 and 5.975 mPa.[118,120-126] The tears have a pseudoplastic character with a yield value of about 0.032 Pa at 33°C.[123] The force needed to move eyelids during a normal blink is about 0.2 N and for a forceful blink, 0.8 N. A force exercised by the eyelid which is greater than 0.9 N is painful.[8] This pain may elicit reflex blinks and reflex tear, eliminating the solution on the eye surface very quickly. The pseudoplastic character of the precorneal film is very important. Between each blink the film is submitted to the gravity force. When the film has a yield value greater than the gravity, no flow occurs and the film is not moved. During a blink the lid moves at a high velocity and the film is submitted to a high rate of shear.[127]

The instillation of an ophthalmic solution should influence the pseudoplastic character of the precorneal tear film as little as possible. This is made possible by the use of a viscous solution with pseudoplastic properties. It may be assumed that the tear film-instilled solution mixture will be pseudoplastic.

The useful viscosity range of the ophthalmic solution is, however, limited. The force to move the tear film-instilled solution mixture at high shear rates must be lower than the pain threshold (or 0.9 N).[8] The use of solutions with high viscosity will elicit reflex tears and reflex blinks resulting in very fast elimination of the mixture from the eye surface. However, solutions containing viscolyzers that also have viscoelastic properties could be used at higher viscosities.[128] A viscoelastic substance exhibits elastic recovery after the deformation that occurs during the shear movement. Viscosity and viscoelasticity are not synonymous, although viscoelasticity is a property that is related to viscosity as well as to molecule length, molecule configuration, and intra- and interchain molecule reactions. Long-chain molecules tend to be more elastic than short-chain molecules.[128]

Ophthalmic solutions may stay at the eye surface for a longer time due to viscosity increase. However, the lacrimal glands continue to secrete fresh tears, which can result in an excess of fluid on the eye surface. This excess must be eliminated by the drainage system. The mixture must flow through the puncti (small openings about 0.3 mm in diameter), which lead to the canaliculi (with variable diameters but generally considered to be about 0.5 mm).[129] The mixture in the puncti and the canaliculi is submitted to lower shear rates than on the eye surface during a blink. The viscosity of an instilled solution should not be too high; it should not obstruct the puncti and the canaliculi. To flow easily through the puncti, thus at a low shear rate, the viscosity of the mixture should not be higher than 40 to 50 mPa.[130]

G. SUSPENDED DRUGS

Suspensions are widely used in ocular drug therapy to administer sparingly soluble drugs, or complexes of soluble drugs, or to obtain a slow dissolution and a prolonged release of the drug. A suspended drug, however, has a lower therapeutic activity than a dissolved drug.[131] The therapeutic activity of an indomethacin suspension, for example, is only 67% compared to that of the saturated solution.[132] To obtain the same effect, the dissolution rate of the particle must be greater than the clearance rate from the cul-de-sac and must be approximately equal to the absorption rate.[133,134]

Ophthalmic suspensions are generally gently deposited in the cul-de-sac. The solid particles remain mainly on the eye surface and do not penetrate the cornea or the anterior chamber, as in the case of particles of glass, wood, or metal propelled by moving machinery or dust and sand blown by the wind.[135,136] The drug particles deposited on the eye surface will be moved by the eyelids at each blink and could cause an abrasion of the outer epithelium layers.[137] They may also cause irritation of sensory nerves in the epithelium.[138] Because the suspended drug is a foreign particle, the irritation could elicit reflex blinks and reflex lacrimation to eliminate the particle. Some particles could also penetrate into the upper layers of the epithelium and dissolve very slowly, building a saturated solution on their surface. This high concentration could be irritant. The irritant power of a particle is determined by its shape, size, and composition.[139] Forms with sharp angles and edges are more irritant than isometric particles with obtuse angles and edges.[140] The length of the needles or the prisms is mainly responsible for the irritation.[141] By preparing small particles by recrystallization or milling, polymorph particles will be obtained. With time the reconversion of the polymorphs to stable forms should lead to larger particles with sharp angles and edges.[142]

It is very difficult to give upper limits of particle size required. Though the tear film has a thickness of about 7 to 8 μm, some ophthalmologists give an upper particle size limit of 50 μm while others propose 30 μm.[143,144] Most pharmacopoeiae give limits of particle size for ophthalmic preparations. The European Pharmacopoeia requires that "on 10 μg solid phase not more than twenty particles have a maximum diameter greater than 25 μm, not more than two particles have a maximum diameter greater than 50 μm and no particle has a maximum diameter greater than 90 μm''.

IV. METHODS TO PROLONG THE RESIDENCE OF THE SOLUTION

The eye may not be irritated by the drugs and adjuvants dissolved nor by the properties of the solution. In many cases it will be necessary to adapt the formulation. The instilled volume must be limited so that it can remain on the eye surface. At the administration, the instilled solution may be spread on the total eye surface and remain there for a long time. The outflow through the puncti must be delayed. The administration technique will be very important.

A. FORMULATION OF THE SOLUTION

1. Drugs

The irritation elicited by a drug may be due to its chemical structure and its concentration in the solution. It is very difficult to correlate the irritation power and the chemical structure. Different substances with similar chemical structures may have a different irritation power. Oxybuprocaine has a much higher transient irritation power than procaine and proparacaine with a similar chemical structure.[145] For the formulation it may be preferable to replace the prescribed drug with another that has the same therapeutic activity but with or without lower irritation properties.

The irritation may also be influenced by the concentration of the drug. The instillation of a 2% carbachol (parasympathomimetic) is more irritant than at 1% and a 0.1 M solution of oxybuprocaine is more irritant than a 0.01 M solution.[145,146] Eye drops containing 1% of pilocarpine solution are irritant.[27,147] When a drop (30 μl) of this solution is instilled and mixed with 7 μl of tears present, the concentration of pilocarpine in the mixture will be 0.8% and is irritant. When Ocusert® Pilo-20 with a release of 20 μg·h^{-1} is placed in the cul-de-sac, the concentration of pilocarpine in the lacrimal fluid will be 0.057% and is not irritant.

Many ophthalmic solutions seem to possess irritant properties. This may be due to the high concentration of the drug. Solutions with lower concentrations are less irritant and are eliminated slowly from the eye. The most appropriate concentration must be determined for each substance and for each formulation. One is advised to use the lowest concentration, because these solutions have the lowest systemic resorption and the least adverse reactions.

2. Adjuvants

Most pharmacopeiae require that aqueous preparations supplied in multidose containers contain antimicrobial preservatives at appropriate concentrations, except when the preparation itself has adequate antimicrobial properties. The preservative must destroy or prevent the growth of microorganisms accidentally introduced in the solution during the instillation.[148,149] If the solution is used on different patients (e.g., in a clinic or in a doctor's office) for the examination of the eyes, a cross-contamination may take place. A patient may be contaminated by pathogenic microorganisms from another patient.[150] In this case the preservative should be bactericidal and should kill the microorganisms in a short period of time. If the solution is used by one person, the solution may be contaminated by the microorganisms of his own eyes. The preservative must not be bactericidal, because the solution will be reinstilled in the same contaminated eye.[151] Thus the preservative must only prevent the growth of the microorganisms. The bactericidal or bacteriostatic activity depends on the concentration of the preservative, but its irritation power also depends on its concentration in the preparation.[152] At high concentrations, when a preservative exerts a bactericidal activity, it will be irritant and will elicit reflex lacrimation.[27,153] However, at lower concentrations, when it is bacteriostatic, it will be well tolerated. Ophthalmic solutions that need a bactericidal concentration of a preservative should, whenever possible, be delivered without a preservative in single-dose containers.

Surfactants are often used in ophthalmic solutions to improve the dispersion of suspended drugs and to increase the resorption of the drugs. Substances such as benzalkoniumchloride, chlorhexidine, sodium lauryl sulfate, and the nonionic surfactants are irritant and elicit reflex lacrimation.[27,56,154] The irritation power depends on their concentration in the solution.[56] The Food and Drug Administration requires that ophthalmic solutions contain no more than 1% Tween 20 or Tween 80. The use of surfactants in solutions coming into contact with the eye should be minimized.

Viscolyzers are used to increase the retention of ophthalmic solutions at the eye surface and to increase the bioavailability of the drug. Different viscolyzers have surface activity properties. This lowering of the surface tension could be irritant and elicit reflex tears and reflex blinks annulling the effect of viscosity increase. Solutions with low or high molecular weight of hydroxypropylmethylcellulose, hydroxypropylcellulose, or polyvinylalcohol have surface tensions lower than 50 mN·m^{-1}.[117,156] Solutions with low or high molecular weight of dextran, hydroxyethylcellulose, or polyvinylpyrrolidone have surface tensions higher than 57 mN·m^{-1}.[117,156] Viscous solutions with low surface tensions are irritant and will be eliminated rapidly from the eye surface. For formulation, viscolyzers with high surface tension should be chosen. Viscous solutions or gels containing carbomer (Carbopol® 940) are pseudoplastic. After instillation, the viscosity decreases dramatically because of an interaction of the carbomer solution with the ions present in the tears.[157,158] At the instillation a pain sensation at the inner canthusis is reported.[158] This may be attributed to some drainage difficulties of the high-molecular-weight polymer through the puncti into the lacrimal drainage system. Sodium hyaluronate seems to have mucoadhesion properties. Its solutions are also viscoelastic and are not irritant.[159-164] If a viscous ophthalmic solution is to be formulated, nonirritant substances with mucoadhesive properties must be chosen.

B. INSTILLED VOLUME

The ophthalmic solutions and suspensions are generally administered by means of a plastic squeeze bottle with an attached dropper tip, and seldom by means of a separate dropper fitted on a glass bottle.

The maximum volume of a solution that can be added into the lower eyelid sack is 30 μl.[2] This must be the maximum volume delivered by both systems. The delivered drop volume can be calculated approximately with the equation of Tates, obtained from semiempirical considerations,[165]

$$V = \frac{2 \cdot \pi \cdot r \cdot \sigma}{g \cdot \rho \cdot f}$$

where V = volume of the drop, r = outer radius of the surface of the dropper tip, σ = dynamic surface tension of the solution,[166] g = gravity, ρ = density of the solution, and f = dimensionless factor to correct the volume, because after the detachment of the drop, several tiny droplets follow the main drop. It is estimated as a function of r/V$^{1/3}$.[167]

The drop size is influenced by the outer diameter of the dropper-tip surface. Several eyedroppers with small outer diameters have been proposed to obtain drops smaller than 30 μl.[168,169] Nevertheless, the drop size is also influenced by the density and the dynamic surface tension of the solution. The ophthalmic solutions generally contain low concentrations of drugs and adjuvants. The density of the solutions is, in general, the same as water. The dynamic surface tension is used, because the formation of a drop occurs in less than 10 s.[170] The viscosity of the solution seems not to influence the drop size.[167] No standard dropper can be used for all solutions. The selection of the outer diameter depends on the composition and the dynamic surface tension of each solution.

A great variation in drop sizes obtained with one dropper is caused by the design of the dropper tip. After detachment of the drop the solution remaining in the dropper must be sucked completely into the plastic bottle. The drop size of the following drop will not be influenced by the solution present in the dropper tip. Also, the solution in the dropper, which was contaminated during the instillation, will be aspirated into the bottle and mixed with the solution containing a preservative. The concentration of the bacteria will be diluted and the preservative will act more easily.[171]

C. ADMINISTRATION OF THE SOLUTION

To maximize the ocular contact time and presumably the drug penetration, and to minimize a rapid flow through the canaliculi and a systemic adsorption, the following administration technique has been proposed.[172-175]

- The head is lightly tilted back and the lower eyelid gently grasped between the thumb and index finger. It is slightly pulled forward to create a small pocket.
- One drop (maximum 30 μl) of an ophthalmic solution is instilled into the pocket without touching the ocular or periocular tissues. The drop must fall on the conjunctiva and not directly on the cornea. The cornea possesses more nerve endings and is more sensitive than the conjunctiva.[176] Because a cold solution (4°C) seems to have a short anesthetic effect vs. a warm (20°C) solution, it seems preferable to instill a cold solution to obtain a slightly delayed irritation.[177]
- The lid is held forward for a few seconds until the drop settles into the lower cul-de-sac. The patient will continue to look forward to avoid a contact between the cornea and the solution and to delay reflex reactions.
- The lower lid is then brought upward until it touches the eye. The lid is then released and the eyelids are gently closed for a minimum of 3 min. During this time the patient does not blink or squeeze the lids. With closed eyelids, the patient rolls his eyes to spread the solution on the eye surface.[175]
- During the time when the eyelids are closed and a few minutes more, gentle pressure is applied on the puncti to prevent drainage of solution through the canaliculi and systemic absorption.

This administration technique would increase the bioavailability and should be used by the nurses in hospitals. Patients and their families should be instructed by physicians and pharmacists. In the case of self-administration, several aids are proposed to instill the solution easily and to control the administration visually.[178,179]

REFERENCES

1. **Sørensen, B. and Jensen, F. T.,** Tear flow in human eyes. Determination by means of radioisotope and gamma camera, *Acta Ophthalmol. (Copenhagen),* 57, 564, 1979.
2. **Mishima, S., Gasset, A., Klyce, S. O., and Baum, J. L.,** Determination of tear volume and tear flow, *Invest. Ophthalmol.,* 5, 264, 1966.
3. **Wright, P.,** Normal tear production and drainage, *Trans. Ophthalmol. Soc. U.K.,* 104, 351, 1985.
4. **Farris, R. L., Stuchell, R. N., and Mandel, I. D.,** Basal and reflex tear analysis. I. Physical measurements: osmolarity, basal volumes and reflex rate, *Ophthalmology (Rochester),* 88, 852, 1981.
5. **Doane, M. G.,** Dynamics of the human eyeblink, *Ivnest. Ophthalmol. Vis. Sci.,* 18 (Suppl.), 198, 1979.

6. **Doane, M. G.,** Interaction of eyelids and tears in corneal wetting and the dynamics of the normal eyeblink, *Am. J. Ophthalmol.,* 89, 507, 1980.

7. **Dudinski, O., Finnin, B. C., and Reed, B. L.,** Acceptability of thickened eye drops to human subjects, *Curr. Ther. Res.,* 33, 322, 1933.

8. **Hung, G., Hsu, F., and Stark, S.,** Dynamics of the human eye blink, *Am. J. Optom. Physiol. Opt.,* 54, 678, 1977.

9. **Drew, G. C.,** Variations in reflex blink-rate during visual-motor tasks, *Q. J. Exp. Psychol.,* 3, 73, 1951.

10. **Walsh, F. B. and Hoyt, W. F.,** The neurology of eyelid closure: orbicularis oculi, blinking and associated aspects of facial innervation, in *Clinical Neuroophthalmology,* Vol. 1, 3rd ed., Walsh, F. B. and Hoyt, W. F., Eds., Williams & Wilkins, Baltimore, 1969, 326.

11. **Benedetto, D. A., Shah, D. O., and Kaufman, H. E.,** The instilled fluid dynamics and surface chemistry of polymers in the preocular tear film, *Invest. Ophthalmol.,* 14, 887, 1975.

12. **Ludwig, A. and Van Ooteghem, M.,** The influence of the dropsize on the elimination of an ophthalmic solution from the precorneal area of human eyes, *Pharm. Acta Helv.,* 62, 56, 1987.

13. **Chrai, S. S., Patton, T. F., Mehta, A., and Robinson, J. R.,** Lacrimal and instilled fluid dynamics in rabbit eyes, *J. Pharm. Sci.,* 62, 1112, 1973.

14. **Zaki, I., Fitzgerald, P., Hardy, J. G., and Wilson, C. G.,** A comparison of the effect of viscosity on the precorneal residence of solution in rabbit and man, *J. Pharm. Pharmacol.,* 38, 463, 1986.

15. **Maurice, D. M.,** Kinetics of topically applied ophthalmic drugs, in *Ophthalmic Drug Delivery: Biopharmaceutical, Technological and Clinical Aspects,* Vol. 11, (Fidia Research Series), Saettone, M. F., Bucci, M., and Speiser, P., Eds., Springer-Verlag, Berlin, 1987, 19.

16. **Mishima, S.,** Pharmacology of ophthalmic solutions, *Asian-Pacific J. Ophthalmol.,* 1, 2, 1989.

17. **Miller, K., Brown, R. H., Lynch, M. G., Eto, C. Y., Lue, J. C., and Novack, G. D.,** Does drop size influence the efficacy of a topical beta blocker?, *Invest. Ophthalmol. Vis. Sci.,* Suppl. 27, 161, 1986.

18. **File, R. R. and Patton, T. F.,** Topically applied pilocarpine: human pupillary response as a function of drop size, *Arch. Ophthalmol.,* 98, 112, 1980.

19. **Charap, A. D., Shin, D. H., Petursson, G., Cinotti, D., Wortham, E., Brown, H., Silverstone, D. E., Atkins, J. M., Eto, C. Y., Lue, J. C. and Novack, G. D.,** Effect of varying drop size on the efficacy and safety of a topical beta blocker, *Ann. Ophthalmol.,* 21, 351, 1989.

20. **Shell, J. W.,** Pharmacokinetics of topically applied ophthalmic drugs, *Surv. Ophthalmol.,* 26, 207, 1982.

21. **Coombs, R. R. A. and Gell, P. G. H.,** Classification of allergic reactions responsible for clinical hypersensitivity and disease, in *Clinical Aspects of Immunology,* Gell, P. H. G., Coombs, R. R. A., and Lachmann, P. J., Eds., Blackwell Scientific, London, 1975, 761.

22. **Easty, D. L.,** Allergic disorders of the eye, *Practitioner,* 220, 581, 1978.

23. **Wilson, F. M.,** Adverse external ocular effects of topical ophthalmic medications, *Surv. Ophthalmol.,* 24, 57, 1979.

24. **Scoville, B., Krieglstein, G. K., Then, E., Yokoyoma, S., and Yokoyama, T.,** Measuring drug-induced eye irritation: a simple new clinical essay, *J. Clin. Pharmacol.,* 25, 210, 1985.

25. **Draize, J. H., Woodard, G., and Calvery, H. O.,** Methods for the study of irritation and toxicity of substances applied topically to the skin and mucous membranes, *J. Pharmacol. Exp. Ther.,* 82, 377, 1944.

26. **Lippa, E. A., Von Deffer, H. A., Hofman, H. M., and Brunner-Ferber, F. L.,** Local tolerance and activity of MK-927, a novel topical carbonic anhydrase inhibitor, *Arch. Ophthalmol.,* 106, 1694, 1988.

27. **Frauenfelder, F. T. and Meyer, S. M.,** *Drug Induced Ocular Side Effects and Drug Interactions,* 3rd ed., Lea & Febiger, Philadelphia, 1989, 1–489.

28. **Hätinen, A., Taräsvirta, M., and Fräki, J. E.,** Contact allergy to components in topical ophthalmic preparations, *Acta Ophthalmology (Copenhagen),* 63, 424, 1985.

29. **Kruyswijk, M. R. L., Van Driel, L. M. J., Polak, B. C. P., and Go-Sennema, A. A.,** Contact allergy following administration of eye drops and eye ointments, *Doc. Ophthalmol.,* 48, 251, 1979.

30. **Polak, B. C. P.,** Bijwerkingen van geneesmiddelen in de oogheelkunde, in *Vorderingen in de Geneeskunde II,* Dees, J., Lambrechts, L. J., and Polak, B. C. P., Eds., Stafleu, Alphen a/d Rijn and Brussels, 1988, 71.

31. **Burstein, N. L.,** The effects of topical drugs and preservatives on the tears and corneal epithelium in dry eye, *Trans. Ophthalmol. Soc. U.K.,* 104, 402, 1985.

32. **Bourrinet, P. and Rodde, D.,** Vérification de la tolérance de quelques conservateurs et bactéricides, *Labo-Pharma Probl. Tech.,* 240, 121, 1975.

33. **Gasset, A. R.,** Benzalkonium chloride toxicity to the human cornea, *Am. J. Ophthalmol.,* 84, 169, 1977.

34. **Boer, Y.,** Irritation by eyedrops containing 2-phenyl-ethanol, *Pharm. Weekbl. Sci. Ed.,* 3, 826, 1981.

35. **Van Haeringen, N. J.,** Allergische en toxische reacties bij gebruik van oog-druppels, *Pharm. Weekbl.,* 122, 1101, 1987.

36. **Ludwig, A. and Van Ooteghem, M.,** Evaluation of sodium hyaluronate of viscous vehicle for eye drops, *J. Pharm. Belg.,* 44, 391, 1989.

37. **Crandall, D. C. and Leopold, I. H.**, The influence of systemic drugs on tear constituents, *Ophthalmology (Rochester)*, 86, 115, 1979.
38. **Polak, B. C. P.**, Side effects of drugs on tear secretion, *Doc. Ophthalmol.*, 67, 115, 1987.
39. **Norn, M.**, The effects of drugs on tear flow, *Trans. Ophthalmol. Soc. U.K.*, 104, 410, 1985.
40. **Krupin, T., Cross, D. A., and Becker, B.**, Decreased basal tear production associated with general anesthesia, *Arch. Ophthalmol.*, 95, 107, 1977.
41. **Egger-Büssing, C. H. and Zirm, M.**, Ein neuer Aspekt beim sekretorischer Verhalten der Tränendrüse, *Klin. Monatsbl. Augenheilkd.*, 176, 85, 1980.
42. **Holly, F. J. and Lemp, M. A.**, Wettability and wetting of corneal epithelium *Exp. Eye Res.*, 11, 239, 1971.
43. **Lemp, M. A., Holly, F. J., Iwata, S., and Dohlman, C. H.**, The precorneal tear film. 1. Factors in spreading and maintaining a tear film over the corneal surface, *Arch. Ophthalmol.*, 83, 89, 1970.
44. **Tiffany, J. M.**, Measurement of the wettability of the corneal epithelium. I. Particle attachment method, *Acta Ophthalmol. (Copenhagen)*, 69, 175, 1990.
45. **Tiffany, J. M.**, Measurement of the wettability of corneal epithelium. II. Contact angle method, *Acta Ophthalmol. (Copenhagen)*, 68, 182, 1990.
46. **Tiffany, J. M., Winter, N., and Bliss, G.**, Tear film stability and tear surface tension, *Curr. Eye Res.*, 8, 507, 1989.
47. **Miller, D.**, Measurement of surface tension of tears, *Arch. Ophthalmol.*, 82, 368, 1969.
48. **Holly, F. J.**, Surface chemical evaluation of artificial tears and their ingredients. II. Interaction with a superficial lipid layer, *Cont. Intraoc. Lens Med. J.*, 4, 52, 1978.
49. **Pfister, R. R. and Burstein, N. L.**, The effects of ophthalmic drugs, vehicles and preservatives on corneal epithelium: A scanning electron microscopic study, *Invest. Ophthalmol.*, 15, 245, 1976.
50. **Norn, M. S. and Opauszki, A.**, Effects of ophthalmic vehicles on the stability of the precorneal tear film *Acta Ophthalmol. (Copenhagen)*, 35, 23, 1977.
51. **Wilson, W. S., Duncan, A. J., and Jay, J. L.**, Effect of benzalkonium chloride on the stability of the precorneal tear film in rabbit and man, *Br. J. Ophthalmol.*, 59, 1667, 1975.
52. **Marsh, R. J. and Maurice, D. M.**, The influence of non-ionic detergents and other surfactants on human corneal permeability, *Exp. Eye Res.*, 11, 43, 1977.
53. **Ludwig, A. and Van Ooteghem, M.**, Influence of the surface tension of eye drops on the retention of a tracer in the precorneal area of human eyes, *J. Pharm. Belg.*, 43, 157, 1988.
54. **Lin, S. P. and Brenner, H.**, Marangoni convection in a tear film *J. Colloid. Interface Sci.*, 85, 59, 1982.
55. **Van Abbé, N. J.**, Eye irritation: studies relating to responses in man and laboratory animals, *J. Soc. Cosmet. Chem.*, 24, 685, 1973.
56. **Etter, J. C. and Wildhaber, A.**, Développement d'un test objectif d'irritation oculaire sur la souris: Intérêt en pharmacie galénique et biopharmacie. Première partie: les tensioactifs, *Pharm. Acta Helv.*, 59, 8, 1984.
57. **Bessière, E., Duquety, M., Magimel, R., and Mirande, B.**, Utilisation en instillations oculaires de produits non ioniques dans certains oedèmes cornéens, *Bull. Soc. Ophtalmol. Fr.*, 14, 230, 1960.
58. **Keller, N., Moore, D., Carper, D., and Longwell, A.**, Increased corneal permeability by the dual effects of transient tear film acidification and exposure to benzalkonium chloride, *Exp. Eye Res.*, 30, 203, 1980.
59. **Burstein, N. L.**, Preservative alteration of corneal permeability in humans and rabbits, *Invest. Ophthalmol. Vis. Sci.*, 25, 1450, 1984.
60. **Green, K. and Downs, S.**, Prednisolone phosphate penetration into and through the cornea, *Invest. Ophthalmol.*, 13, 316, 1974.
61. **Green, K. and Downs, S.**, Ocular penetration of pilocarpine in rabbits, *Arch. Ophthalmol.*, 93, 1165, 1975.
62. **Tønjum, A. M.**, Permeability of the rabbit corneal epithelium to horseradish peroxidase after the influence of benzalkonium chloride, *Acta Ophthalmol. (Copenhagen)*, 54, 335, 1975.
63. **Singh, T. and Maurice, D.**, A test for acute corneal toxicity, *Invest. Ophthalmol. Vis. Sci.*, Suppl. 26, 175, 1985.
64. **Holly, F. J. and Esquivel, E. D.**, Colloid osmotic pressure of artificial tears, *J. Ocular Pharmacol.*, 1, 327, 1985.
65. **Terry, J. E. and Hill, R. M.**, Human tear osmotic pressure, diurnal variations and the closed eye, *Arch. Ophthalmol.*, 96, 120, 1978.
66. **Benjamin, W. J. and Hill, R. M.**, Human tears: osmotic characteristics, *Invest. Ophthalmol. Vis. Sci.*, 24, 1624, 1983.
67. **Gilbard, P. J., Farris, R. L., and Santamaria, J.**, Osmolarity of tear microvolumes in keratoconjunctivitis sicca, *Arch. Ophthalmol.*, 96, 677, 1978.
68. **Farris, R. L., Stuchell, R. N., and Mandel, I. D.**, Basal and reflex human tear analysis. I. Physical measurements: osmolarity, basal volumes, and reflex flow rate, *Ophthalmology (Rochester)*, 88, 852, 1981.

69. **Benjamin, W. J. and Hill, R. M.**, Tonicity of human tear fluid sampled from the cul-de-sac, *Br. J. Ophthalmol.*, 73, 624, 1989.
70. **Gilbard, J. P. and Farris, R. L.**, Tear osmolarity and ocular surface disease in keratoconjunctivitis sicca, *Arch. Ophthalmol.*, 97, 1642, 1979.
71. **Gilbard, J. F. and Farris, R. L.**, Ocular surface drying and tear film osmolarity in thyroid disease, *Acta Ophthalmol. (Copenhagen)*, 61, 108, 1983.
72. **Maurice, D. M.**, Influence on corneal permeability of bathing with solutions of differing reaction and tonicity, *Br. J. Ophthalmol.*, 39, 463, 1955.
73. **Duke-Elder, S. and Gloster, J.**, The sensitivity of the cornea, in *The Physiology of the Eye and of Vision, Vol. IV System of Ophthalmology*, Duke-Elder, S., Ed., H. Kimpton, London, 1968, 414.
74. **Mishima, S.**, Some physiological aspects of the precorneal tear film, *Arch. Ophthalmol.*, 73, 223, 1965.
75. **Gilbard, J. F., Carter, J. B., Sang, D. N., Refojo, M. F., Hanninen, L. A., and Kenyon, K. R.**, Morphologic effect of hyperosmolarity on rabbit corneal epithelium *Ophthalmology (Rochester)*, 91, 1205, 1984.
76. **Bisantis, C., Squeri, C. A., Colosi, P., Provenzano, P., and Trombetta, C.**, Sur l'usage des collyres hypo-, iso-, et hyper-osmotiques, acides ou alcalins, dans le diagnostic et le traitement des anomalies de la sécrétion des larmes, *Bull. Mem. Soc. Fr. Ophtalmol.*, 94, 75, 1982.
77. **Riegelman, S. and Vaughan, D. G.**, Ophthalmic solutions, *J. Am. Pharm. Assoc.*, pract. ed., 8, 474, 1958.
78. **Trolle-Lassen, C.**, Investigations into the sensitivity of the human eye to hypo- and hypertonic solutions as well as solutions with unphysiological hydrogen ion concentrations, *Pharm. Weekbl.*, 93, 148, 1958.
79. **Maurice, D. M.**, The tonicity of an eye drop and its dilution by tears, *Exp. Eye Res.*, 11, 30, 1971.
80. **Ludwig, A. and Van Ooteghem, M.**, The influence of the osmolality on the precorneal retention of ophthalmic solutions, *J. Pharm. Belg.*, 42, 259, 1987.
81. **Holly, F. J. and Lamberts, D. W.**, Effect of nonisotonic solutions on tear film osmolality, *Invest. Ophthalmol. Vis. Sci.*, 20, 236, 1981.
82. **Barendsen, H., Oosterhuis, J. A., and Van Haeringen, N. J.**, Concentration of fluorescein in tear fluid after instillation of eye-drops. I. Isotonic eye-drops, *Ophthalmic Res.*, 11, 73, 1979.
83. **Coles, W. H. and Jaros, P. A.**, Dynamics of ocular surface pH, *Br. J. Ophthalmol.*, 68, 549, 1984.
84. **Norn, M. S.**, Function of meibomian glands and tear pH, *Acta Ophthalmol. (Copenhagen)*, 65 (Suppl. 182), 48, 1987.
85. **Fischer, F. H. and Wiederholt, M.**, Human precorneal tear film pH measured by microelectrodes, *Graefes Arch. Clin. Exp. Ophthalmol.*, 218, 168, 1982.
86. **Norn, M. S.**, Hydrogen ion concentration of tear fluid, *Acta Ophthalmol. (Copenhagen)*, 46, 189, 1968.
87. **Hind, H. W. and Goyan, F. M.**, The hydrogen ion concentration and osmotic properties of lacrimal fluid, *J. Am. Pharm. Assoc., Sci. Ed.*, 38, 477, 1949.
88. **Hudelo, A. and Mergier, J.**, Etude du pH lacrimal en fonction de l'état local et de l'état général, *Ann. Ocul.*, 185, 764, 1952.
89. **Carney, L. G. and Hill, R. M.**, Human tear pH; diurnal variations, *Arch. Ophthalmol.*, 94, 821, 1976.
90. **Abelson, M. B., Udell, I. J., and Weston, J. H.**, Normal human tear pH by direct measurement, *Arch. Ophthalmol.*, 99, 301, 1981.
91. **Norn, M. S.**, Tear fluid pH in normals, contact lens wearers, and pathological cases, *Acta Ophthalmol. (Copenhagen)*, 66, 485, 1988.
92. **Carney, L. G. and Hill, R. M.**, Hydrogen ion concentrations of human tears: effects of prolonged eye closure, *Arch. Ophtalmol. (Paris)*, 36, 835, 1976.
93. **Holden, B. A., Ross, R., and Jenkins, J.**, Hydrogel contact lenses impede carbon dioxide efflux from the human cornea, *Curr. Eye Res.*, 6, 1283, 1987.
94. **Holden, B. A.**, The ocular response to contact lens wear, *Optom. Vis. Sci.*, 66, 717, 1989.
95. **Browning, D. J.**, Tear pH in ocular rosacea, *Invest. Ophthalmol. Vis. Sci.*, Suppl. 25, 41, 1984.
96. **Dahl, H. and Dahl, C.**, Hydrogen ion concentration of tear fluid in newborn infants, *Acta Ophthalmol. (Copenhagen)*, 63, 692, 1985.
97. **Norn, M.**, Tear pH: a survey, *Acta Ophthalmol. (Copenhagen)*, 68 (Suppl. 195), 62, 1990.
98. **Thygesen, J. E. M. and Jensen, O. L.**, pH Changes of the tear fluid in conjunctival sac during postoperative inflammation of the human eye, *Acta Ophthalmol. (Copenhagen)*, 65, 134, 1987.
99. **Carney, L. G., Mauger, T. F., and Hill, R. M.**, Buffering in human tears: pH responses to acid and base challenge, *Invest. Ophthalmol. Vis. Sci.*, 30, 747, 1989.
100. **Carney, L. G., Mauger, T. F., and Hill, R. M.**, Tear buffering in contact lens wearers, *Acta Ophthalmol. (Copenhagen)*, 68, 75, 1990.
101. **Parrish, C. M. and Chandler, J. W.**, Corneal trauma, in *The Cornea*, Kaufman, H. E., Barron, B. A., McDonald, M. B., and Waltman, S. R. Eds., Churchill Livingstone, New York, 1988, 599.

102. **Lemp, M. A.**, Cornea and sclera, *Arch. Ophthalmol.*, 92, 158, 1974.
103. **Norn, M.**, Tear pH after instillation of buffer *in vivo, Acta Ophthalmol. (Copenhagen)*, 63 (Suppl. 173), 32, 1985.
104. **Longwell, A., Birss, S., Keller, N., and Moore, D.**, Effect of topically applied pilocarpine on tear film pH, *J. Pharm. Sci.*, 65, 1654, 1976.
105. **Basu, P. K., Avaria, M., and Hasany, S. M.** Effect of acidic lake water on the eye, *Can. J. Ophthalmol.*, 17, 74, 1982.
106. **Swan, K. C.**, Use of methylcellulose in ophthalmology, *Arch. Ophthalmol.*, 33, 378, 1945.
107. **Mueller, W. H. and Deardorff, D. L.**, Ophthalmic vehicles: The effect of methylcellulose on the penetration of homatropine hydrobromide through the cornea, *J. Am. Pharm. Assoc., Sci. Ed.*, 45, 334, 1956.
108. **Blaug, S. M. and Canada, A. T.**, Relationship of viscosity, contact time and prolongation of action of methylcellulose containing ophthalmic solutions, *Am. J. Hosp. Pharm.*, 22, 662, 1965.
109. **Linn, M. L. and Jones, L. T.**, Rate of lacrimal excretion of ophthalmic vehicles, *Am. J. Ophthalmol.*, 65, 76, 1968.
110. **Adler, C. A., Maurice, D. M., and Paterson, M. E.**, The effect of viscosity of the vehicle on the penetration of fluorescein into the human eye, *Exp. Eye Res.*, 11, 34, 1971.
111. **Hardberger, R., Hanna, C., and Boyd, C. M.**, Effects of drug vehicles on ocular contact time, *Arch. Ophthalmol.*, 93, 42, 1975.
112. **Trueblood, J. H., Rossomondo, R. M., Carlton, W. H., and Wilson, L. A.**, Corneal contact times of ophthalmic vehicles: evaluation and microscintigraphy, *Arch. Ophthalmol.*, 93, 127, 1975.
113. **Melis-Decerf, C. and Van Ooteghem, M.**, An *in vitro* method simulating drug release from viscous eye drops in rabbit and man, *J. Pharm. Pharmacol.*, 31, 12, 1979.
114. **Marquard, R. and Christ, T.**, Untersuchungen zur Verweildauer von Tränenersatzmitteln, *Klin. Monatsbl. Augenheilkd.*, 189, 254, 1986.
115. **Folk, J. C., Kumar, V., Piper, J. G., Barcellos, W. A., Schoenwald, R. D., and Chien, D. S.**, Aqueous versus viscous phenylephrine. II. Mydriatic effects, *Arch. Ophthalmol.*, 104, 1192, 1986.
116. **Hon-Kin Li, V. and Robinson, J. R.**, Solution viscosity effects on the ocular dispositioh of cromolyn sodium in the albino rabbit, *Int. J. Pharm.*, 53, 219, 1989.
117. **Ludwig, A. and Van Ooteghem, M.**, The evaluation of viscous ophthalmic vehicles by slit lamp fluorophotometry in humans, *Int. J. Pharm.*, 54, 95, 1989.
118. **Kalachandra, S. and Shah, D. O.**, Lubrication properties of tear substitutes, in *The Preocular Tear Film in Health, Disease and Contact Lens Wear*, Holly, F. J., Ed., Dry Eye Institute, Lubbock TX, 1986, 733.
119. **Kalachandra, S. and Shah, D. O.**, Lubrication and surface chemical properties of ophthalmic solutions, *Ann. Ophthalmol.*, 17, 808, 1985.
120. **Duke-Elder, S. and Gloster, J.**, The lubrication of the eye: the physico-chemical properties of tears, in *The Physiology of the Eye and of Vision, Vol. IV System of Ophthalmology*, Duke-Elder, S., Ed. H. Kimpton, London, 1968, 420.
121. **Liotet, S. and Cochet, P.**, Notions concernant les larmes humaines: origine, physiologie et composition, *Arch. Ophtalmol. (Paris)*, 27, 251, 1967.
122. **Schuller, W. O., Young, W. H., and Hill, R. M.**, Clinical measurement of the tears: viscosity, *J. Am. Optom. Assoc.*, 43, 1358, 1972.
123. **Hamano, H. and Mitsunaga, S.**, Measurement of the viscosity of tears, *Folia Ophthalmol. Jpn.*, 24, 435, 1973.
124. **Hamano, H.**, Viscosity of tears, *Acta Soc. Ophthalmol. Jpn.*, 77, 704, 1973.
125. **Hamano, H. and Mitsunaga, S.**, Viscosity of rabbit tears, *Jpn. J. Ophthalmol.*, 17, 290, 1973.
126. **Kaura, R. and Tiffany, J. M.**, The role of mucous glycoproteins in the tear film in *The Preocular Tear Film in Health, Disease and Contact Lens Wear*, Holly, F. J., Ed. Drye Eye, Lubbock, TX, 1986, 728.
127. **Bron, A. J.**, Prospects for the dry eye, *Trans. Ophthalmol. Soc. U.K.*, 104, 801, 1985.
128. **Liesegang, T. J.**, Viscoelastic substances in ophthalmology, *Surv. Ophthalmol.*, 34, 268, 1990.
129. **Doane, M. G.**, Blinking and the mechanisms of the lacrimal drainage system, *Ophthalmology (Rochester)*, 88, 844, 1981.
130. **Steiger-Trippi, K.**, Viskositätserhöhende Hilfsstoffe für die Arzneiformung, *Schweiz. Apoth. Ztg.*, 51, 961, 1958.
131. **Lippman, O.**, Local irritating effect caused by topical use of steroids in the eye, *Arch. Ophthalmol.*, 57, 339, 1957.
132. **Van der Graaf, H.**, Oogheelkundige toepassing van indomethacine, *Pharm. Weekbl.*, 117, 1117, 1982.
133. **Hui, H. W. and Robinson, J.**, Effect of particle dissolution rate on ocular drug bioavailability, *J. Pharm. Sci.*, 75, 280, 1986.
134. **Bisrat, M., Nyström, C., and Edman, P.**, Influence of dissolution rate of sparingly soluble drugs on corneal permeability *in vitro, Int. J. Pharm.*, 63, 49, 1990.

135. **Duke-Elder, S. and Mac Paul, P.** Retained foreign bodies, in *Injuries, Vol. XIV, System of Ophthalmology,* Duke-Elder S., Ed., H. Kimpton, London, 1968, 451.

136. **Gombos, G. M.,** *Handbook of Ophthalmic Emergencies,* Gombos, G. M., Ed., Medical Examination Publishing, Flushing, NY, 1973, 99.

137. **Parrish, C. M. and Chandler, B. A.,** Corneal trauma, in *The Cornea,* Kaufman, H. E., Barron, B. A., McDonald, M. B., and Waltman, S. R., Eds., Churchill Livingstone, New York, 1988, 599.

138. **Millodot, M.,** A review of research on the sensitivity of the cornea, *Ophthalmol. Physiol. Opt.,* 4, 305, 1984.

139. **Müller, F. and Seidel, H.,** Untersuchung der Teilchengrösse in Augensalben, *Pharmazie,* 18, 803, 1963.

140. **Jaensch, P. A.,** *Augenschädigungen in Industrie und Gewerbe,* Wiss.-Verlag, Stuttgart, 1958, 153.

141. **Speiser, P.,** Dispersions et préparations ophtalmiques, *Il Farmaco, pract. ed.,* 23, 181, 1967.

142. **Borka, L.,** Nakrystaller i øyesalver-litt om polymorfi, *Nor. Apotekerforen. Tidsskr.,* 85, 440, 1977.

143. **Doden, W. and Böker, W.,** Über die Teilchengrösse in Augensalben inkorporierter Medikamente, *Klin. Monatsbl. Augenheilkd.,* 135, 305, 1959.

144. **Speiser, P.,** Teilchengrösse in Augensalben, *A.P.V. Informationsdienst,* 8, 87, 1962.

145. **Wildhaber, A. and Etter, J. C.,** Développement d'un test objectif d'irritation oculaire sur la souris: Intérêt en pharmacie galénique et biopharmacie, Deuxième partie: Les anesthésiques locaux en instillations uniques et itératives, *Pharm. Acta Helv.,* 63, 257, 1988.

146. **Scoville, B., Krieglstein, G. K., Then, E., Yokoyama, S., and Yokoyama, T.,** Measuring drug-induced eye irritation: a simple new clinical assay, *J. Clin. Pharmacol.,* 25, 210, 1985.

147. **Krejci, L. and Harrison, R.,** Antiglaucoma drug effects on corneal epithelium. A comparative study in tissue culture, *Arch. Ophthalmol.,* 84, 766, 1970.

148. **Waylward, G. and Wilson, R. S.,** Contamination of dropper bottles with tear fluid in an ophthalmic outpatient, *Br. Med. J.,* 294, 1587, 1987.

149. **Høvding, G. and Sjursen, H.,** Bacterial contamination of drops and dropper tips in-use multidose eye drop bottles, *Acta Ophthalmol. (Copenhagen),* 60, 213, 1982.

150. **Älund, B., Olson, O. T., and Sandell, E.,** Studies on in-use microbial contamination of eye drops, *Acta Pharm. Suec.,* 15, 389, 1978.

151. **Miestereck, H.,** Konservierung von Augentropfen, *Referate des Symposions "Konservierung pharmazeutischer und kosmetischer Produkte",* Concept 4, Heidelberg, 21, 1981.

152. **Brewitt, H.,** Rasterelektronenmikroskopische Untersuchungen zur lokalen Hornhautverträglichkeit von Betablokeraugentropfen mit und ohne Konservierungsstoffe, *Ophthalmologica,* 201, 152, 1990.

153. **Barkman, R., Germanis, M., Karpe, G., and Malmborg, A. S.,** Preservatives in eye drops, *Acta Ophthalmol. (Copenhagen),* 47, 461, 1969.

154. **Green, K., Cheeks, L., and Chapman, J. M.,** Surfactant pharmacokinetics in the eye, in *Ophthalmic Drug Delivery, Biopharmaceutical, Technological and Clinical Aspects,* Vol. 11, (Fidia Research Series), Saettone, M. S., Bucci, G., and Speiser, P., Eds., Springer-Verlag, Berlin, 1987, 171.

155. **Robinson, J. R. and Goshman, L. M.,** Topical drug delivery systems (eye, ear, nose), in *Pharmaceutics and Pharmacy Practice,* Banker, G. and Chalmers, R., Eds., Lippincott, Philadelphia, 1982, 312.

156. **Saettone, M. F., Giannaccini, B., Teneggi, A., Savigni, P., and Tellini, N.,** Vehicle effects on ophthalmic bioavailability: The influence of different polymers on the activity of pilocarpine in rabbits and man, *J. Pharm. Pharmacol.,* 34, 464, 1982.

157. **Ünlü, N., Ludwig, A., Van Ooteghem, M., and Hincal, A.,** Formulation of Carbopol 940 ophthalmic vehicles, and *in vitro* evaluation of the influence of simulated lacrimal fluid on their physico-chemical properties, *Pharmazie,* 46, 784, 1991.

158. **Ludwig, A., Ünlü, N. and Van Ooteghem, M.,** Evaluation of viscous ophthalmic vehicles containing carbomer by slit-lamp fluorophotometry in humans, *Int. J. Pharm.,* 61, 15, 1990.

159. **Hui, H. W. and Robinson, J.,** Ocular delivery of progesterone using a bioadhesive polymer, *Int. J. Pharm.,* 26, 203, 1985.

160. **Saettone, M. F., Monti, D., Torracca, M. T., Chetoni, P., and Giannaccini, B.,** Mucoadhesive liquid ophthalmic vehicles — evaluation of macromolecular ionic complexes of pilocarpine, *Drug Dev. Ind. Pharm.,* 15, 2475, 1989.

161. **Madsen, K., Schenholm, M., Jahnke, G., and Tengblad, A.,** Hyaluronate binding to intact corneas and cultured endothelial cells, *Invest. Ophthalmol. Vis. Sci.,* 30, 2132, 1989.

162. **Ludwig, A. and Van Ooteghem, M.,** Evaluation of sodium hyaluronate as viscous vehicle for eye drops, *J. Pharm. Belg.,* 44, 391, 1989.

163. **Saettone, M. F., Giannaccini, B., Chetoni, P., Torracca, M. T., and Monti, D.,** Evaluation of high- and low-molecular weight fractions of sodium hyaluronate and an ionic complex as adjuvants for topical ophthalmic vehicles containing pilocarpine, *Int. J. Pharm.,* 72, 131, 1991.

164. **Middleton, D. L. and Robinson, J.,** Design and evaluation of an ocular bioadhesive delivery system, *S. T. P. Pharma Sci.,* 3, 200, 1991.

165. **Münzel, K., Büchi, J., and Schultz, O.-E.,** *Galenisches Praktikum* , Wissenschaft.-Verlag, Stuttgart, 1959, 54.

166. **Chattoraj, D. K. and Birdi, K. S.,** *Adsorption and the Gibbs Surface Excess,* Plenum Press, New York, 1984, 24.

167. **Harkins, W. D. and Brown, F. E.,** The measurement of surface tension and weight of falling drops, *J. Am. Chem. Soc.,* 41, 499, 1919.

168. **Veikko Pirilä, H.,** Tip part of a dosage vessel, U.S. Patent 4,936,498, 1990.

169. **Brown, R. H., Hotchkiss, M. L., and Davis, E. B.,** Creating smaller eyedrops by reducing eyedropper tip dimensions, *Am. J. Ophthalmol.,* 99, 460, 1985.

170. **Tadros, T. F.,** Spreading and retention of aqueous solution droplets of fluorocarbon and hydrocarbon surfactants and their mixtures on wheat leaves, in *Wetting, Spreading and Adhesion,* Padday, J. F., Ed., Academic Press, London, 1978, 455.

171. **Georgieff, T.,** Shared use of ophthalmic solutions, *Can. J. Hosp. Pharm.,* 43, 89, 1990.

172. **Frauenfelder, F. T.,** Extraocular fluid dynamics: how best to apply topical ocular medication, *Trans. Am. Ophthalmol. Soc.,* 74, 457, 1976.

173. **Kass, M. A., Hodapp, E. Gordon, M., Kolker, A. E., and Goldberg, I.,** Patient administration of eyedrops: observations, *Ann. Ophthalmol.,* 14, 889, 1982.

174. **Lisi, D. M. and Fazoi, A.,** Instructions provided by manufacturers for proper use of nonprescription ophthalmic drops, *Am. J. Hosp. Pharm.,* 48, 987, 1981.

175. **Van Ooteghem, M.,** Augenpräparate, in *Hagers Handbuch der Pharmazeutischen Praxis, Vol 2: Methoden,* Nürnberg, E. and Surmann, P., Eds., Springer-Verlag, Berlin, 633, 1991.

176. **Draeger, J.,** Topography of the corneal sensitivity, in *Corneal Sensitivity,* Draeger J., Ed., Springer-Verlag, Vienna 1984, 40.

177. **Mansour, A. M.,** Tolerance to topical preparations: cold or warm?, *Ann. Ophthalmol.,* 23, 21, 1991.

178. **Ritch, R. and Astrove, E.,** A positioning aid for eyedrop administration, *Ophthalmology (Rochester),* 89, 284, 1982.

179. **Letocha, C. E.,** Methods for self-administration of eyedrops, *Ann. Ophthalmol.,* 17, 768, 1985.

Chapter 3

THE EFFECTS OF PRESERVATIVES ON CORNEAL PERMEABILITY OF DRUGS

Keith Green

TABLE OF CONTENTS

I.   Corneal Anatomy 44

II.   Corneal Physiology 44

III.   Influence of Factors Other Than Preservatives 44

IV.   Preservatives 46
        A.   Surfactants 46
                1.   Benzalkonium Chloride 46
                2.   Cetylpyridinium Chloride 48
                3.   Other Surfactants 48
        B.   Thimerosal 48
        C.   Chlorobutanol 49
        D.   Methyl- and Propylparaben (Esters of Parahydroxybenzoic
                Acid) 49
        E.   Chlorhexidine Digluconate 50
        F.   Hydrogen Peroxide (H$_2$O$_2$) 50
        G.   Sorbic Acid 51
        H.   Sodium Bisulfite 51
        I.   Ethylenediaminetetraacetic Acid 51

V.   Conclusions 52

Acknowledgments 53

References 53

I. CORNEAL ANATOMY

Any consideration of drug permeation through the cornea must take into account the structure of this tissue[1] that forms the focus of this review. The outermost-facing membrane is a five-cell layer epithelium that is 35 to 60 μm thick in mammals. More keratinized cells are at the superficial aspect; they desquamate and are freed from the underlying cells by the upper lid as it crosses the cornea during each blink. Underlying the two-cell layer superficial cells are the wing cells which are two to three cell layers thick. Finally, passing posteriorly, there is a single layer of tall, columnar basal cells that are attached by hemidesmosomes either to Bowman's membrane or to a thin basement membrane.

Under the epithelium is the largest portion of the cornea (>80%), the stroma, which contains collagen fibrils (oriented so that the cornea is transparent when at normal thickness), glycosaminoglycans, and keratocytes, stromal cells that occupy between 4 and 10% of the stromal volume. Passing posteriorly, Descemet's membrane, the basement membrane of the endothelium, is next. The endothelium is a single layer of squamous cells approximately 5 μm thick, with a characteristic hexagonal shape when seen from the anterior chamber, that forms the posterior border of the cornea.

II. CORNEAL PHYSIOLOGY

Physiologically, the epithelium is relatively impermeant to polar or hydrophilic compounds with a relative molecular weight greater than 60 to 100 Da. Glucose (M_r 180 Da), for example, does not pass the epithelium.[2] Lipophilic compounds pass the epithelium due to solubilization in the lipid cell membranes.[3,4] The major resistance to the movement of ions[5,6] or water[7] across the epithelium is at the inner superficial cell layer or the outermost wing cell layer. Access of nutrients to the epithelium occurs through the endothelium and stroma[8,9] rather than from the tear film. The stromal permeability is high and even high-molecular-weight substances diffuse with ease.[10-14] Although the endothelium is the site of active ion transport systems that regulate corneal thickness,[15-17] large molecules (up to 70,000 Da) can traverse this membrane.[10,12-14,18-23]

The influence of several preservatives on both epithelial and endothelial permeability will be discussed. These compounds include: benzalkonium chloride, cetylpyridium chloride, thimerosal and methyl mercury compounds, chlorobutanol, methylparaben and propylparaben, chlorhexidine digluconate, and sodium bisulfite; other chemicals such as hydrogen peroxide and sorbic acid, that have been suggested as preservatives or have limited use in ophthalmic practice thus far; and chemicals such as ethylenediaminetetraacetic acid (EDTA) that are listed as preservatives in ophthalmic solutions, but are chelating agents. Because benzalkonium chloride is a surfactant, corneal permeability effects of other surfactants will be discussed. These compounds may gain access to the eye surface through their use in shampoos.[24-26]

III. INFLUENCE OF FACTORS OTHER THAN PRESERVATIVES

It is prudent to briefly indicate the effects of ambient pH,[27,28] vehicle tonicity, age, and the use of vehicle viscosity-enhancing materials[29] on corneal permeability. This has relevance because sometimes the permeability effects of certain preservatives may be influenced by their combination with one or more other factors. It is important to remember these variables when comparing data obtained under different experimental conditions in order to interpret preservative effects alone.

The corneal epithelium is extremely tolerant of large variations in pH and tonicity.[30] The sodium permeability of the epithelium is unchanged from pH 4 to 10.[30] Outside this range epithelial permeability increases, especially when bathed with more alkaline solutions. Variations from slightly hypotonic to extremely hypertonic are tolerated without change in epithelial permeability, although an increase to about ten times normal occurs in more hypotonic solutions. Exposure to hypertonic solutions of 10% NaCl (about 1250 to 1500 mOsm) for 10 min did not alter permeability.[30]

Ramselaar et al.[31] found that human corneal fluorescein permeability was unaffected in a pH range from 4.5 to 7, and tonicity ranging from isotonic (270 mOsm) to hypertonic (620 mOsm). The inulin permeability of rabbit cornea was sensitive to the pH of instilled eye drops, but the increase in permeability at acid pH occurred despite greater lacrimation at this pH.[32] The effect, therefore, is truly one of pH rather than a side effect of the pH change.[33] Other studies[34] showed that rabbit corneal epithelial inulin permeability was enhanced threefold after the addition of a pH 4-buffered eye drop onto the cornea, compared to the permeability after a pH 7-buffered eye drop. These studies demonstrated that one drop of an acidic ophthalmic preparation reduced tear pH for 10 to 15 min due to the weak buffering capacity of rabbit tears. Increasing the delivery vehicle pH promoted increased corneal pilocarpine and glycerin permeation.[35,36] The increase in penetration of both glycerin, a nonionizable compound, and pilocarpine is due to the smaller pH-induced lacrimation at pH 7 or 8 compared to that induced at pH 4 or 5. A direct effect of pH on pilocarpine was ruled out.

The corneal endothelium is far more sensitive to changes in both pH and tonicity. The optimum endothelial pH is 7.4 to 7.5; below pH 6.7 and above pH 8.5 the electrical potential difference (PD) across the endothelium is zero.[15] Corneal swelling occurred outside of the pH range. Outside the pH range 6.5 to 8.2 both structural and functional alterations occurred to human and rabbit endothelia.[37] The endothelium can withstand variations in tonicity from 200 to 400 mOsm[38] as long as essential ions are present. Perfusion of rabbit or human endothelia with solutions of differing tonicity caused the cornea to swell or deswell quickly to a new steady-state thickness, and structural changes occurred only outside the tolerance limits. The composition of the bathing solution is important for the maintenance of the *in vitro* endothelium. Certain ions are essential (sodium, potassium, calcium, chloride, and bicarbonate) as well as reduced glutathione and adenosine.[15,39-41] Compounds such as chondroitin sulfate, that are used in corneal preservative solutions prior to transplantation, have been shown to sustain higher transendothelial PD with maximums at 1% and PD reductions at lower or higher concentrations.[42] Local anesthetics may also influence corneal permeability.[43,44]

Viscosity-enhancing materials added to ophthalmic solutions enhance corneal epithelial permeability by allowing more drug uptake by ocular tissues.[45] The viscosity enhancers decrease the solution drainage rate from the ocular surface.[35,46-54] Several studies, in both man and rabbit, have shown that methylcellulose increases drug penetration through the cornea by increasing contact time.[55-58] Methylcellulose, 0.4%, was nontoxic to the endothelium and had no effect on corneal thickness (and by inference endothelial permeability).[59]

Age may influence permeability characteristics.[24,60,61] Younger eyes show greater drug penetration despite the use of smaller drop sizes and lesser total mass of drug applied to the eye.[24] Drug kinetics also differ, with tissues of young eyes taking up more drug and releasing it more quickly than adult eye tissues.

Drugs may be directly toxic to cells. Direct cytotoxic effects of phenylephrine have been noted on the rabbit corneal endothelium after topical application to de-epithelialized corneas.[62] The effects were minimal in the intact cornea, but the responses of endothelial vacuolization and loss of cellular adhesion were confirmed in tissue culture.[63] Swelling of corneal endothelial cells was noted after topical application of epinephrine or dipivalyl epinephrine eye drops to rabbit eyes.[64] Gentamicin alone induced corneal endothelial and conjunctival changes,[64] as well as extraocular muscle myopathy,[65] after subconjunctival injection.

IV. PRESERVATIVES

A. SURFACTANTS

This category of preservative agents encompasses anionic, cationic, and neutral chemicals. Cationic surfactants tend to act on microbes indiscriminately by solubilizing cell membranes, while anionic surfactants may act in different ways. In ophthalmic practice one cationic detergent, benzalkonium chloride (BAK), is widely used as a preservative because of its bacteriostatic and bacteriocidal efficacy at a wide range of vehicle pH.[66] Because of its mode of action, it is not surprising that BAK also indiscriminately affects corneal cell membranes.

1. Benzalkonium Chloride

Benzalkonium chloride (BAK) was originally used to increase corneal permeability to carbachol,[67,68] as well as to provide asepsis of ophthalmic solutions.[69-74] BAK concentrations ranging from 0.01 to 0.04% caused some superficial punctate keratitis, increased superficial cell desquamation, inhibited the corneal epithelial healing rate, and caused some conjunctival hyperemia and discomfort. BAK is used in ophthalmic drug preparations at concentrations between 0.004 and 0.02%. The latter concentration is at the threshold of tolerance. Concentrations of this magnitude have been calculated to exist in the tear film after BAK release from either soft or hard contact lenses.[75]

An increase in corneal epithelial permeability may be deduced from morphological changes and from direct permeability determinations. BAK induced dose-dependent morphological changes in the epithelium with low (0.0004 to 0.001%) concentrations causing partial loss of surface microvilli.[76-78] Higher concentrations (0.01 to 0.04%) caused lifting of cell borders with desquamation.[76,79-82] Durand-Cavagna et al.[83] have noted corneal epithelial changes in rabbits but not in dogs, using both slit-lamp and light microscopy after 0.01% BAK in a hydroxyethylcellulose vehicle was applied to the ocular surface. In the absence of hydroxyethylcellulose, BAK had no effect. It was concluded that hydroxyethylcellulose increased vehicle viscosity and hence increased the vehicle contact time, allowing the permeability increase to occur. BAK caused some loss of surface structure in rabbits after topical application.[79,84,85] High concentrations of BAK (0.5 to 2.0%) caused gross corneal and conjunctival changes.[86,87]

Physiological changes in epithelial PD indicate alterations in membrane permeability. Transepithelial PD was disturbed with BAK concentrations of 0.0004[76] or 0.005% *in vitro*, and 0.01% *in vivo*.[80] BAK at 0.0004%[76] caused a slow, inhibitory phase in PD after about 1 h, and 0.001% BAK temporarily increased both PD and short circuit current (SCC) before causing inhibition. A marked inhibition of PD occurred *in vivo* within 1 min after 0.02% BAK addition.[80] The initial hyperpolarization of PD was dose dependent, as was the maximal reduction in PD, and the percentage recovery at 2 h after exposure to BAK.[80] BAK at 0.004 to 0.01% had no influence on epithelial aerobic metabolism.[88]

BAK influence on rabbit epithelial permeability has been demonstrated for fluorescein,[89] pilocarpine,[90,91] prednisolone acetate,[92] chloramphenicol,[93] carbachol,[32] dexamethasone,[91] and sodium chloride,[94] and for prostaglandin $F_{2\alpha}$[95] in pig epithelium. BAK caused dose-dependent increases in epithelial sulforhodamine B permeability of corneas of freshly killed mice.[96]

Keller et al.[34] found no increase in inulin (M_r 5000 Da) permeability across the *in vivo* rabbit cornea with 0.01% BAK at pH 7, but an increase occurred at pH 4. A threefold increase in permeability to inulin was detected with 0.02% BAK at neutral pH. Burstein[97] found that 0.01% BAK increased rabbit corneal fluorescein permeability 1.8 times when measured *in vivo* 30 min after BAK addition to the tear film. In man, 0.01% BAK had no effect, but 0.02% BAK increased anterior chamber fluorescein by 1.23 times. Human corneal epithelial fluorescein permeability was increased by BAK alone, and greater increases occurred in the presence of oxybuprocaine hydrochloride or tetracaine hydrochloride, although the latter did not alone increase permeability.[31] Göbbels and Spitznas[98] found that BAK increased human corneal fluorescein permeability 3.1 times.

BAK increases permeability by separating superficial and wing cells,[89] allowing horseradish peroxidase (M_r >50,000 Da) to penetrate into the wing cell layer of the epithelium.[79] The superficial cell membranes become diffuse and leaky, but the majority of the increase in epithelial permeability is caused by the vast increase in paracellular pathway. BAK effects in man[31,77] are less than those in rabbits and mice.[77,89,96] BAK disturbs the tear film of man and rabbit, also leading to secondary changes in epithelial permeability.[99,100]

Cultured human and rat corneal epithelial cells were partially lysed when incubated for 15 min at low BAK concentrations; 0.01% BAK lysed all cells.[101] These changes suggest that enhanced membrane permeability would occur. The epithelial effects are not surprising since BAK is preferentially absorbed by corneal epithelium and conjunctiva.[25,26,102,103] Corneal exposure to single or multiple drops of BAK leads to epithelial accumulation with little penetration into the rest of the cornea[102] and no penetration into the anterior chamber except in neonatal rabbits.[25]

A 0.02% concentration of BAK impaired the healing of iodine gas lesions in rabbit and guinea pig corneal epithelium.[104] In other experiments with either mechanical lesions (scraping) or chemical lesions (*n*-heptanol) in rabbits, BAK was found to have no effect on the rate of epithelial lesion healing.[105] While some morphological changes were noted in cells covering the denuded area of cornea, the effects of 0.02% BAK were not sufficient to impair cellular mobility, healing, or permeability to sucrose.

Endothelial changes have been noted clinically after topical treatment with BAK-containing solutions.[106] The topical administration of 0.133% BAK to de-epithelialized *in vivo* rabbit corneas (5 doses, given 7 min apart) caused no change in corneal endothelial cell structure or function.[107] No effect was noted from topical 0.005% BAK on rabbit endothelium when applied to normal rabbit eyes.[64] The dose-response curve of corneal swelling after direct endothelial exposure to BAK begins at 0.0001%. This is the threshold for physiological and morphological alterations of rabbit corneal endothelium.[107] BAK exposure for 15 min induces effects without subsequent recovery. Effects of topical BAK on endothelial permeability to prednisolone phosphate have been noted.[92]

Concentrations of 0.05% BAK washed through the rabbit anterior chamber caused permanent endothelial loss.[108,109] This illustrates the extreme damage that BAK may cause, since the rabbit endothelium has a strong capacity for regeneration.[110-112] Collin and Carrol[113] and Collin[114] placed drops of 0.02% BAK hourly onto either normal or keratectomized rabbit corneas caused a slight clarification of endothelial mitochondria; similar data were observed after treatment with 0.01% BAK plus 0.1% EDTA. In keratectomized corneas, however, the majority of endothelial mitochondria were swollen and disrupted. Some changes occurred in stromal cells. BAK can penetrate into the cornea where there is an epithelial defect and cause changes in endothelial permeability.

The use of low concentrations (0.01% or lower) of BAK appears to be acceptable from both a microbiological and toxicological perspective. Knowledge that BAK does not penetrate into the anterior chamber, no matter how much accumulates in the corneal epithelium, is reassuring in that toxic responses would not occur with low concentrations. There will undoubtedly remain some idiosyncratic responses, even to 0.01% BAK, but these must be dealt with individually.

2. Cetylpyridinium Chloride

Cetylpyridinium chloride (CPC) enhanced rabbit corneal penetration of drugs *in vivo*, but this increased drug penetration was ascribed to drug release from protein-binding sites.[115] Studies on isolated rabbit cornea[116] showed that CPC inhibited the transcorneal (transepithelial) PD and caused epithelial ultrastructural changes. Determinations of corneal epithelial penicillin permeability[117] confirmed that CPC increased drug penetration. Dose-related increases of rabbit corneal epithelial fluorescein permeability were found after topical application of more than 100 μg CPC.[118]

A dose-response relationship of rabbit corneal endothelial permeability was found, with 0.01 mM CPC being the threshold for both functional and ultrastructural damage.[107] Exposure to CPC for 15 min caused a permeability increase.

3. Other Surfactants

Marsh and Maurice[119] compared several surfactants regarding human corneal fluorescein permeability. Single drops of nonionic detergents with a hydrophilic/lipophilic balance range of 16 to 17 increased fluorescein permeation. While most detergents followed a pattern of increasing permeability when this balance number was achieved, some detergents did not follow this general rule, suggesting that chemical specificity can play a role. The order of efficacy was Brij 58 > Tween 80 > Brij 25. Increased opacity of isolated bovine cornea was related to anionic and nonionic detergents, but not to cationic detergents.[120]

A cationic surfactant, cetyltrimethylammonium bromide, reduced the electrical resistance, increased potassium exchange, and increased isolated bovine corneal hydration to a greater degree than sodium dodecylsulfate and Tween X-100.[121] Taniguchi et al.[122] found that Tween 80 increased the rate of dexamethasone and dexamethasone valerate penetration across the isolated rabbit cornea. Muir[123,124] showed that lauryl trimethylammonium bromide produced larger effects on the opacity of isolated bovine corneal epithelium than sodium lauryl sulfate and Tween 20.

Sodium lauryl sulfate (SLS), an ingredient in shampoos, penetrates into all ocular and systemic tissues when applied to the eye as a topical drop.[24-26] The SLS effects on corneal epithelial healing rate[105] and on normal epithelial structure would suggest that corneal permeability is enhanced. The sucrose permeability of freshly regenerated epithelium after SLS treatment[105] was increased by 30% compared to normal epithelium.

B. THIMEROSAL

This agent has been used both in topical ophthalmic solutions and contact lens cleaning solutions. Some hypersensitivity has been found[125-127] that is similar to superior limbic keratoconjunctivitis. Thimerosal can cause punctate keratitis, corneal opacities, corneal edema, and subepithelial infiltrates.[128] The concentration needed to induce inflammation is 0.1%,[69] while Gasset et al.[86] found no gross changes after 7 d of 1.0%, and almost no histologic changes in rabbit cornea after 7 d of 2.0% thimerosal. Concentrations of 0.005% were found to have no stinging effects,[129] and 0.004[130] and 0.001%[105] did not interfere with corneal epithelial healing rates. When 0.004% thimerosal was applied to the cornea for 2 d stromal cells were only minimally altered.[114] The corneal endothelium undergoes ultrastructural alteration after the application of 0.004% thimerosal in the presence or absence of 0.1% EDTA. Endothelial cells showed some dilatation of the endoplasmic reticulum and mitochondria with dilated cristae.[131]

Thimerosal at 0.00004% had no effect on corneal epithelial electrical characteristics or ultrastructure,[76,81] although 0.0001% caused some partial denuding of surface microvilli and some inhibition of the PD. Corneal epithelial cells of human and rat cultured *in vitro* show greater than 60% lysis of cells after exposure to 0.004% thimerosal for 15 min.[101] Similarly, 0.0005% killed all rabbit corneal epithelial cells growing in tissue culture after 1 h exposure, and 0.004% thimerosal prevented corneal cell proliferation.[132] The threshold for thimerosal to alter corneal epithelial aerobic metabolism was greater than clinical concentrations.[88]

Direct perfusion of rabbit or human corneal endothelium with 0.0005 or 0.0001% thimerosal for 5 h induced no changes in endothelial structure or function.[133] Concentrations of 0.001 and 0.005% increased corneal thickness and caused irreversible structural changes after 2 h. Concentrations of 0.01 and 0.1% thimerosal caused a rapid increase in corneal thickness and cell death within 1 h.

Capella and Schaefer[134] reported that Adsorbobase containing 0.002% thimerosal and 0.05% EDTA allowed a much greater corneal uptake of fluorescein in man than solutions containing other additives such as 5.0% chlorobutanol or 0.1% BAK. The difference in viscosity enhancers between vehicles primarily influenced the data.

Thimerosal has only a small effect on corneal permeability and would not be anticipated to greatly influence drug penetration at normal concentrations.

C. CHLOROBUTANOL

Although comparisons are difficult because of the use of different vehicles, it appears that 5% chlorobutanol had little effect on fluorescein uptake into human cornea.[134] Later studies by Göbbels and Spitznas[98] indicated that fluorescein uptake into human cornea was increased by chlorobutanol by 1.7 times over controls. Camber and Edman[91] found that 0.05% chlorobutanol increased pilocarpine and dexamethasone entry across pig epithelium. Pfister and Burstein[81] found no effect of topical chlorobutanol on epithelial ultrastructure. Burstein and Klyce,[76] however, reported that 0.1% chlorobutanol caused an initial stimulation of SCC across the cornea, but a decrease in PD within 60 min after exposure. There was also a loss of some epithelial surface cells. At 0.05% there was a decrease in PD across the cornea, but the SCC remained constant, indicating that passive ionic permeability increased. Chlorobutanol had a low level of cell lysis (<10%) in rat and human cultured epithelial cells, and caused the least effects of the preservatives tested (BAK, thimerosal, and chlorhexidine digluconate [CHD]).[101]

Chlorobutanol, when used at concentrations normally found in ophthalmic solutions, increases corneal epithelial permeability to drugs.

D. METHYL- AND PROPYLPARABEN (ESTERS OF PARAHYDROXYBENZOIC ACID)

One study reported 0.3% methylparaben and 0.04% propylparaben effects[135] after subconjunctival injections and examination of corneal endothelium. Cells showed intracellular vacuolization and thickening.

In an interesting study methylparaben was used as a test, nonionic permeant to study corneal permeability. Caprylic acid enhanced the transcorneal penetration of bunazosin, as did increasing the ambient pH, but the corneal permeability to methylparaben was not altered by caprylic acid.[136] Coles[137] noted that mixtures of methylparaben and propylparaben cause swelling of corneas after endothelial perfusion at concentrations of 0.432/0.048 (methylparaben/propylparaben) mg/ml and 0.252/0.028 mg/ml, but not at 0.072/0.008 mg/ml.

Although the data is minimal, it is considered unlikely that the parabens alter corneal epithelial permeability to drugs.

E. CHLORHEXIDINE DIGLUCONATE

Chlorhexidine digluconate (CHD or CDG) is widely used in contact lens solutions and in presurgical scrub solutions used to prepare the skin. Corneal side effects of CHD are punctate keratitis and edema, indicating effects on corneal epithelial permeability. High tear concentrations may be reached after CHD desorption from soft contact lenses,[138] but the adsorption of CHD is so small on hard contact lenses that tear concentrations are low even at maximum values.[139] CHD is normally used at concentrations ranging from 0.0025 to 0.004%.

Studies by Browne et al.[140] tested the rabbit corneal response to CHD either as a 0.1 ml solution or after contact lens wear for 8 h per day with soaking of the lenses in a 0.005% CHD solution for 16 h per day. These processes were continued for 21 d, but no corneal effects were noted. Concentrations of 20 μg CHD per ml perfused across the rabbit endothelium caused corneal swelling, and endothelial cells became rounded and swollen with loss of microvilli.[141] Epithelial perfusion in a protein-free solution resulted in dose-dependent cell sloughing with loss of microvilli. Little or no corneal swelling ensued, however, when oil bathed the endothelium, indicating little or no breakdown of the epithelial permeability barrier. Corneal swelling followed at concentrations of 500 and 1000 μg/ml when the epithelium was perfused with CHD and the endothelium perfused with Ringer. Examination of the endothelium indicated that CHD passed through the cornea to the endothelium where structural changes were noted, undoubtedly accompanied by permeability changes to account for the corneal swelling. The normal tear film CHD concentration after soft contact lens wear would be 60 to 80 μg/ml.

CHD at 2% was nontoxic to the epithelium or endothelium of rabbit cornea when examined with light microscopy,[142] although Dormans and van Logten[82] found exfoliation of corneal epithelial superficial cells after 0.1% CHD exposure. Burstein[78] found that 0.001% or 0.0025% CHD had no effect on either rabbit or cat epithelium, while 0.005% caused some cell borders to lose microvilli. At 0.075% CHD more microvilli were lost, and at 0.1% cell margins were lifted and ruffled. Burstein[97] found that 0.01% CHD increased rabbit corneal fluorescein permeability by 1.5 times over controls, but no effects were seen at 0.02% CHD in humans. Rat and human corneal epithelial cells in culture underwent lysis when exposed to CHD for 15 min at 0.01%; roughly 40% of the cells released ^{51}Cr. The *in vitro* rabbit corneal permeability to sorbitol was increased by about 85% after 0.01% CHD,[143] compared to a 9.6 times increase after corneal de-epithelialization. CHD slightly increased the corneal permeability to pilocarpine and dexamethasone.[91] CHD (0.01%) also increased human corneal fluorescein permeability,[31] although the increase was less than that caused by BAK.

Several reports have indicated that corneal edema, indicative of an alteration in corneal epithelial permeability, can occur after the accidental spillage of Hibiclens (a solution containing CHD) on the eye.[144-146]

Overall, therefore, it appears that CHD can cause increased corneal permeability to drugs, and would be expected to enhance permeation when included in ophthalmic preparations.

F. HYDROGEN PEROXIDE (H_2O_2)

This chemical was introduced as a contact lens cleaner in 1983. Concentrations of 30 ppm (about 1 mM) to 100 ppm (about 3 mM) were presented to cultured human corneal epithelial cells.[147] At 1 mM cell retraction occurred with cessation of cell movement and mitotic activity in 7 to 8 h, while at about 2 mM cell movement stopped instantly with cell death at 4 or 5 h. At 3 mM cell death occurred within a few minutes of exposure to H_2O_2. These results indicate epithelial effects of H_2O_2 that could result in significant permeability alterations. The data, however, were collected upon continuous exposure to H_2O_2, or, at least, with an initial concentration as denoted. Because of the intracellular protective enzyme systems, catalase and the glutathione redox cycle, the H_2O_2 concentration in the bathing medium would decrease.[148]

Perfusion of isolated rabbit corneal epithelium with a 10 min pulse of H_2O_2 concentrations as high as about 6 mM gave no significant swelling. With sustained perfusion for 150 min, however, significant stromal swelling occurred with 2 and 5 mM (72 and 153 ppm, respectively) H_2O_2.[149,150] Residual H_2O_2 at the epithelial surface in current contact lens disinfection is well below concentrations needed to induce corneal swelling. These findings are substantiated by clinical experience.[151,152] Given the exposure of the cornea to 50 to 80 ppm H_2O_2, a change in corneal permeability caused by H_2O_2 is unlikely. Recent studies have also shown that corneas with intact epithelia allow no H_2O_2 to cross the cornea when contact lenses containing 20 mM H_2O_2 are placed on the anterior corneal surface.[153]

The corneal endothelium is normally exposed to aqueous humor H_2O_2 at concentrations from 20 to 80 μM.[154-157] The endothelium is more sensitive to H_2O_2 than the epithelium. The threshold for endothelial damage is 0.3 to 0.4 mM in the presence of glucose,[158] and 50 μM in the absence of glucose[159] in isolated rabbit cornea. Above these thresholds dose-dependent corneal swelling ensues, accompanied by ultrastructural changes. Inhibition of active transport processes are first affected,[160] followed, at higher concentrations of H_2O_2, by disturbance of passive permeability.[158]

The endothelium has protective mechanisms that degrade peroxide and can be inhibited with 3-aminotriazole[161,162] and BCNU (1,3-bis-(2-chloroethyl)-1-nitrosourea)[163,164] or BSO (buthionine sulfoximine).[157] The protective systems can normally handle H_2O_2 that reaches the endothelium when used as a preservative.[164]

It is unlikely that H_2O_2, in concentrations normally occurring on the epithelial surface, has any effect on corneal epithelial permeability.

G. SORBIC ACID

A 0.1% concentration of sorbic acid delayed the proliferation of rabbit corneal epithelial cells in tissue culture, and decreased the lifespan of the cells.[132] The concentration was equal to that used in the care of contact lenses. Whether these results indicate changes in epithelial permeability *in vivo* due to the possible suppression of the replacement of desquamated superficial cells remains to be studied.

H. SODIUM BISULFITE

The *in vitro* perfusion of rabbit corneal endothelium with diluted epinephrine solutions caused corneal swelling that was determined to be related to the antioxidant, sodium bisulfite, included in the solution.[165] This was confirmed in a later study[166] that lead to the development of a sulfite-free solution for intraocular use.[167]

Direct intracameral injections of mixtures of either 0.02% sodium bisulfite and 0.1% chlorobutanol, or 0.1% sodium bisulfite and 0.5% chlorobutanol had no effect on cat corneal endothelial cell density.[168] Subconjunctival injections of 0.2% sodium bisulfite caused intracellular vacuolization and thickening of rabbit endothelium that persisted for up to 5 d.[135] The subconjunctival injection of 1.0 mg sodium bisulfite had no effect on rabbit corneal endothelium upon examination at 7 d.[64] Waltman et al.[169] attributed human endothelial cell density reductions, after long-term application of a commercial epinephrine preparation (Glaucon), to the presence of sodium bisulfite in the solution.

I. ETHYLENEDIAMINETETRAACETIC ACID

Ethylenediamine-tetraacetic acid (EDTA) is a chelating agent that binds divalent cations such as calcium and magnesium. Ashton et al.[143] showed that EDTA increased rabbit corneal epithelial permeability to sorbitol by 2.9 times compared to a 9.6 times increase found after de-epithelialization. Rabbit corneal permeability *in vivo* to polar compounds was increased in the presence of 0.5% EDTA.[170] EDTA has been shown, using fluorescence and confocal microscopic technologies, to act not only on cell junctions, but also through disruption of the plasma membrane of rabbit corneal epithelial cells.[171] Marsh and Maurice[119] found that neither 0.34 nor 1.0% EDTA eye drops had any influence on the anterior chamber fluorescein concentration in man.

The *in vivo* administration of 0.1% EDTA to normal or keratectomized corneas for 2 d caused morphological changes in stromal cells,[114] and both 0.01 and 0.1% EDTA also caused condensation of the mitochondria of endothelial cells.[113] Greater changes occurred in the absence of the epithelium.

V. CONCLUSIONS

From the foregoing, it is apparent that there is a range of preservatives that may be used in topical drug formulations. While there has been a trend toward the development of unit dose preparations that are preservative-free, these preparations are primarily used in surgical or immediately post-surgical environments, and the mainstay of outpatient topical medications will remain as preservative-containing solutions. This is especially true when solutions are used at low dosing frequencies rather than the high frequency of use with dry eye solutions.

Wherever preservatives are employed their use must be evaluated on a risk to benefit ratio. The most obvious benefit of preservatives is that of acting as a bactericide for the solution to prevent microbial growth should the container come in contact with a potentially contaminating surface during drug application. There is a broad conjunctival flora which could potentially be damaging to an eye if a solution became contaminated and sustained growth of the bacteria occurred. The next, but less evident, benefit of certain preservatives is to increase corneal epithelial permeability.[172] This factor, which may occur because of the bactericidal action of the preservative, may play an important role in drug bioavailability since the latter has corneal penetration as a major contributing factor.[173] BAK, for example, is an excellent bactericide that also induces increased drug permeation across the cornea,[172] and because of the lack of penetration of this compound beyond the corneal epithelium, BAK has a markedly diminished potential toxicity to internal ocular structures. Use of this compound at concentrations less than 0.01% appears to be appropriate to satisfy bactericidal, toxicological, and pharmaceutical considerations.

Each preservative must be evaluated in relation to its potential use and with regard to long-term safety and toxicological considerations. Although it has not been examined in great detail, the use of thimerosal, with the potential for mercuric involvement of tissues, is probably not one of the better choices of preservative. This is especially true when one considers the range of preservatives available. Chlorobutanol is effective and also increases corneal permeability at concentrations widely used at present; one must also keep in mind, however, its volatility and escape from plastic containers which render it a liability for long-term shelf-life. Chlorhexidine has its limitations as a preservative because of the development of sensitivity of ocular tissues (as with thimerosal). The parabens appear to be nontoxic and offer a viable preservative. Hydrogen peroxide can be unstable in certain solutions; otherwise it has excellent qualities, including the ability to be metabolized by eye tissues and thus, to a great extent, is automatically regulated in eye tissues. Sorbic acid appears to have excellent qualities, but sodium bisulfite and EDTA are undesirable even when labeled as antioxidants.

The ideal preservative probably does not exist, although low concentrations of benzalkonium chloride (<0.01%), the parabens, and hydrogen peroxide probably approach utopia.

As with many other situations in life, the choice of preservative is a balance of risk vs. benefit, and for those preservatives listed immediately above, the balance is on the side of benefit given adherence to certain concentrations and a mode of utilization.

ACKNOWLEDGMENTS

Studies in the author's laboratory were supported in part by National Eye Institute Research Grant EYO4558 and in part by an Unrestricted Departmental Award from Research to Prevent Blindness, Inc. I thank Brenda Sheppard for her valuable secretarial assistance and Lisa Cheeks for her diligent editorial assistance.

REFERENCES

1. **Hogan, M. J., Alvarado, J. A., and Weddell, J. E.,** *Histology of the Human Eye. An Atlas and Textbook,* W. B. Saunders, Philadelphia, 1971.
2. **Bachman, W. G. and Wilson, G.,** Essential ions for maintenance of the corneal epithelial surface, *Invest. Ophthalmol. Vis. Sci.,* 26, 1484, 1985.
3. **Benson, H.,** Permeability of the cornea to topically applied drugs, *Arch. Ophthalmol.,* 91, 313, 1974.
4. **Swan, K. and White, N.,** Corneal permeability. I. Factors affecting penetration of drugs into the cornea, *Am. J. Ophthalmol.,* 25, 1043, 1942.
5. **Klyce, S. D.,** Electrical profiles in the corneal epithelium, *J. Physiol.,* 226, 407, 1972.
6. **Marshall, W. S. and Klyce, S. D.,** Cellular and paracellular pathway resistances in the "tight" Cl^--secreting epithelium of rabbit cornea, *J. Membr. Biol.,* 73, 275, 1983.
7. **Green, K.,** Anatomic study of water movement through rabbit corneal epithelium, *Am. J. Ophthalmol.,* 67, 110, 1969.
8. **Maurice, D. M.,** Nutritional aspects of corneal grafts and prostheses, in *Corneo-Plastic Surgery,* Rycroft, P. V., Ed., Pergamon Press, New York, 1969, 197.
9. **Maurice, D. M.,** The structure and transparency of the cornea, *J. Physiol.,* 136, 263, 1957.
10. **Maurice, D. M.,** The use of permeability studies in the investigation of submicroscopic structure, in *The Structure of the Eye,* Smelser, G. K., Ed., Academic Press, New York, 1961, 381.
11. **Maurice, D. M. and Watson, P. G.,** The distribution and movement of serum albumin in the cornea, *Exp. Eye Res.,* 4, 355, 1965.
12. **Green, K., Laughter, L., and Hull, D. S.,** Rabbit corneal endothelial permeability in the presence and absence of adenosine and glutathione, *Curr. Eye Res.,* 2, 797, 1983.
13. **Green, K., Berdecia, R., and Cheeks, L.,** Mussel adhesive protein: permeability characteristics when used as a basement membrane, *Curr. Eye Res.,* 6, 835, 1987.
14. **Green, K., DeBarge, L. R., Cheeks, L., and Phillips, C. I.,** Centripetal movement of fluorescein dextrans in the cornea: relevance to arcus, *Acta Ophthalmol.,* 65, 538, 1987.
15. **Fischbarg, J. and Lim, J. J.,** Role of cations, anions and carbonic anhydrase in fluid transport across rabbit corneal endothelium, *J. Physiol.,* 241, 647, 1974.
16. **Hodson, S. and Miller, F.,** The bicarbonate ion pump in the endothelium which regulates the hydration of rabbit cornea, *J. Physiol.,* 263, 563, 1976.
17. **Huff, J. W. and Green, K.,** Characteristics of bicarbonate, sodium and chloride fluxes in the rabbit corneal endothelium, *Exp. Eye Res.,* 36, 607, 1983.
18. **Mishima, S. and Trenberth, S. M.,** Permeability of the corneal endothelium to nonelectrolytes, *Invest. Ophthalmol.,* 7, 34, 1968.
19. **Kim, J. H., Green, K., Martinez, M., and Paton, D.,** Solute permeability of the corneal endothelium and Descemet's membrane, *Exp. Eye Res.,* 12, 231, 1971.
20. **Hull, D. S., Green, K., Boyd, M., and Wynn, H. R.,** Corneal endothelium bicarbonate transport and the effect of carbonic anhydrase inhibitors on endothelial permeability and fluxes and corneal thickness, *Invest. Ophthalmol. Vis. Sci.,* 16, 883, 1977.
21. **Hull, D. S., Berdecia, R., and Green, K.,** Corneal storage in MK medium and K-Sol: effect on ionic and non-ionic fluxes, *Invest. Ophthalmol. Vis. Sci.,* 28, 2088, 1987.
22. **Maurice, D. M.,** The cornea and sclera, in *The Eye, Vol 1, Vegetative Physiology and Biochemistry,* 3rd ed., Davson, H., Ed., Academic Press, New York, 1984, 1.

23. **Maurice, D. M.,** Structures and fluids involved in the penetration of topically applied drugs, *Int. Ophthalmol. Clin.,* 20, 7, 1980.
24. **Clayton, R. M., Green, K., Wilson, M., Zehir, A., Jack, J., and Searle, L.,** The penetration of detergents into adult and infant eyes: possible hazards of additives to ophthalmic preparations, *Fd. Chem. Toxicol.,* 23, 239, 1985.
25. **Green, K., Chapman, J., Cheeks, L., and Clayton, R. M.,** Surfactant penetration into the eye, in *Concepts in Toxicology. Drug-Induced Ocular Side Effects and Ocular Toxicology,* Hockwin, O., Ed., S. Karger, Basel, 1987, 126.
26. **Green, K., Chapman, J. M., Cheeks, L., Clayton, R. M., Wilson, M., and Zehir, A.,** Detergent penetration into young and adult rabbit eyes: comparative pharmacokinetics, *J. Toxicol. Cutan. Ocular Toxicol.,* 6, 89, 1987.
27. **Hind, H. and Goyan, F.,** A new concept of the role of hydrogen ion concentration and buffer systems in the preparation of ophthalmic solutions, *J. Am. Pharm. Assoc. Sci. Ed.,* 36, 33, 1947.
28. **Martin, F. N. and Mims, J. L.,** Preparation of ophthalmic solutions with special reference to hydrogen ion concentration and tonicity, *Arch. Ophthalmol.,* 44, 561, 1950.
29. **Norn, M. S.,** Role of the vehicle in local treatment of the eye, *Acta Ophthalmol.,* 42, 727, 1964.
30. **Maurice, D. M.,** Influence on corneal permeability of bathing with solutions of differing reaction and tonicity, *Br. J. Ophthalmol.,* 39, 463, 1955.
31. **Ramselaar, J. A. M., Boot, J. P., van Haeringen, N. J., van Best, J. A., and Oosterhuis, J. A.,** Corneal epithelial permeability after instillation of ophthalmic solutions containing local anaesthetics and preservatives, *Curr. Eye Res.,* 7, 947, 1988.
32. **Smolen, V. F., Clevenger, J. M., Williams, E. J., and Bergdolt, M. W.,** Biophasic availability of ophthalmic carbachol. I. Mechanisms of cationic polymer- and surfactant-promoted miotic activity, *J. Pharm. Sci.,* 62, 958, 1973.
33. **Conrad, J. M., Reay, W. A., Polcyn, R. E., and Robinson, J. R.,** Influence of tonicity and pH on lacrimation and ocular drug bioavailability, *J. Parenter. Drug Assoc.,* 32, 149, 1978.
34. **Keller, N., Moore, D., Carper, D., and Longwell, A.,** Increased corneal permeability induced by the dual effects of transient tear film acidification and exposure to benzalkonium chloride, *Exp. Eye Res.,* 30, 203, 1980.
35. **Sieg, J. W. and Robinson, J. R.,** Vehicle effects on ocular drug bioavailability. I. Evaluation of fluorometholone, *J. Pharm. Sci.,* 64, 931, 1975.
36. **Sieg, J. W. and Robinson, J. R.,** Vehicle effects on ocular drug bioavailability. II. Evaluation of pilocarpine, *J. Pharm. Sci.,* 66, 1222, 1977.
37. **Gonnering, R., Edelhauser, H. F., Van Horn, D. L., and Durant, W.,** The pH tolerance of rabbit and human corneal endothelium, *Invest. Ophthalmol. Vis. Sci.,* 18, 373, 1979.
38. **Edelhauser, H. F., Hanneken, A. M., Pederson, H. J., and Van Horn, D. L.** Osmotic tolerance of rabbit and human corneal endothelium, *Arch. Ophthalmol.,* 99, 1281, 1981.
39. **Dikstein, S. and Maurice, D. M.,** The metabolic basis to the fluid pump in the cornea, *J. Physiol.,* 221, 29, 1972.
40. **Anderson, E. I., Fischbarg, J., and Spector, A.,** Fluid transport, ATP level and ATPase activities in isolated rabbit corneal endothelium, *Biochim. Biophys. Acta,* 307, 557, 1973.
41. **Edelhauser, H. F., Van Horn, D. L., Hyndiuk, R. A., and Schultz, R. O.,** Intraocular irrigating solutions. Their effect on the corneal endothelium, *Arch. Ophthalmol.,* 93, 648, 1975.
42. **Koniarek, J. P., Lee, H. B., Rosskothen, H. D., Liebovitch, L. S., and Fischbarg, J.,** Use of trans-endothelial electrical potential difference to assess the chondroitin sulfate effect in corneal preservation media, *Invest. Ophthalmol. Vis. Sci.,* 29, 657, 1988.
43. **Harnisch, J. P., Hoffmann, F., and Dumitrescu, L.,** Side-effects of local anesthetics on the corneal epithelium of the rabbit eye, *Albrecht von Graefe's Arch. Klin. Exp. Ophthalmol.,* 197, 71, 1975.
44. **Mishima, S.,** Clinical pharmacokinetics of the eye, *Invest. Ophthalmol. Vis. Sci.,* 21, 504, 1981.
45. **Burstein, N. L. and Anderson, J. A.,** Review: corneal penetration and ocular bioavailability of drugs, *J. Ocular Pharmacol.,* 1, 309, 1985.
46. **Chrai, S. S. and Robinson, J. R.,** Ocular evaluation of methylcellulose vehicle in albino rabbits, *J. Pharm. Sci.,* 63, 1218, 1974.
47. **Patton, T. F. and Robinson, J. R.,** Ocular evaluation of polyvinyl alcohol vehicle in rabbits, *J. Pharm. Sci.,* 64, 1312, 1975.
48. **Grass, G. M. and Robinson, J. R.,** Relationship of chemical structure to corneal penetration and influence of low-viscosity solution on ocular bioavailability, *J. Pharm. Sci.,* 73, 1021, 1984.
49. **Camber, O. and Edman, P.,** Sodium hyaluronate as an ophthalmic vehicle: some factors governing its effect on the ocular absorption of pilocarpine, *Curr. Eye Res.,* 8, 563, 1989.
50. **Saettone, M. F., Giannaccini, B., Savigni, B., and Wirth, A.,** The effect of different ophthalmic vehicles on the activity of tropicamide in man, *J. Pharm. Pharmacol.,* 32, 519, 1980.

51. **Kupferman, A., Ryan, W. J., and Leibowitz, H. M.,** Prolongation of anti-inflammatory effect of prednisolone acetate. Influence of formulation in high-viscosity gel, *Arch. Ophthalmol.*, 99, 2028, 1981.
52. **Schoenwald, R. D., Ward, R. L., DeSantis, L. M., and Roehrs, R. E.,** Influence of high-viscosity vehicles on miotic effect of pilocarpine, *J. Pharm. Sci.*, 67, 1280, 1978.
53. **Lee, V. H. and Robinson, J. R.,** Mechanistic and quantitative evaluation of precorneal pilocarpine disposition in albino rabbits, *J. Pharm. Sci.*, 68, 673, 1979.
54. **Hardberger, R. E., Hanna, C., and Goodart, R.,** Effects of drug vehicles on ocular uptake of tetracycline, *Am. J. Ophthalmol.*, 80, 133, 1975.
55. **Mueller, W. H. and Deardorff, D. L.,** Ophthalmic vehicles: the effect of methylcellulose on the penetration of homatropine hydrobromide through the cornea, *J. Am. Pharm. Assoc. Sci. Ed.*, 45, 334, 1956.
56. **Rosenblum, C., Dengler, R. E., and Geoffroy, R. F.,** Ocular absorption of dexamethasone phosphate disodium by the rabbit, *Arch. Ophthalmol.*, 77, 234, 1967.
57. **Waltman, S. R. and Patrowicz, T. C.,** Effects of hydroxypropyl methylcellulose and polyvinyl alcohol on intraocular penetration of topical fluorescein in man, *Invest. Ophthalmol.*, 9, 966, 1970.
58. **Adler, C. A., Maurice, D. M., and Paterson, M. E.,** The effect of viscosity of the vehicle on the penetration of fluorescein into the human eye, *Exp. Eye Res.*, 11, 34, 1971.
59. **MacRae, S. M., Edelhauser, H. F., Hyndiuk, R. A., Burd, E. M., and Schultz, R. O.,** The effects of sodium hyaluronate, chondroitin sulfate, and methylcellulose on the corneal endothelium and intraocular pressure, *Am. J. Ophthalmol.*, 95, 332, 1983.
60. **Miller, S. C. and Patton, T. F.,** Age-related differences in ophthalmic drug disposition. I. Effect of size on the intraocular tissue distribution of pilocarpine in albino rabbits, *Biopharm. Drug Dispos.*, 2, 215, 1981.
61. **Miller, S. C. and Patton, T. F.,** Age-related differences in ophthalmic drug disposition. II. Drug-protein interactions of pilocarpine and chloramphenicol, *Biopharm. Drug Dispos.*, 3, 115, 1982.
62. **Edelhauser, H. F., Hine, J. E., Pederson, H., Van Horn, D. L., and Schultz, R. O.,** The effect of phenylephrine on the cornea, *Arch. Ophthalmol.*, 97, 937, 1979.
63. **Staatz, W. D., Van Horn, D. L., Edelhauser, H. F., and Schultz, R. O.,** Effects of phenylephrine on bovine corneal endothelium in culture, *Ophthalmic Res.*, 12, 244, 1980.
64. **Sasamoto, K., Akagi, Y., Kodama, Y., and Itoi, M.,** Corneal endothelial changes caused by ophthalmic drugs, *Cornea*, 3, 37, 1984.
65. **Chapman, J. M., Abdelatif, O. M. A., Cheeks, L., and Green, K.,** Subconjunctival gentamicin induction of extraocular muscle myopathy, *Ophthalmic Res.*, in press, 1992.
66. **Mullen, W., Shepherd, W., and Labovitz, J.,** Ophthalmic preservatives and vehicles, *Surv. Ophthalmol.*, 17, 469, 1973.
67. **O'Brien, C. S. and Swan, K.,** Doryl in the treatment of glaucoma simplex, *Trans. Am. Ophthalmol. Soc.*, 39, 175, 1941.
68. **O'Brien, C. S. and Swan, K. C.,** Carbaminoylcholine chloride in treatment of glaucoma simplex, *Arch. Ophthalmol.*, 27, 253, 1942.
69. **Thompson, R., Isaacs, M. L., and Khorazo, D.,** A laboratory study of some antiseptics with reference to ocular application, *Am. J. Ophthalmol.*, 20, 1087, 1937.
70. **Swan, K. C.,** Reactivity of the ocular tissues to wetting agents, *Am. J. Ophthalmol.*, 27, 1118, 1944.
71. **Leopold, I.,** Local toxic effect of detergents on ocular structures, *Arch. Ophthalmol.*, 34, 99, 1945.
72. **Ginsburg, M. and Robson, J. M.,** Further investigations on the action of detergents on the eye, *Br. J. Ophthalmol.*, 33, 574, 1949.
73. **Dabezies, O. H., Naugle, T., and Reich, L.,** Evaluation of a stronger concentration of preservative (benzalkonium chloride) in contact lens soaking solution, *Eye Ear Nose Throat Mon.*, 45, 78, 1966.
74. **Barkman, R., Germanis, M., Karpe, G., and Malmborg, S.,** Preservatives in eye drops, *Acta Ophthalmol.*, 47, 461, 1969.
75. **Chapman, J. M., Cheeks, L., and Green, K.,** Interactions of benzalkonium chloride with soft and hard contact lenses, *Arch. Ophthalmol.*, 108, 244, 1990.
76. **Burstein, N. L. and Klyce, S. D.,** Electrophysiologic and morphologic effects of ophthalmic preparations on rabbit cornea epithelium, *Invest. Ophthalmol. Vis. Sci.*, 16, 899, 1977.
77. **Burstein, N. L.,** Corneal cytotoxicity of topically applied drugs, vehicles and preservatives, *Surv. Ophthalmol.*, 25, 15, 1980.
78. **Burstein, N. L.** Preservative cytotoxic threshold for benzalkonium chloride and chlorhexidine digluconate in cat and rabbit corneas, *Invest. Ophthalmol. Vis. Sci.*, 19, 308, 1980.
79. **Tønjum, A. M.,** Effects of benzalkonium chloride upon the corneal epithelium studied with scanning electron microscopy, *Acta Ophthalmol.*, 53, 358, 1975.
80. **Green, K. and Tønjum, A. M.,** The effect of benzalkonium chloride on the electropotential of the rabbit cornea, *Acta Ophthalmol.*, 53, 348, 1975.

81. **Pfister, R. R. and Burstein, N.**, The effects of ophthalmic drugs, vehicles, and preservatives on corneal epithelium: a scanning electron microscope study, *Invest. Ophthalmol.*, 15, 246, 1976.
82. **Dormans, J. A. and van Logten, M. J.**, The effects of ophthalmic preservatives on corneal epithelium of the rabbit: a scanning electron microscopical study, *Toxicol. Appl. Pharmacol.*, 62, 251, 1982.
83. **Durand-Cavagna, G., Delort, P., Duprat, P., Bailly, Y., Plazonnet, B., and Gordon, L. R.**, Corneal toxicity studies in rabbits and dogs with hydroxyethyl cellulose and benzalkonium chloride, *Fundam. Appl. Toxicol.*, 13, 500, 1989.
84. **Tønjum, A. M.**, Permeability of rabbit corneal epithelium to horseradish peroxidase after the influence of benzalkonium chloride, *Acta Ophthalmol.*, 53, 335, 1975.
85. **Maudgal, P. C., Cornelis, M., and Missotten, L.**, Effects of commercial ophthalmic drugs on rabbit corneal epithelium. A scanning electron microscopic study, *Albrecht von Graefes Arch. Klin, Exp. Ophthalmol.*, 216, 191, 1981.
86. **Gasset, A. R., Ishii, Y., Kaufman, H. E., and Miller, T.**, Cytotoxicity of ophthalmic preservatives, *Am. J. Ophthalmol.*, 78, 98, 1974.
87. **Gasset, A. R.**, Benzalkonium chloride toxicity to the human cornea, *Am. J. Ophthalmol.*, 84, 169, 1977.
88. **Burton, G. D. and Hill, R. M.**, Aerobic responses of the cornea to ophthalmic preservatives, measured in vivo, *Invest. Ophthalmol. Vis. Sci.*, 21, 842, 1981.
89. **Green, K. and Tønjum, A. M.**, Influence of various agents on corneal permeability, *Am. J. Ophthalmol.*, 72, 897, 1971.
90. **Green, K. and Downs, S. J.**, Ocular penetration of pilocarpine in rabbits, *Arch. Ophthalmol.*, 93, 1165, 1975.
91. **Camber, O. and Edman, P.**, Influence of some preservatives on the corneal permeability of pilocarpine and dexamethasone in vitro, *Int. J. Pharm.*, 39, 229, 1987.
92. **Green, K. and Downs, S.**, Prednisolone phosphate penetration into and through the cornea, *Invest. Ophthalmol.*, 13, 316, 1974.
93. **Green, K. and MacKeen, D. L.**, Chloramphenicol retention on, and penetration into, the rabbit eye, *Invest. Ophthalmol.*, 15, 220, 1976.
94. **Barlosova, D., Obenberger, J., and Bibr, B.**, Vliv detergentnich latek na permeabilitu rohovky, *Cesk. Oftalmol.*, 35, 421, 1979.
95. **Camber, O. and Edman, P.**, Factors influencing the corneal permeability of prostaglandin $F_{2\alpha}$ and its isopropyl ester in vitro, *Int. J. Pharm.*, 37, 27, 1987.
96. **Maurice, D. and Singh, T.**, A permeability test for acute corneal toxicity, *Toxicol. Lett.*, 31, 125, 1986.
97. **Burstein, N. L.**, Preservative alteration of corneal permeability in humans and rabbits, *Invest. Ophthalmol. Vis. Sci.*, 25, 1453, 1984.
98. **Göbbels, M. and Spitznas, M.**, Influence of artificial tears on corneal epithelium in dry-eye syndrome, *Albrecht von Graefs Arch. Klin. Exp. Ophthalmol.*, 227, 139, 1989.
99. **Wilson, W. S., Duncan, A. J., and Jay, J. L.**, Effect of benzalkonium chloride on the stability of the precorneal tear film in rabbit and man, *Br. J. Ophthalmol.*, 59, 667, 1975.
100. **Burstein, N. L.**, The effects of topical drugs and preservatives on the tears and corneal epithelium in dry eye, *Trans. Ophthalmol. Soc. UK*, 104, 402, 1985.
101. **Neville, R., Dennis, P., Sens, D., and Crouch, R.**, Preservative cytotoxicity to cultured corneal epithelial cells, *Curr. Eye Res.*, 5, 367, 1986.
102. **Green, K. and Chapman, J. M.**, Benzalkonium chloride kinetics in young and adult albino and pigmented rabbit eyes, *J. Toxicol. Cutan. Ocular Toxicol.*, 5, 133, 1986.
103. **Champeau, E. J. and Edelhauser, H. F.**, Effect of ophthalmic preservatives on the ocular surface: conjunctival and corneal uptake and distribution of benzalkonium chloride and chlorhexidine digluconate, in *The Preocular Tear Film in Health, Disease and Contact Lens Wear*, Holly, F. J., Lambert, D. W., and MacKeen, D. L., Eds., Dry Eye Institute, Lubbock, TX, 1986, 292.
104. **Kossendrup, D., Wiederholt, M., and Hoffmann, F.**, Influence of cyclosporin A, dexamethasone, and -benzalkonium chloride (BAK) on corneal epithelial wound healing in the rabbit and guinea pig eye, *Cornea*, 4, 177, 1985.
105. **Green, K., Johnson, R. E., Chapman, J. M., Nelson, E., and Cheeks, L.**, Surfactant effects on the rate of rabbit corneal epithelial healing, *J. Toxicol. Cutan. Ocular Toxicol.*, 8, 253, 1989.
106. **Lemp, M. A. and Zimmerman, L. E.**, Toxic endothelial degeneration in ocular surface disease treated with topical medications containing benzalkonium chloride, *Am. J. Ophthalmol.*, 105, 670, 1988.
107. **Green, K., Hull, D. S., Vaughn, E. D., Malizia, A. A., and Bowman, K.**, Rabbit endothelial response to ophthalmic preservatives, *Arch. Ophthalmol.*, 95, 2218, 1977.
108. **Maurice, D. and Perlman, M.**, Permanent destruction of the corneal endothelium in rabbits, *Invest. Ophthalmol. Vis. Sci.*, 16, 646, 1977.
109. **Jumblatt, M. M., Maurice, D. M., and McCulley, J. P.**, Transplantation of tissue-cultured corneal endothelium, *Invest. Ophthalmol. Vis. Sci.*, 17, 1135, 1978.

110. **Khodadoust, A. A. and Green, K.,** Physiological function of regenerating endothelium, *Invest. Ophthalmol.,* 15, 96, 1976.

111. **Van Horn, D. L., Sendele, D. D., Seideman, S., and Buco, P. J.,** Regenerative capacity of the corneal endothelium in rabbit and cat, *Invest. Ophthalmol. Vis. Sci.,* 16, 597, 1977.

112. **Yee, R. W., Geroski, D. H., Matsuda, M., Champeau, E. J., Myer, L. A., and Edelhauser, H. F.,** Correlation of corneal endothelial pump site density, barrier function, and morphology in wound repair, *Invest. Ophthalmol. Vis. Sci.,* 26, 1191, 1985.

113. **Collin, H. B. and Carroll, N.,** Ultrastructural changes to the corneal endothelium due to benzalkonium chloride, *Acta Ophthalmol.,* 64, 226, 1986.

114. **Collin, H. B.,** Ultrastructural changes to corneal stromal cells due to ophthalmic preservatives, *Acta Ophthalmol.,* 64, 72, 1986.

115. **Mikkelson, T. J., Chrai, S. S., and Robinson, J. R.,** Competitive inhibition of drug-protein interaction in eye fluids and tissues, *J. Pharm. Sci.,* 62, 1942, 1973.

116. **Green, K.,** Electrophysiological and anatomical effects of cetylpyridinium chloride on the rabbit cornea, *Acta Ophthalmol.,* 54, 145, 1976.

117. **Godbey, R. E. W., Green, K., and Hull, D. S.,** Influence of cetylpyridinium chloride on corneal permeability to penicillin, *J. Pharm. Sci.,* 68, 1176, 1979.

118. **Green, K., Bowman, K. A., Elijah, R. D., Mermelstein, R., and Kilpper, R. W.,** Dose-effect response of the rabbit eye to cetylpyridinium chloride, *J. Toxicol. Cutan. Ocular Toxicol.,* 4, 13, 1985.

119. **Marsh, R. J. and Maurice, D. M.,** The influence of non-ionic detergents and other surfactants on human corneal permeability, *Exp. Eye Res.,* 11, 43, 1971.

120. **Igarashi, H. and Northover, A. M.,** Increases in opacity and thickness induced by surfactants and other chemicals in the bovine isolated cornea, *Toxicol. Lett.,* 39, 249, 1987.

121. **Carter, L. M., Duncan, G., and Rennie, G. K.,** Effects of detergents on the ionic balance and permeability of isolated bovine cornea, *Exp. Eye Res.,* 17, 409, 1973.

122. **Taniguchi, K., Itakura, K., Morisaki, K., and Hayashi, S.,** Effects of Tween 80 and liposomes on the corneal permeability of anti-inflammatory steroids, *J. Pharmacobiodyn.,* 11, 685, 1988.

123. **Muir, C. K.,** Opacity of bovine cornea *in vitro* induced by surfactants and industrial chemicals compared with ocular irritancy *in vivo, Toxicol. Lett.,* 24, 157, 1985.

124. **Muir, C. K.,** Surfactant-induced opacity of bovine isolated cornea: an epithelial phenomenon? *Toxicol. Lett.,* 38, 51, 1987.

125. **Wilson, L. A., McNatt, J., and Rietschel, R.,** Delayed hypersensitivity to thimerosal in soft contact lens wearers, *Ophthalmology,* 88, 804, 1981.

126. **Rietschel, R. L. and Wilson, L. A.,** Ocular inflammation in patients using soft contact lenses, *Arch. Dermatol.,* 118, 147, 1982.

127. **Mondino, B. J., Salamon, S. M., and Zaidman, G. W.,** Allergic and toxic reactions of soft contact lens wearers, *Surv. Ophthalmol.,* 26, 337, 1982.

128. **Fraunfelder, F. T.,** *Drug-Induced Ocular Side Effects and Drug Interactions,* 3rd ed., Lea & Febiger, Philadelphia, 1989.

129. **Klein, M., Millwood, E. G., and Walther, W. W.,** On the maintenance of sterility in eye drops, *J. Pharm. Pharmacol.,* 6, 725, 1954.

130. **Rucker, I., Kettrey, R., Bach, F., and Zeleznick, L.,** A safety test for contact lens wetting solutions. Evaluation of commercially available solutions, *Ann. Ophthalmol.,* 4, 1000, 1972.

131. **Collin, H. B. and Carroll, N.,** In vivo effects of thimerosal on the rabbit corneal endothelium: an ultrastructural study, *Am. J. Optom. Physiol. Opt.,* 64, 123, 1987.

132. **Simmons, P. A., Clough, S. R., Teagle, R. H., and Jaanus, S. D.,** Toxic effects of ophthalmic preservatives on cultured rabbit corneal epithelium, *Am. J. Optom. Physiol. Opt.,* 65, 867, 1988.

133. **Van Horn, D. L., Edelhauser, H. F., Prodanovich, G., Eiferman, R., and Pederson, H. J.,** Effect of the ophthalmic preservative thimerosal on rabbit and human corneal endothelium, *Invest. Ophthalmol. Vis. Sci.,* 16, 273, 1977.

134. **Capella, J. A. and Schaefer, I. M.,** Comparison of ophthalmic vehicles using fluorescein uptake technique, *Eye Ear Nose Throat Mon.,* 53, 23, 1974.

135. **Weinreb, R. N., Wood, I., Tomazzoli, L., and Alvarado, J.,** Subconjunctival injections. Preservative-related changes in the corneal endothelium, *Invest. Ophthalmol. Vis. Sci.,* 27, 525, 1986.

136. **Kato, A. and Iwata, S.,** Studies on improved corneal permeability to bunazosin, *J. Pharmacobiodyn.,* 11, 330, 1988.

137. **Coles, W. H.,** Effects of antibiotics on the in vitro rabbit corneal endothelium, *Invest. Ophthalmol.,* 14, 246, 1975.

138. **MacKeen, D. L. and Green, K.,** Chlorhexidine kinetics of hydrophilic contact lenses, *J. Pharm. Pharmacol.,* 30, 678, 1978.

139. **MacKeen, D. L. and Green, K.,** Chlorhexidine kinetics in hard contact lenses, *J. Pharm. Pharmacol.,* 31, 714, 1979.
140. **Browne, R. K., Anderson, A. N., Charvez, B. W., and Azzarello, R. J.,** Ophthalmic response to chlorhexidine digluconate in rabbits, *Toxicol. Appl. Pharmacol.,* 32, 621, 1975.
141. **Green, K., Livingston, V., Bowman, K., and Hull, D. S.,** Chlorhexidine effects on corneal epithelium and endothelium, *Arch. Ophthalmol.,* 98, 1273, 1980.
142. **Gasset, A. R. and Ishii, Y.,** Cytotoxicity of chlorhexidine, *Can. J. Ophthalmol.,* 10, 98, 1975.
143. **Ashton, P., Diepold, R., Platzer, A., and Lee, V. H.,** The effect of chlorhexidine acetate on the corneal penetration of sorbitol from an arnolol formulation in the albino rabbit, *J. Ocular Pharmacol.,* 6, 37, 1990.
144. **MacRae, S. M., Brown, B., and Edelhauser, H. F.,** The corneal toxicity of presurgical skin antiseptics, *Am. J. Ophthalmol.,* 97, 221, 1984.
145. **Phinney, R. B., Mondino, B. J., Hofbauer, J. D., Meisler, D. M., Langston, R. H., Forstot, S. L., and Benes, S. C.,** Corneal edema related to accidental Hibiclens exposure, *Am. J. Ophthalmol.,* 106, 210, 1988.
146. **Tabor, E., Bostwick, D. C., and Evans, C. C.,** Corneal damage due to eye contact with chlorhexidine gluconate, *JAMA,* 261, 557, 1989.
147. **Tripathi, B. J. and Tripathi, R. C.** Hydrogen peroxide damage to human corneal epithelial cells in vitro. Implications for contact lens disinfection systems, *Arch. Ophthalmol.,* 107, 1516, 1989.
148. **Polansky, J. R., Fauss, D. J., Hydorn, T., and Bloom, E.,** Cellular injury from sustained vs. acute hydrogen peroxide exposure in cultured human corneal endothelium and human lens epithelium, *CLAO J.,* 16 (Suppl.), 23, 1990.
149. **Wilson, G.,** Effect of hydrogen peroxide on epithelial light-scattering and stromal deturgescence, *CLAO J.,* 16 (Suppl.), 11, 1990.
150. **Wilson, G. S. and Chalmers, R. L.,** Effect of H_2O_2 concentration and exposure time on stromal swelling: an epithelial perfusion model, *Optom. Vis. Sci.,* 67, 252, 1990.
151. **Holden, B.,** A report card on hydrogen peroxide for contact lens disinfection, *CLAO J.,* 16 (Suppl.), 61, 1990.
152. **McNally, J. J.,** Clinical aspects of topical application of dilute hydrogen peroxide solutions, *CLAO J.,* 16 (Suppl.), 46, 1990.
153. **Riley, M. V. and Kast, M.,** Penetration of hydrogen peroxide from contact lenses or tear-side solutions into the aqueous humor, *Optom. Vis. Sci.,* 68, 546, 1991.
154. **Bhuyan, K. C. and Bhuyan, D. K.,** Regulation of hydrogen peroxide in eye humors: effect of 3-amino-1H-1,2,4-triazole on catalase and glutathione peroxidase of rabbit eye, *Biochim. Biophys. Acta,* 497, 641, 1977.
155. **Spector, A. and Garner, W. H.,** Hydrogen peroxide and human cataract, *Exp. Eye Res.,* 33, 673, 1981.
156. **Costarides, A., Recasens, J. F., Riley, M. V., and Green, K.,** The effects of ascorbate, 3-aminotriazole, and 1,3-bis(2-chloroethyl)-1-nitrosourea on hydrogen peroxide levels in the rabbit aqueous humor, *Lens Eye Tox. Res.,* 6, 167, 1989.
157. **Costarides, A., Riley, M. V., and Green, K.,** Roles of catalase and the glutathione redox cycle in the regulation of anterior chamber hydrogen peroxide, *Ophthalmic Res.,* 23, 284, 1991.
158. **Hull, D. S., Csukas, S., Green, K., and Livingston, V.,** Hydrogen peroxide and corneal endothelium, *Acta Ophthalmol.,* 59, 409, 1981.
159. **Riley, M. V. and Giblin, F. J.,** Toxic effects of hydrogen peroxide on corneal endothelium, *Curr. Eye Res.,* 2, 451, 1982.
160. **Hull, D. S., Green, K., Thomas, L., and Alderman, N.,** Hydrogen peroxide mediated corneal endothelial damage: induction by oxygen free radical, *Invest. Ophthalmol. Vis. Sci.,* 25, 1246, 1984.
161. **Csukas, S., Costarides, A., Riley, M. V., and Green, K.,** Hydrogen peroxide in the rabbit anterior chamber: effects on glutathione, and catalase effects on peroxide kinetics, *Curr. Eye Res.,* 6, 1395, 1987.
162. **Birnbaum, D. B., Csukas, S., Costarides, A., Forbes, E., and Green, K.,** 3-amino-triazole effects on the eye of young and adult rabbits in the presence and absence of hydrogen peroxide, *Curr. Eye Res.,* 6, 1403, 1987.
163. **Riley, M.,** Pump and leak in regulation of fluid transport in rabbit cornea, *Curr. Eye Res.,* 4, 371, 1985.
164. **Riley, M. V.,** Physiologic neutralization mechanisms and the response of the corneal endothelium to hydrogen peroxide, *CLAO J.,* 16 (Suppl.), 16, 1990.
165. **Hull, D. S., Chemotti, M. T., Edelhauser, H. F., Van Horn, D. L., and Hyndiuk, R. A.,** Effect of epinephrine on the corneal endothelium, *Am. J. Ophthalmol.,* 79, 245, 1975.
166. **Edelhauser, H. F., Hyndiuk, R. A., Zeeb, A., and Schultz, R. O.,** Corneal edema and the intraocular use of epinephrine, *Am. J. Ophthalmol.,* 93, 327, 1982.
167. **Slack, J.W., Edelhauser, H. F., and Helenek, M. J.,** A bisulfite-free intraocular epinephrine solution, *Am. J. Ophthalmol.,* 110, 77, 1990.

168. **Olson, R. J., Kolodner, H., Riddle, P., and Escapini, H.,** Commonly used intraocular medications and the corneal endothelium, *Arch. Ophthalmol.,* 98, 2224, 1980.

169. **Waltman, S. R., Yarian, D., Hart, W., and Becker, B.,** Corneal endothelial changes with long-term topical epinephrine therapy, *Arch. Ophthalmol.,* 95, 1357, 1977.

170. **Grass, G. M., Wood, R. W., and Robinson, J. R.,** Effects of calcium chelating agents on corneal permeability, *Invest. Ophthalmol. Vis. Sci.,* 26, 110, 1985.

171. **Rojanasakul, Y., Liaw, J., and Robinson, J. R.,** Mechanisms of action of some penetration enhancers in the cornea: laser scanning confocal microscopic and electrophysiology studies, *Int. J. Pharm.,* 66, 131, 1990.

172. **Green, K.,** The role of surfactants as bactericides in topical drug delivery, *STP Pharma Sciences,* 2, 34, 1992.

173. **Keister, J. C., Cooper, E. R., Missel, P. J., Lang, J. C., and Hager, D. F.,** Limits on optimizing ocular drug delivery, *J. Pharm. Sci.,* 80, 50, 1991.

Chapter 4

SOLID POLYMERIC INSERTS/DISKS AS DRUG DELIVERY DEVICES

Marco Fabrizio Saettone

TABLE OF CONTENTS

I.   Introduction 62

II.   Soluble Inserts 63
      A.   Inserts Based on Synthetic and Semisynthetic Polymers 64
      B.   Inserts Based on Naturally Occurring Polymers 68
      C.   Soluble Inserts Utilizing Particular Approaches 69
            1.   The Muco-Adhesive Approach 69
            2.   The Prodrug Approach 70
            3.   The Drug Carrier Approach 70

III. Insoluble Inserts 70
      A.   Hydrogel Contact Lenses 70
      B.   Membrane-Controlled Reservoir Inserts 71
      C.   Other Insoluble Devices 73

IV.   Conclusions 73

References 74

0-8493-7296-8/93/$0.00 + $.50

61

I. INTRODUCTION

This review is focused on solid devices delivering drugs to the anterior part of the eye; those used for the posterior part of the eye (scleral buckling materials) and implantable devices will not be treated. Even with this limitation, the present text makes no pretension at exhaustivity. Its main purpose is to provide a general overview of the field, to outline the most recent research trends, and, possibly, to stimulate further thought. The interested readers will find additional information in the many excellent reviews that have been dedicated, entirely or in part, to solid ophthalmic medications.[1-13]

Since the character of this review is primarily technological/biopharmaceutical, a number of papers dealing with pharmacological and clinical evaluations of inserts, but not disclosing any basic data about the devices (such as physical properties and components), have not been included. By an analogous line of reasoning, the patent literature on ophthalmic inserts, which might deserve a specialized review, has been mentioned only sparingly. The sincerest apologies are presented to the authors of the work, which forcibly, but in some cases inadvertently, has not been mentioned.

Throughout the text it will be assumed that the reader has at least a working knowledge of the problems and intricacies of ocular anatomy and physiology, ocular drug delivery, pharmacokinetics, and bioavailability. A basic knowledge of the principles of drug release from polymeric devices is also assumed. Thus, this background information will be dispensed with. The reader willing to expand his/her knowledge will find adequate information in reviews, chapters in books (including the present one), and other publications, some of which are mentioned in the References section.[5,6,11,14-17]

Some definitions and brief historical notes should be of relevance here. All solid medications mentioned in this review are indicated by the general name *inserts*. This word is self-explanatory, and originates from the latin *inserere,* to introduce. Solid medications have been applied to the eye for many centuries. The term collyrium, now reserved exclusively for liquid ocular medications (eye drops), originates from the Greek word κολλυριον, indicating a poultice, or a dry medicinal paste formed as a flat, small pancake or cylinder, which could also be used as a suppository. In time, only ocular medications, either liquid, solid, or semisolid, were denominated collyria. As the Roman physician Oribasius (325–403) put it, *"quae collyria proprie dicuntur, ea oculis adhibentur"* (all things used for the eye are denominated collyria). A clearer distinction between dry and liquid collyria evolved during the middle ages, when the former were denominated, using Arab words, *Sief* or *Alkohl.* The latter word originally indicated a very fine antimony powder, used to paint the eyelids. The dry collyria, consisting of mixtures of minerals, herbs, and/or animal secretions, were molded into the form of small pyramids, or tablets the size and shape of a lentil. For use, these could be placed under the eyelids or insufflated onto the eye as a fine powder.[18]

In the sixteenth century, the celebrated French physician and surgeon Ambroise Paré (1517–1590) stated that "...there are three types of collyria: viz., aqueous ones, properly said collyria, others having the consistency of honey, and dry ones, also called *sief*".

Medications strongly resembling some of the present insoluble inserts, the so-called "collyres secs gradués, or papiers médicamenteux" (graded dry collyria, or medicated papers), are described in a French nineteenth century pharmacy manual.[19] These consisted of squares of dry filter paper, previously impregnated with drug solutions (e.g., atropine sulfate, pilocarpine hydrochloride, etc.). The drug content, in milligrams per square centimeters, was exactly determined. For use, small sections of the paper, corresponding to the desired amount of drug, were cut and applied under the eyelid.

Likewise, the so-called "lamellae", so often referred to as the precursors of the present soluble inserts, consisted of thin, circular plates of glycerinated gelatin containing different ophthalmic drugs. The lamellae were included in different official compendia, including the British Pharmacopoeia, up to the first half of the present century. They came to an end when more stringent requirements for sterility of ophthalmic preparations were enforced.

In conclusion, the concept of applying a solid medication to the eye is by no means new. Even if liquid (or semisolid) collyria have always predominated in medical practice, solid medications have been with greater or lesser success and popularity, inserted into diseased eyes throughout the centuries. Presently we are experiencing a new surge of scientific interest for these ancient, never completely extinct dosage forms. It can be assumed that the revival has been stimulated by the following main factors:

1. Advances in polymer chemistry: availability of improved polymers and biopolymers, sometimes tailored to the specific needs of ocular delivery (e.g., bioadhesive polymers)
2. Advances in ocular pharmacokinetics
3. Better understanding of release kinetics from solid dosage forms
4. Improved approaches in pharmacological evaluation (animal tests) and clinical testing of ophthalmic medications
5. Objective need for improved ophthalmic dosage forms

Concerning point 5, if one accepts the reasonable opinion of Lee and Robinson that "existing ocular delivery systems (i.e., standard eyedrops and ointments) are fairly primitive and inefficient...",[11] ophthalmic inserts might present valuable assets, such as:

1. Increased ocular permanence with respect to standard vehicles, hence a prolonged drug activity and a higher drug bioavailability
2. Accurate dosing (all of the drug is theoretically retained at the absorption site)
3. Possible reduction of systemic absorption, which occurs freely with standard eye drops via the nasal mucosa
4. Better patient compliance resulting from a reduced frequency of medication and a lower incidence of visual and systemic side-effects
5. Possibility of targeting internal ocular tissues through noncorneal (conjunctival-scleral) penetration routes
6. Increased shelf life with respect to eye drops, due to the absence of water
7. Possibility of providing a constant rate of drug release

The actual realization of these goals will be discussed in the following sections, in which the literature on inserts is examined. In the present review, in order to provide a framework for discussion, the different types of inserts have been classified on the basis of their physical characteristics, as follows:

*   *Soluble inserts* (undergoing gradual dissolution and/or surface erosion once placed in the conjunctival cul-de-sac)
*   *Insoluble inserts* (including medicated contact lenses, constant-rate release devices such as the Ocusert®, etc.)

This distinction is useful for practical purposes, even if borderline cases can be found in the literature.

II. SOLUBLE INSERTS

Under this designation have been grouped all monolytic polymeric devices that at the end of their service are no longer present in the eye. They have been further divided, depending on the nature of the polymers, into inserts based on synthetic or semisynthetic polymers and inserts based on natural polymers. Some devices utilizing particular approaches (bioadhesion, prodrugs, drug carriers) have been examined as a separate group.

A polymeric matrix can disappear from the eye as a consequence of two different processes: dissolution and erosion. In some cases these processes may coexist, and a clear-cut definition of the real mechanism is difficult. These devices can also be classified, according to their drug-release characteristics, as swelling-controlled and chemically-controlled; most of the soluble inserts belong to the former type, while erodible ones belong to the latter.[20]

In swelling-controlled devices, the active agent is homogeneously dispersed in a glassy polymer. Since glassy polymers are essentially drug-impermeable, no diffusion through the dry matrix occurs. When the insert is placed in the eye, water from the tear fluid begins to penetrate the matrix, then swelling, and consequently polymer chain relaxation, takes place. The incorporated drug diffuses from the swollen layer. In linear amorphous polymers, dissolution of the matrix follows the swelling process; other polymers (crosslinked, or containing chain entanglements, or partially crystalline ones) may undergo a very slow dissolution or remain undissolved. Thus, some inserts of this type, even if classified as "soluble", may remain in the eye as empty "ghosts" after releasing their drug content. Depending on their structure, and given time, they would presumably undergo complete elimination. Release from these devices will, in general, follow Fickian, "square root of time" kinetics; in some instances, however, known as case II transport, zero order kinetics can be observed.[21]

In chemically controlled, erodible devices, the rate of drug release is controlled by a chemical reaction (hydrolysis) that leads to polymer solubilization, or degradation to small, water-soluble molecules. These polymers, as specified by Heller, may undergo bulk or surface hydrolysis.[22] For optimum activity, erodible inserts should conform to the second case, in which the hydrolytic process is confined to the outer surface, and drug release rate is constant in time (zero order kinetics) provided that the device maintains a constant surface geometry and that the drug is poorly water-soluble. Polymers demonstrating surface erosion characteristics are partially esterified copolymers of vinyl methyl ether and maleic anhydride (PVM/MA), poly(ortho esters), and polyanhydrides.

A. INSERTS BASED ON SYNTHETIC AND SEMISYNTHETIC POLYMERS

Some Russian workers are to be given the credit for reviving soluble inserts, believed extinct after the disappearance of the gelatin "lamellae" in the late forties. Yakovlev and Lenkevich reported in 1966 that polyvinylalcohol (PVA) disks containing pilocarpine provided sustained miosis and intraocular pressure (IOP) reduction.[23] This pioneering work was expanded upon by Maichuk, Khromow, and associates, who eventually developed the so-called SODI (soluble ophthalmic drug insert), subsequently introduced into clinical practice in the U.S.S.R. In a way it is unfortunate that the vast body of technological, pharmacological, and clinical research carried out by these workers had little diffusion and popularity in the Western world.

Maichuk,[24-29] and Maichuk and Tishina,[30] first investigated the properties of eye films made with crosslinked PVA, and containing antibiotics, sulfonamides, idoxuridine, pilocarpine, atropine, etc. These medications, when tested in comparison with standard aqueous and oily vehicles, produced higher and more prolonged drug levels in the tear film. Due to their poor solubility, however, they were not well tolerated by the patients and had to be removed after a few hours of wear. The concomitant work of Khromow and associates led to the development of a new, soluble copolymer of acrylamide, N-vinylpyrrolidone, and ethyl acrylate (ratio, 0.25:0.25:0.5), designated as ABE, which showed the most favorable properties.[31-33] A comparison of medicated eye films prepared with different polymers, showed that ABE produced the highest concentration of drugs in rabbit ocular tissues.[34]

After large-scale preclinical and clinical testing, the ABE copolymer was used for the industrial manufacture of the SODI, in the form of sterile, thin films of oval shape, weighing 15 to 16 mg, color-coded for different drugs (over 20 common ophthalmic drugs, or drug combinations). After introduction into the upper conjunctival sac, a SODI softens in 10 to 15 s, conforming to the shape of the eyeball; in the next 10 to 15 min the film turns into a polymer clot, which gradually dissolves within 1 h, while releasing the drug. The feeling of "extraneous body" in the eye disappears in 5 to 15 min.

Release from these, and from similar soluble inserts to be described later, does not show any vehicle control, and produces a prolonged-pulse entry of the drug. However, due to the capacity of the ocular tissues to act as drug reservoirs, a single SODI application has been reported to replace 4 to 12 drop instillations or 3 to 6 applications of ointment, and to constitute a valid once-a-day therapy even for long-term treatment of glaucoma.[34,35] Attempts to introduce these devices in the Western world have hitherto been unsuccessful, even though they have been in clinical use in the Eastern countries for more than a decade.

In more recent years, Saettone and coworkers have published a series of papers on monolithic polymeric ocular inserts. In a first study it was sought to verify whether simple, commercially available polymers could be used to prepare practical inserts containing pilocarpine (Pi).[36] A series of circular matrices (0.4 mm thickness, 4.0 mm diameter) were prepared, by casting from aqueous solutions, with four different types of PVA and two types of hydroxypropylcellulose (HPC), selected after screening more than 20 commercial polymers. Pi was dispersed in the matrices as the nitrate (PiN) or as a polyacrylic acid salt (Pi/PAA). When tested for miotic activity in rabbits, the latter inserts significantly increased the drug bioavailability when compared with Pi eye drops, or with PVA inserts containing PiN. The activity pattern of all inserts corresponded to a prolonged-pulse release, with higher activity peaks and increased duration with respect to the activity induced by Pi eye drops. Clinical tests on glaucoma patients, carried out with PVA inserts containing PiN or Pi/PAA, showed that both types could effectively control the intraocular pressure (IOP) for a 24-h period after a single administration. However, the IOP reduction observed with the Pi/PAA inserts was significantly greater.[37]

The synthesis of specific polymeric acidic materials, designed to form salts or polyanionic complexes with Pi base, was subsequently attempted.[38] The following copolymers and terpolymers, all containing acrylic acid (AA) in different proportions, were prepared: AA-methyl acrylate; AA-vinyl acetate; AA-hydroxyethyl acrylate; AA-acrylamide; AA-acrylamide-vinylpyrrolidone; AA-acrylamide-vinyl acetate; and AA-methyl acrylate-hydroxyethyl acrylate. Some of these polymers were used to prepare inserts containing Pi base. When tested for miotic activity in rabbits, these inserts did not significantly increase the drug bioavailability with respect to PiN eye drops, presumably because of their high solubility, which resulted in rapid elimination of the polymer-bound drug from the eye. The addition of PVA to the inserts, however, resulted in a significantly increased bioavailability and duration of activity. This effect was attributed to a decreased solubility of the matrices in the tear fluid. The study pointed to the importance of a proper balance between insert solubility, that could be modulated by addition of PVA, and drug diffusivity, that could be controlled by salifying Pi base with the acidic polymer.

In a subsequent investigation by Saettone et al.,[39] a series of partial esters (ethyl, 2-methoxyethyl, n-butyl) of (maleic acid-alkyl vinyl ether) copolymers with ethyl or n-butyl as alkyl substituents were synthesized, and used to prepare ocular inserts containing ionically bound Pi base. When tested in rabbits, all inserts produced moderate increases in the duration of activity and bioavailability of Pi with respect to PiN eye drops, and no significant differences were detected among the various matrices, in spite of rather dissimilar chemical structures. On the basis of physicochemical and *in vitro* release tests, this behavior was attributed to a fast hydration and partial dissolution of the matrices, and to an incomplete release of the ionically bound drug.

The previously described matrices were all prepared by casting from aqueous or organic solutions. The application of a standard tabletting (compression) technique to the preparation of Pi inserts was described by Saettone et al. in 1990.[40] Suitable mixtures containing PiN and HPC plus varying proportions of lactose and glyceryl palmito-stearate were compressed in the form of thin disks (5 mm diameter, 0.3 mm thickness). One side of the matrices was then coated with a methacrylic, water-impermeable polymer (Eudragit® RS), so that release could occur only from the opposite side. Animal tests showed that increasing the lipophilic character of the matrices resulted in augmented Pi bioavailability and duration of action. One-sided coating of the matrices also led to an increased bioavailability of Pi with respect to uncoated samples, presumably as the consequence of reduction of systemic, transconjunctival absorption. The study, although requiring a further validation with other ophthalmic drugs, supported the possibility of using the compression technique for preparing Pi inserts exhibiting a sustained miotic activity.

A more recent communication by Saettone et al. dealt with an evaluation of polymeric (hydroxypropylmethylcellulose, PVA, xanthan gum, etc.) Pi matrices prepared by extrusion, having the form of small cylinders (1.5 mm diameter, 3 mm length).[41] The cylindrical shape, patterned after that of the Lacrisert® device mentioned at the end of this section, may ensure a better retention in the conjunctival sac. The inserts were coated with a mixture of methacrylic polymers (Eudragit® RL + RS) in order to modify the drug-release characteristics. The coated matrices released the drug *in vitro* at a constant rate for 6 to 8 h, and in rabbit tests provided a much longer duration of miotic activity and an increased bioavailability with respect to the noncoated ones.

Another unusual technique, compression molding at a relatively high (150°C) temperature, has been described by Harwood and Schwartz for the preparation of HPC films containing Pi.[42] These workers incorporate in their matrices, besides PiN, Pi pamoate, a water-insoluble salt. *In vitro* tests showed that the release rate, which followed "square root" kinetics, was dramatically lower when the matrices contained PI pamoate. The release was also influenced by the polymer type; it was faster for matrices prepared with low-viscosity grades of HPC.

Extensive and rigorous investigations of soluble and erodible inserts have been published in the last decade by a group of Finnish scientists, notably Salminen, Urtti and co-workers. In the first study,[43] a soluble polyvinylpyrrolidone (PVP) insert containing Pi (0.85 mg), which released *in vitro* 80% of its Pi content in 35 min, was tested for miotic activity in albino rabbits in comparison with other Pi vehicles. The peak response and bioavailability were in the order: insert (0.85 mg Pi) > oily solution (1.00 mg Pi) > aqueous solution (2.30 mg Pi) > aqueous solution (0.85 mg Pi). The authors concluded that the soluble insert, however, produced, at most, a prolonged-pulse entry of the drug.

In subsequent studies, the effects of hydrophilicity of Pi matrices containing HPC of medium and high molecular weight and PVP were investigated *in vitro*, by examining their drug release characteristics,[44] and *in vivo* (miotic activity in rabbits).[45] An increased concentration of PVP in the matrices increased their hydrophilicity and the release rate, which in general followed Fickian kinetics. However, different release rates did not correspond to significant differences in miotic activity, and this was attributed to the rod shape and to the small size of the matrices, and to possible systemic, rather than intraocular, absorption.

Another series of investigations by the same group was dedicated to an extensive evaluation of matrices prepared with alkyl (ethyl, propyl, and butyl) half-esters of poly(vinyl methyl ether/maleic anhydride), PVM/MA, a polymer whose structure is indicated below:

$$OCH_3$$
$$|$$
$$[-CH_2-CH-CH-CH-]_n$$
$$|\quad\ |$$
$$HOOC\quad COOR$$

A preliminary *in vitro* investigation,[46] demonstrated that Pi was released at a constant rate for bout 7 h from the butyl half-ester matrices. This was attributed to Case II transport, i.e., to the constant rate of solvent-induced polymer relaxation in the matrices, rather than to erosion-controlled kinetics, as reported by other authors for release of hydrocortisone, a poorly water-soluble drug, from analgous matrices.[47] The same PVM/MA butyl ester matrices, as well as HPC matrices, proved capable of reducing, in rabbits, the systemic absorption of Pi, with respect to an aqueous solution of the drug. The $(AUC_{0-6\ h}/AUC_{0-6\ h,\ i.v.})$ values were 0.72, 0.67, and 0.41 for the aqueous solution, the HPC insert, and the butyl PVM/MA insert, respectively.[48]

Further investigations on PVM/MA half-ester matrices dealt with the chemical variables influencing *in vitro* release of timolol (Ti),[49,50] and with the effects induced on the ocular and systemic absorption of Ti in rabbits by the presence of a buffering agent (disodium phosphate) and of a vasoconstrictor (methaoxedrine) in the matrices.[51] The effect of the vasoconstrictor was to decrease the peak Ti concentration in plasma about three times, and increase about twofold that in the tear fluid. When compared with the unbuffered matrices, the buffered ones (independently of the presence of vasoconstrictor) at least doubled the concentration ratio of iris/ciliary body to plasma; the best ratios were achieved with the buffered matrices containing methaoxedrine. In conclusion, these studies showed that ocular inserts, besides being capable of increasing the ocular bioavailability, can significantly reduce the systemic absorption of a drug.

Evaluations of the ocular delivery of Pi in rabbits from soluble inserts prepared with PVA, PAA, and MC have also been reported by other authors.[52,53] Another recent paper dealt with the effect of administration of dexamethasone in different polymeric films on the drug disposition in different eye tissues; the polymeric materials were PVA, different methacrylic polymers (Eudragit®), cellulose acetate phthalate (CAP), hydroxypropylcellulose (HPC), ethyl cellulose (EC), and gelatin, plus suitable plasticizers (PEG 400 or glycerol).[54] All inserts produced a considerable increase in ocular absorption of the steroid, when compared with a suspension dosage form.

An unconventional application of ophthalmic soluble inserts was recently described by a group of French investigators, who evaluated the possibility of "ophthalmosystemic" administration of morphine by HPC inserts prepared by direct compression.[55] When compared with an aqueous solution, the inserts significantly modified the plasma concentration profiles of morphine. Although the drug dose administered with the inserts was only 16% higher, the AUC was increased by 52%, the T_{max} was increased from 16.8 to 135 min, and the C_{max} was reduced from 105.5 to 36.6 ng/l.

Finally, mention should be made of the so-called "soluble artificial tear inserts", or "slow release artificial tears" (SRAT), unmedicated inserts based on cellulose derivatives (in particular, HPC) or on natural polymers. The stability of the precorneal tear film can be altered by defects in the corneal surface, and by qualitative/quantitative changes of the film itself. The slow solubilization of a suitable polymeric insert may provide a continuous flow of polymer into the tear film, thus stabilizing the film more efficiently than the intermittent therapy with conventional tear substitutes.[56] Several investigations have eventually led to the development of the Lacrisert® (Merck Sharp & Dohme), an HPC cylindrical insert used in the treatment of patients with keratitis sicca.[57-59] Of particular interest is a paper by Katz and Blackman, reporting on the effect of the size and shape of the inserts on tolerance and retention by human volunteers.[57] Expulsion of rod-shaped units was significantly ($p < 0.01$) less frequent than expulsion of oval, flat inserts.

B. INSERTS BASED ON NATURALLY OCCURRING POLYMERS

The use of biopolymers for the manufacture of soluble ophthalmic inserts has attracted the interest of several workers. These materials (in particular polypeptides, polysaccharides, etc.) are considered by some authors potentially less toxic for outer ocular tissues than synthetic polymers, even if the danger of sensitization and antigen-antibody reactions cannot be discounted *a priori*. It is unfortunate that many reports on the use of devices of this type have been reported in ophthalmological and clinical journals, where full details on the composition are usually not given.

In 1972 Dohlman described a polypeptide matrix, crosslinked to provide a slow dissolution rate, for the delivery of hydrocortisone acetate. The matrix delivered the steroid at the rate of 2 or 9 μg/h; its greater efficacy with respect to hydrocortisone eye drops was proved on an ocular inflammatory model in rabbits.[60] A similar matrix releasing hydrocortisone at a rate of 10 μg/h was tested in 1975 by Allansmith et al.[61] on human volunteers with an experimental model of ocular inflammation, with reportedly good results; the dose of steroid delivered by the inserts was only $1/_{34}$ of the dose that would have been delivered by conventional eye drops instilled 4 times daily. Polypeptide elliptical matrices delivering steroids (hydrocortisone acetate and prednisolone acetate) at a constant rate (10 μg/h) were also tested by Keller and co-workers, with analogous results, on an experimental model of conjunctivitis induced in rabbits by immunization with bovine serum albumin.[62] Polypeptide matrices delivering idoxuridine at constant rate (30 μg/h) have been successfully used for the treatment of acute herpes simplex keratitis in rabbits.[63]

Another biopolymer that has attracted the attention of insert prospectors is collagen. An investigation on the possible use of collagen as a solid vehicle for Pi delivery was reported in 1975 by Rubin et al.[64] In the same year Kitazawa described clinical trials, on glaucoma patients, of rod-shaped and flat inserts made with solubilized collagen, containing, respectively, 2 and 4 mg of Pi.[65] Bloomfield and colleagues have described solubilized collagen inserts for the treatment of tear film abnormalities (SRAT) and for delivery of gentamycin.[66,67] Solubilization of collagen was obtained by succinylation prior to casting into membranes; crosslinking by ultraviolet light was used when it was desired to prolong the dissolution time.

A recent paper by Vasantha et al. was concerned with the preparation and *in vitro* testing of collagen inserts for delivery of Pi.[68] Pepsin-treated calf-skin collagen films containing Pi (either entrapped or coupled to collagen hydrazide) were prepared by casting from aqueous solution; modulation of release was obtained by crosslinking with glutaraldehyde. Depending on the modifications made on the collagen carrier, a 5 to 15 d constant-rate release of Pi was reported.

Collagen shields should also be mentioned as an interesting example of the use of this biopolymer in ocular drug delivery.[13] Fabricated with porcine scleral tissue, and originally developed as a corneal bandage, these devices, once softened by the tear fluid, form a thin, pliable film that conforms exactly to the corneal surface, and undergoes dissolution in 12, 24, or 72 h. Drug loading of collagen shields can be effected by soaking in drug solutions prior to application, as will be described in the next section for medicated contact lenses. Although these devices have been tested for the delivery of several drugs, the results reported to the present date do not appear superior to those reported for other soluble inserts.[69-72] Collagen shields, however, which are available on the market (Bio-Cor®, Bausch & Lomb Pharmaceuticals), are well accepted by ophthalmologists, and are undoubtedly more effective than eye drops for delivering drugs to the eye, may in time find a place among ophthalmic drug vehicles.

Alginic (1,4,-β,D-mannuronic) acid as solid carrier for Pi has been evaluated in a series of papers by Loucas and Haddad.[73-75] Administration of Pi as the alginate in the form of disks (0.3 mm thickness, 3 to 7 mm diameter, 3.1 to 7.8 mg) was found to prolong the duration of miotic activity in rabbits to a greater degree (7.5 vs. 3.5 h) than solutions of Pi alginate and of PiHCl in the presence of MC, both of the same viscosity (72 cps).

The use of chitin [poly(N-acetyl-D-glucosamine)], an important structural component of the outer skeleton of invertebrates, as a matrix material for Pi inserts was described in a patent by Capozza.[76] Chitin, which is insoluble, was converted enzymatically to a decomposed, soluble form, which is slowly degraded by the lysozyme contained in the tears. These inserts produced a prolonged (6 h) pupillary response in rabbits.

Another biomaterial, fibrin, prepared from human plasma, has been evaluated as a carrier for Pi by Miyazaki and co-workers.[77] Fibrin film, which is a flexible, nontoxic, sterilizable, and absorbable material, was soaked in PiHCl solutions (5.0 or 10%) for 24 h, then dried, crushed in a mortar, and heat-pressed to produce circular inserts. These were tested for release *in vitro* and for miotic activity in rabbits. The authors stated that the use of fibrin film as an ocular delivery system may present substantial advantages over liquid dosage forms.

C. SOLUBLE INSERTS UTILIZING PARTICULAR APPROACHES
1. The Muco-Adhesive Approach

Muco-adhesive polymeric formulations, capable of adhering to the mucin-epithelial surfaces existing on the eye surface (cornea, sclera, conjunctiva), are nowadays actively investigated for their potential to increase the residence time of ocular medications, hence the overall drug bioavailability. Some synthetic polymers, such as PAA, polycarbophil, etc., and biopolymers, notably hyaluronic acid (HA), an ubiquitous component of animal extracellular tissues, have shown a prolonged retention in ocular tissues.[78,79]

The possibility of improving the inherent good ocular retention properties of inserts by introducing muco-adhesive properties was reported in 1989 by Saettone and co-workers.[80] A series of PAA and HA matrices prepared by compression and by casting, and containing Pi or tropicamide (Tr), were evaluated for muco-adhesion, for ocular retention, and for biological activity in rabbits. The muco-adhesive properties were investigated *in vitro* using a tensile apparatus with mucin-coated surfaces, while the ocular retention was estimated visually using a fluorescent marker. Good to excellent muco-adhesive properties were detected in the HA preparations; the bioavailability enhancing effect, however, was better for Tr than for Pi, probably because of the high solubility and diffusivity of the latter drug. The study, while confirming the good bioadhesive properties of HA, evidenced the relevance of the physicochemical characteristics of the drug to the efficacy of a muco-adhesive ocular delivery system.

A recent report by Benedetti et al. dealt with a preliminary evaluation of HA containing covalently bound methylprednisolone (MP).[81] The polymer-drug was administered ocularly to rabbits as microspheres and as circular inserts prepared by casting. The AUCs for MP concentration in the tear fluid after administration of the microspheres, the inserts, and a standard MP aqueous suspension were 204.6, 203.8 and 48.6, respectively. The authors attributed these results to the muco-adhesive properties of the polymer.

2. The Prodrug Approach

Prodrugs are labile chemical derivatives of existing drugs, capable of enhancing the absorption, decreasing the side-effects, and/or prolonging the duration of action of the parent drug.[82] The observations that (1) some timolol (Ti) ester prodrugs are less absorbed systemically, while being absorbed ocularly equally well or better than Ti;[83] and (2) erodible inserts have been shown capable of reducing the systemic absorption of Pi and Ti while promoting their ocular absorption,[48,51] stimulated Lee and co-workers to investigate whether administration of Ti prodrugs in erodible inserts could further reduce the systemic absorption of the drug and improve its ocular bioavailability.[84] PVA, HPC, or PVM/MA inserts containing Ti or different Ti prodrugs were tested in rabbits, and the concentrations of Ti in blood, corneal epithelium, and iris-ciliary body were determined. When compared with Ti inserts, the prodrug inserts reduced the plasma Ti concentration, but apparently did not increase the drug concentration in the ocular tissues. However, separate tests showed that the prodrug-containing inserts were more active than Ti inserts in reducing the IOP of ocularly hypertensive rabbits. This observation has led to the hypothesis that the inserts might promote absorption of the prodrug through noncorneal (scleral) routes.[85]

3. The Drug Carrier Approach

Poly(alkylcyanoacrylate) nanoparticles have been shown to increase the bioavailability of Pi, possibly as a result of adhesion to the ocular mucosae and sustained release of the adsorbed drug.[86] Jacob-La Barre and Kaufman have investigated the possibility of incorporating poly(butylcyanoacrylate) nanoparticles containing Pi into 24-h collagen shields, as an attempt to develop a sustained-delivery device for this drug.[72] The nanoparticle-loaded shields, when tested in rabbits in a preliminary study, showed superior retention and activity characteristics with respect to the controls, which were unencapsulated drug in shields, drug in nanoparticles but not in shields, and Pi solution.

III. INSOLUBLE INSERTS

Under this heading have been grouped all those devices that, by virtue of their chemical structure, are absolutely insoluble and need removal from the eye after deliverance of the drug. For convenience they will be divided into three main categories: (1) drug-presoaked contact lenses; (2) membrane-controlled reservoir inserts (e.g., the Ocusert® system); and (3) other experimental insoluble devices.

A. HYDROGEL CONTACT LENSES

The first and most widely used contact lens material is poly(2-hydroxyethyl methacrylate) (HEMA), cross-linked with a small amount of ethylene glycol dimethacrylate (EGDMA). HEMA-PVP copolymers, such as hefilcon-A, or PHP (80% HEMA and 20% PVP) are also in use. Depending on their composition, amount of hydroxyl groups, and the degree of crosslinking, these polymers can absorb up to 80% water.[87]

Thus, the rationale for using hydrogel contact lenses in ocular drug delivery is their capacity to absorb large quantities of drug solution, and subsequently, to release the absorbed drug to the ocular tissues by diffusion. Release of drugs from these systems can be calculated by two equations,[20,88] the first of which, known as the "early time approximation", describes the first 60% of the process, while the second one, the "late time approximation", describes the remaining 40%.

$$dM_t/dt = 2M_\infty (D/\pi l^2 t)^{1/2} \tag{1}$$

$$dM_t/dt = (8DM_\infty/l^2) \exp(-\pi^2 Dt/l^2) \tag{2}$$

Medicated contact lenses, which usually induce a prolonged-pulse entry of the drug, have been found valid for some therapeutic treatments.[89,90] However, as pointed out by Shell in the case of pilocarpine, since 90% of the drug is released during the first 20 min, administration of the drug dose necessary to achieve a full day of hypotensive therapy produces significant side-effects, such as increased miosis and myopia.[4]

Sedlacek is credited for first suggesting, in 1965, the use of hydrogel contact lenses for ophthalmic drug delivery.[91] Several investigators were subsequently attracted by the potential advantages of this simple delivery system. Waltman and Kaufman, using Bionite® and Soflens® contact lenses, investigated the uptake and subsequent ocular delivery of fluorescein, used as a model drug.[92] Subsequently, Kaufman et al. investigated the potential of Bionite® lenses for delivery of idoxuridine, polymyxin B, and Pi, and discussed the advantages of lens soaking vs. drug instillation over the lens.[93] Even if instillation of a drug solution over an unmedicated contact lens has been found significantly more effective than instillation of a more concentrated drug solution in the absence of the lens,[94] presoaked lenses are considered a more efficient and reliable delivery system.[95] These devices have been tested clinically with a number of drugs, including antibiotics, corticosteroids, antiglaucoma drugs, etc.[94-100]

The use of drug-impregnated hydrogel lenses seems to be restricted to a few clinical applications, such as the treatment of acute ocular inflammations and infections, and, in particular, of corneal problems.[90]

Hydrogel inserts showing a constant rate of release of erythromycin estolate have been investigated by Ozawa et al.[101] These authors used ternary copolymers of PVP, vinyl acetate, and glycidyl methacrylate, or PVP, methyl methacrylate, and ethyl acrylate, with water contents ranging from 23 to 78%, developed by Hosaka et al.[102] The inserts were loaded with the drug by soaking them in a solution of erythromycin estolate in dioxane; they were subsequently freeze-dried after removing the solvent by elution with an artificial tear solution. *In vivo* tests in rabbit eyes showed that the drug concentration in the tear film could be maintained at an almost constant level for 6 d, with an elution rate of 240 to 290 $\mu g/cm^2$ per day.

B. MEMBRANE-CONTROLLED RESERVOIR INSERTS

The Ocusert® therapeutic system, developed by Alza Corporation, has probably been the first practical realization of the dreams and endeavors of all insertologists: a device releasing the drug at a rigorously constant and reproducible rate for over one week. The issue of constant rate vs. pulsed or prolonged-pulse release had been examined in a fundamental paper by Lerman and Reininger in 1971.[103] These authors demonstrated for the first time in glaucoma patients that sustained release of Pi (simulated by continuous instillation of microdrops) provided good IOP control with a fraction of the drug dose administered by conventional eye drop therapy. As a consequence, both the ocular and systemic unwanted side-effects of the drug were greatly reduced. The report pointed to zero-order as the ideal delivery pattern for Pi, and possibly for other potentially toxic ophthalmic drugs.

Two types of Ocusert®, first marketed in the U.S. in 1974, are available: the Pilo-20 and Pilo-40. The former delivers the drug at a rate of 20 $\mu g/h$ for 7 d, and the latter at a rate of 40 μg/h. This device, which is certainly familiar to most readers of this review, has been exhaustively described and discussed in a series of specialized paper and book chapters.[1-10,104,105] Briefly, it consists of a reservoir containing Pi alginate (refer to References 73 to 75) enclosed above and below by thin ethylene-vinyl acetate (EVA) membranes. The whole device is encircled by a retaining ring of the same material, impregnated with titanium dioxide. The dimensions of the elliptical device are (for the 20 μg/h system): major axis, 13.4 mm; minor axis, 5.7 mm; thickness, 0.3 mm. The membranes are the same in both systems. To obtain a higher release rate, the reservoir of the 40–μg/h system contains about 90 mg of di(2-ethylhexyl)phthalate as flux enhancer. The release rate from the system is described by simplified equation

$$dM/dt = (Dp \ Km \ Cs)/\delta m \tag{3}$$

which assumes infinite sink conditions in the eye, and the presence of a saturated Pi solution (with saturation solubility Cs) in the reservoir. The release rate should remain constant until the drug concentration in the reservoir, Cs, remains constant.

The release kinetics of the Ocusert® have been discussed in detail,[6,106] and several papers describing clinical trials have been published.[107-109]

Another experimental device that can be classified as a membrane-controlled reservoir insert was developed and investigated by Urtti and co-workers.[110,111] The device consisted of a thin silicone tubing (1.45 × 1.94 × 0.24 mm; internal diameter × outside diameter × wall thickness) cut in 15-mm sections and sealed at both ends with Silastic® adhesive. The sealed cylinders could be filled with different Ti solutions using a syringe fitted with a 25-gauge needle. Release rate and release patterns from these inserts could be modulated by changing the drug concentration and the pH in the reservoir, and the storage time. Zero-order release rates *in vitro* of Ti of 0.7 to 7.3 mg/h for 8 h were obtained; in inserts with a core pH of 8.64 the rate increased linearly with increasing drug concentration from 2.5 to 20 mg/ml. Release from a cylindrical-reservoir device of this type should obey the equation:

$$dM/Dt = \frac{2\pi hD \ K \ \Delta C}{\ln (r_o/r_i)} \tag{4}$$

where h is the length of the cylinder, r_o and r_i are the outer and inner radii, respectively, and the other symbols have the usual meaning.[87] Zero-order drug release is achieved when ΔC, the concentration gradient of the drug across the membrane, remains constant.

In subsequent studies on these cylindrical inserts, the effect of the administration site (inferior vs. superior conjunctival sac) on ocular absorption of Ti in rabbits, and the ocular vs. systemic absorption in the same animals were investigated.[112,113] Administration of Ti as eye drops produced very nearly equal concentrations in the inferior and superior portions of ocular tissues, while the cylindrical device produced higher concentrations in the parts of the eye closer to the application site. When compared with application in the inferior conjunctival sac, placement of the devices in the upper sac resulted in increased corneal and total ocular absorption of Ti. When the insert was placed in the inferior sac the drug concentration in the aqueous humor was very low, indicating a possible absorption via a noncorneal route. Administration of Ti with the controlled-release system resulted in a twofold increase in ocular bioavailability with respect to eye drops, and a much lower plasma concentration (<1.0 ng/ml vs. 17.16 ng/ml). The latter finding is of particular interest, since it delineates the possibility of improving the ocular to systemic concentration ratio of Ti, and of other β-blockers used in glaucoma therapy, by the use of appropriate delivery systems.

C. OTHER INSOLUBLE DEVICES

An osmotically driven monolithic device for release of Pi and epinephrine (Ep) at a controlled rate was patented in 1979 by Alza.[114] The system comprises a formulation consisting of a Pi or Ep osmotic solute dispersed through a polymer matrix (e.g., polyethylene, EVA, ethylene-methyl acrylate, etc.), such that the formulation is surrounded by the polymer as discrete small domains. Upon placement in the cul-de-sac, the matrix is imbibed by the tears as a result of the osmotic pressure gradient created by the drug formulation. The drug is consequently leached out and released from the matrix at a constant rate. The drug release rate can be controlled by modulating different parameters, such as polymer type and degree of cross-linking, osmotic properties of the drug formulation, surface area of the insert, etc.

Biological data on matrices of this type, releasing Ep or β-blockers, have been reported.[115,116]

Another water-activated system, consisting of a flat silicone reservoir device for constant rate release of ophthalmic drugs, was more recently described by Sutinen and associates.[117] Solid propranolol or sotalol hydrochloride plus osmotic or buffering additives were entrapped between two silicone membranes containing mannitol as a pore-forming material. *In vitro* studies demonstrated that the polar solid salts did not partition into the polymer walls of the device during storage, thus avoiding the initial burst of drug release observed with the silicone cylindrical inserts.[109,110] Drug release was activated by water, and the constant rate of release could be controlled over a wide range with pH-adjusting agents in the core.

An evaluation of an ethylene-vinyl alcohol (EVAl) hydrophilic copolymer as matrix material for a long-acting delivery system for Pi HCl was reported in 1985 by Hou et al.,[118] the same group who had previously investigated fibrin film as an ophthalmic drug carrier.[77] Different types of EVAl (15 to 81% ethylene content) were used to prepare thin films and spherical beads containing different concentrations of the drug (15, 20, and 25% w/w). *In vitro* release tests showed that, after a burst effect, the release rate was approximately linear with $t^{1/2}$, while in rabbits a prolongation of the miotic effect with respect to administration of eye drops was observed. These results are substantially in line with those reported for many soluble inserts and hydrogel devices.

IV. CONCLUSIONS

After over 20 years of investigations on solid ophthalmic drug delivery devices, the following points seem well established:

1. Soluble inserts may constitute an improved drug delivery system, provided that adequate measures be taken to control release of very soluble drugs, such as pilocarpine. This can be realized by adequately modulating the rate of swelling/erosion of the matrices, by using insoluble drug salts or complexes, or by ionically binding the drug to the polymer. The possibility of incorporating suitable drug carriers into the inserts (see, for example, the nanoparticle approach described in Reference 72) should also be considered. Even if many soluble inserts release the drug with a declining rate, they provide a saturation of the corneal/scleral tissues surrounding the application site, which then act as reservoir for subsequent transcorneal (or trans-scleral) absorption of the drug. The overall effect is a prolonged-pulse entry of the drug into the eye. This can be considered satisfactory for many therapeutic treatments, even if there is a risk of undesirable concentration peaks in the aqueous humor. The possibility of a once-a-day therapy with soluble inserts vs. multiple instillations of conventional eye drops has been amply demonstrated. Thus, these simple and low-cost devices might constitute a valid alternative to the traditional ocular medications.

2. The possibility of realizing soluble/erodible inserts displaying constant drug release rates for several hours has been demonstrated. Further investigations in this direction might allow reduction of the negative effect produced by the pulse-entry of the drug into the eye.

3. Suitably formulated inserts, both soluble and insoluble, have been shown capable of diminishing the systemic absorption of ocularly applied drugs, as a result of a decreased drainage into the nasal cavity, which is one of the major systemic absorption sites of topical ocular medications.[118] This is particularly important if one considers the potential systemic toxicity of some recently introduced drugs, such as the β-blockers. Another potential advantage of insert therapy is the possibility of promoting noncorneal drug penetration, thus increasing the efficacy of some hydrophilic drugs which are poorly absorbed through the cornea.[13]

4. The slow, constant-rate release pattern realized by inserts of the Ocusert® type can be considered as the most desirable condition for long-term therapy, both in view of its efficacy and the reduction of ocular and systemic side-effects. The Ocusert®, however, is not the ultimate insert; some properties of devices of this type (e.g., their ocular retention) might be subject to improvement.

5. Particular applications of inserts might be foreseen, such as their use for ophthalmo-systemic delivery of proteins and peptides.[120]

On consideration of their potential and the advantages that have been cited in the introduction, it is surprising that solid polymeric devices, either soluble or insoluble, have not yet gained a wider popularity. The Ocusert® and the Lacrisert® systems are the only inserts marketed in the Western countries, and the acceptance of these devices has been, to the present date, far from enthusiastic. This has been attributed to psychological factors, such as the reluctance of ophthalmologists and patients to abandon the traditional liquid and semisolid medications, to price factors, and to occasional therapeutic failures (e.g., unnoticed expulsion from the eye, membrane rupture, etc.). In the opinion of other authors, inserts will be accepted only when capable of delivering drugs at least on a monthly basis.[11] It is hoped that such a pessimistic view will be disproved by future development, and that improved inserts for once-a-day, once-a-week, or (why not?) once-a-month treatment will eventually find wide acceptance and diffusion.

REFERENCES

1. **Richardson, K. T.,** Ocular microtherapy: membrane-controlled drug delivery, *Arch. Ophthalmol.*, 93, 74, 1975.
2. **Pavan-Langston, D.,** New drug delivery systems, in *Symposium on Ocular Therapy*, Vol. 9, Leopold, I. H. and Burns, R. P., Eds., John Wiley & Sons, New York, 1976, chap. 2.
3. **Lamberts, D. W.,** Solid delivery devices, in *Clinical Pharmacology of the Anterior Segment, Int. Ophthalmol. Clin.* 20, 3, 1980.
4. **Shell, J. W.,** New ophthalmic drug delivery systems, in *Ophthalmic Drug Delivery Systems*, Robinson, J. R., Ed., American Pharmaceutical Association, Washington, D.C., 1980, chap. 4.
5. **Chiou, G. and Watanabe, K.,** Drug delivery to the eye, *Pharm. Ther.*, 17, 269, 1982.
6. **Chien, Y. W.,** Ocular controlled drug administration, in *Novel Drug Delivery Systems*, Marcel Dekker, New York, 1982, chap. 2.
7. **Ueno, N. and Refojo, M. F.,** Ocular pharmacology of drug release devices, in *Controlled Drug Delivery, Vol. 2 — Clinical Applications*, Bruck, S. D., Ed., CRC Press, Boca Raton, FL, 1983, chap. 4.
8. **Mikkelson, T. J.,** Ophthalmic drug delivery, *Pharm. Technol.*, 8, 90, 1984.

9. **Shell, J. W.**, Ophthalmic drug delivery systems, *Surv. Ophthalmol.*, 29, 117, 1984.

10. **Buri, P.**, Voie oculaire, in *Formes Pharmaceutiques Nouvelles,* Buri, P., Puisieux, F., Doelker, E., and Benoit, J. P., Eds., Lavoisier, Paris, 1985.

11. **Lee, V. H. L. and Robinson, J. R.**, Review: topical ocular drug delivery: recent development and future challenges, *J. Ocular Pharmacol.*, 2, 67, 1986.

12. **Salminen, L.**, Pilocarpine inserts: experimental and clinical experiences, in *Ophthalmic Drug Delivery — Biopharmaceutical, Technological and Clinical Aspects,* Vol. 11, (Fidia Research Series), Liviana Press, Padua, Italy, 1987.

13. **Lee, V. H. L.**, Review: new directions in the optimization of ocular drug delivery, *J. Ocular Pharmacol.*, 6, 157, 1990.

14. **Greaves, J. L.**, Ocular drug delivery, in *Physiological Pharmaceutics — Biological Barriers to Drug Absorption* , Wilson, C. G. and Washington, N., Eds., Ellis Horwood, London, 1989, chap. 8.

15. **Mishima, S.**, Clinical pharmacokinetics of the eye, *Invest. Ophthalmol. Vis. Sci.*, 21, 504, 1981.

16. **Maurice, D. M. and Mishima, S.**, Ocular pharmacokinetics, in *Pharmacology of the Eye,* Sears, M. L., Ed., Springer-Verlag, Berlin, 1984, chap. 2.

17. **Van Ooteghem, M. M.**, Factors influencing the retention of ophthalmic solutions on the eye surface, in *Ophthalmic Drug Delivery — Biopharmaceutical, Technological and Clinical Aspects,* Vol. 11, (Fidia Research Series), Saettone, M. F., Bucci, G., and Speiser, P., Eds., Liviana Press, Padua, Italy, 1987.

18. **Antonibon, A.**, *Storia dei Colliri,* V. Idelson, Naples, Italy, 1939.

19. **Deschamps, M.**, *Compendium de Pharmacie Pratique,* Germer Baillière, Paris, 1868, 521.

20. **Heller, J.**, Controlled drug release from monolithic systems, in *Ophthalmic Drug Delivery — Biopharmaceutical, Technological and Clinical Aspects,* Vol. 11, (Fidia Research Series), Saettone, M. F., Bucci, G., and Speiser, P., Eds., Liviana Press, Padua, Italy, 1987.

21. **Korsmeyer, R. W. and Peppas, N. A.**, Macromolecular and modeling aspects of swelling-controlled systems, in *Controlled Release Delivery Systems,* Roseman, T. J. and Mansdorf, S. Z., Eds., Marcel Dekker, New York, 1983, chap. 4.

22. **Heller, J.**, Controlled release of biologically active compounds from bioerodible polymers, *Biomaterials*, 1, 51, 1980.

23. **Yakovlev, A. A. and Lenkevich, M. M.**, Use of pilocarpine-impregnated PVA films in the treatment of glucomatous patients, *Vestn. Oftal'mol.*, 79, 40, 1966.

24. **Maichuk, Y. F.**, Polyvinyl alcohol as ophthalmic vehicle for antibiotics, *Oftal'mol. Zh.*, 5, 350, 1964.

25. **Maichuk, Y. F.**, Polyvinyl alcohol films with antibiotics in the therapy of eye infections, *Antibiotiki*, 5, 435, 1967.

26. **Maichuk, Y. F.**, Polymeric ophthalmic inserts with antibiotics, in *Proc. Conf. Ophthalmologists,* Moscow, 1967, 403.

27. **Maichuk, Y. F.**, Polymeric drug delivery systems in ophthalmology, in *Ocular Therapy,* Leopold, I. H. and Burns, R. P., Eds., John Wiley & Sons, New York, 1976, 1.

28. **Maichuk, Y. F.**, Ophthalmic drug inserts, *Invest. Ophthalmol.*, 14, 87, 1975.

29. **Maichuk, Y. F.**, Soluble ophthalmic drug inserts, *Lancet*, 1, 173, 1975.

30. **Maichuk, Y. F. and Tishina, I. F.**, Polyacrylamide, prolongating vehicle for eyedrops, *Vestn. Oftal'mol.*, 6, 60, 1971.

31. **Khromow, G. L., Davydov, A. B., and Demina, L. V.**, Synthesis and modification of water-soluble elastic polymers based on poly(acrylamide) and other vinyl compounds, in *Trans. 17th All-Union Conf. High Molecular Weight Compounds,* Moscow, 1969.

32. **Khromow, G. L., Starunova, L. N., Maichuk, Y. F., Davydov, A. B., and Kondratyeva, T. S.**, Primary assessment of the long-acting properties of biologically compatible polymers, *Khim. Farm. Zh.*, 6, 24, 1974.

33. **Khromow, G. L., Davydov, A. B., Maichuk, Y. F., and Tishina, I. F.**, Base for ophthalmological medicinal preparations and an ophthalmological medicinal film, U.S. Patent 3,935,303, 1976.

34. **Maichuk, Y. F.**, Medicated eye films, *Medexport,* Moscow, 1985, 1.

35. **Maichuk, Y. F. and Erichev, V. P.**, Soluble ophthalmic drug inserts with pilocarpine, experimental and clinical study, *Glaucoma*, 3, 329, 1981.

36. **Saettone, M. F., Giannaccini, B., Chetoni, P., Galli, G., and Chiellini, E.**, Vehicle effects in ophthalmic bioavailability: an evaluation of polymeric inserts containing pilocarpine, *J. Pharm. Pharmacol.*, 36, 229, 1984.

37. **Odello, G., Saettone, M. F., Giannaccini, B., Mastrojeni, L., and Meucci, G.**, Efficacia e durata dell'effetto di nuovi inserti congiuntivali contenenti pilocarpina, *Proc. 10th Conv. Soc. Oftalm. Sicil., Mazara del Vallo,* February 22 to 24, 1985, 201.

38. **Saettone, M. F., Giannaccini, B., Marchesini, G., Galli, G., and Chiellini, E.**, Polymeric inserts for sustained ocular delivery of pilocarpine, in *Polymers in Medicine II,* Chiellini, E., Giusti, P., Migliaresi, C., and Nicolais, L., Eds., Plenum Press, New York, 1986, 409.

39. **Saettone, M. F., Giannaccini, B., Leonardi, G., Monti, D., Chetoni, P., Galli, G., and Chiellini, E.,** Inserts for sustained ocular delivery of pilocarpine: evaluation of a series of partial esters of (maleic acid-alkyl vinyl ether) alternating copolymers, in *Polymers in Medicine III,* Migliaresi, C., Nicolais, L., Giusti, P., and Chiellini, E., Eds., Elsevier, Amsterdam, 1988, 209.

40. **Saettone, M. F., Chetoni, P., Torracca, M. T., Giannaccini, B., Naber, L., Conte, U., Sangalli, M. E., and Gazzaniga, A.,** Application of the compression technique to the manufacture of pilocarpine ophthalmic inserts, *Acta Pharm. Technol.,* 36, 15, 1990.

41. **Saettone, M. F., Torracca, M. T., Giannaccini, B., Pagano, A., Rodriguez, L., and Cini, M.,** Evaluation of new polymeric ophthalmic matrices prepared by extrusion, *Proc. 10th Pharm. Technol. Conf.,* Bologna, 1991.

42. **Harwood, R. J. and Schwartz, J. B.,** Drug release from compression molded films: preliminary studies with pilocarpine, *Drug Dev. Ind. Pharm.,* 8, 663, 1982.

43. **Salminen, L., Urtti, A., Kujari, H., and Juslin, M.,** Prolonged pulse entry of pilocarpine with a soluble drug insert, *Albrecht von Graefes Arch. Klin. Exp. Ophthalmol.,* 221, 96, 1983.

44. **Urtti, A., Juslin, M., and Miinalainen, O.,** Pilocarpine release from hydroxypropyl cellulose-polyvinylpyrrolidone matrices, *Int. J. Pharm.,* 25, 165, 1985.

45. **Urtti, A., Periviita, L., Slaminen, L., and Juslin, M.,** Effects of hydrophilicity of polymer matrix on in vitro release rate of pilocarpine and on its miotic activity in rabbit eyes, *Drug Dev. Ind. Pharm.,* 11, 257, 1985.

46. **Urtti, A.,** Pilocarpine release from matrices of alkyl half-esters of poly(vinyl methyl ether/maleic anhydride), *Int. J. Pharm.,* 26, 45, 1985.

47. **Heller, J., Baker, R. W., Gale, R. M., and Rodin, J. O.,** Controlled drug release by polymer dissolution. I. Partial esters of maleic anhydride copolymers — properties and theory, *J. Appl. Polym. Sci.,* 22, 1991, 1978.

48. **Urtti, A., Salminen, L., and Miinalainen, O.,** Systemic absorption of ocular pilocarpine is modified by polymer matrices, *Int. J. Pharm.,* 23, 147, 1985.

49. **Finne, U., Kyyrönen, K., and Urtti, A.,** Drug release from monoisopropyl ester of poly(vinyl methyl ether-maleic anhydride) can be modified by basic salts in the polymer matrix, *J. Controlled Release,* 10, 189, 1989.

50. **Finne, U., Rönkkö, K., and Urtti, A.,** Timolol release from matrices of monoesters of polyvinyl methyl ether-maleic anhydride): effects of polymer molecular weight and a basic additive, *J. Pharm. Sci.,* 80, 670, 1991.

51. **Finne, U., Väisänen, V., and Urtti, A.,** Modification of ocular and systemic absorption of timolol from ocular inserts by a buffering agent and a vasoconstrictor, *Int. J. Pharm.,* 65, 19, 1990.

52. **Grass, G. M., Cobbly, J., and Makoid, M. C.,** Ocular delivery of pilocarpine from erodible matrices, *J. Pharm. Sci.,* 73, 618, 1984.

53. **Habib, F. S. and Attia, M. A.,** Ocular delivery of pilocarpine hydrochloride from water-soluble polymeric inserts, *Acta Pharm. Technol.,* 32, 133, 1986.

54. **Attia, M. A., Kassem, M. A., and Safwat, S. M.,** In vivo performance of [³H]dexamethasone ophthalmic film delivery systems in the rabbit eye, *Int. J. Pharm.,* 47, 21, 1988.

55. **Dumortier, G., Zuber, M., Chast, F., Sandouk, P., and Chaumeil, J. C.,** Systemic absorption of morphine after ocular administration: evaluation of morphine salt insert in vitro and in vivo, *Int. J. Pharm.,* 59, 1, 1990.

56. **Bloomfield, S. E, Dunn, M. W., Miyata, T., Stenzel, K. H., Randle, S. S., and Rubin, A. L.,** Soluble artificial tear inserts, *Arch. Ophthalmol.,* 95, 247, 1977.

57. **Katz, I. M. and Blackman, W. M.,** A soluble sustained-release ophthalmic delivery unit, *Am. J. Ophthalmol.,* 83, 728, 1977.

58. **Gautheron, P. D., Lotti, V. J., and Le Douarec, J. C.,** Tear film breakup time prolonged with unmedicated cellulose polymer inserts, *Arch. Ophthalmol.,* 97, 1944, 1979.

59. **Arrata, M. and Sfeir, T.,** Traitement de la secheresse oculaire par implants solubles, *Bull. Soc. Fr. Ophthalmol.,* 92, 134, 1981.

60. **Dohlman, C. H., Pavan-Langston, D., and Rose, J.,** A new ocular insert for continuous constant-rate delivery of medication to the eye, *Ann. Ophthalmol.,* 4, 823, 1972.

61. **Allansmith, M. R., Lee, J. R., McClellan, B. H., and Dohlman, C. H.,** Evaluation of a sustained-release hydrocortisone ocular insert in humans, *Trans. Am. Acad. Ophthalmol. Otolaryngol.,* 79, OP128, 1975.

62. **Keller, N., Longwell, A. M., and Birss, S. A.,** Intermittent vs. continuous steroid administration, *Arch. Ophthalmol.,* 94, 644, 1976.

63. **Pavan-Langston, D., Langston, R. H. S., and Geary, P. A.,** Idoxuridine ocular insert therapy, *Arch. Ophthalmol.,* 93, 1349, 1975.

64. **Rubin, A. L., Stenzel, K. H., Miyata, T., White, M. J., and Dunn, M.**, Collagen as a vehicle for drug delivery, preliminary report, *J. Clin. Pharmacol.*, 13, 309, 1973.
65. **Kitazawa, Y.**, Problems of primary open-angle glaucoma, *Acta Soc. Ophthalmol. Jpn.*, 79, 1715, 1975.
66. **Bloomfield, S. E., Miyata, M. W., Dunn, M. W., Bueser, N., Stenzel, K. H., and Rubin, A. L.**, Soluble artificial tear inserts, *Arch. Ophthalmol.*, 95, 247, 1977.
67. **Bloomfield, S. E., Miyata, M. W., Dunn, M. W., Bueser, N., Stenzel, K. H. and Rubin, A. L.**, Soluble gentamycin ophthalmic inserts as drug delivery systems, *Arch. Ophthalmol.*, 96, 885, 1978.
68. **Vasantha, R., Sehgal, P. K., and Panduranga Rao, K.**, Collagen ophthalmic inserts for pilocarpine drug delivery system, *Int. J. Pharm.*, 47, 95, 1988.
69. **Sawusch, M. R., O'Brien, T. P., Dick, J. D., and Gottsch, J. D.**, Use of collagen corneal shields in the treatment of bacterial keratitis, *Am. J. Ophthalmol.*, 106, 279, 1988.
70. **Eswein, M. B., O'Brien, T. P., Osato, M. S., and Jones, D. B.**, Antimicrobial efficacy of antiseptic-containing collagen corneal shields, *Invest. Ophthalmol. Vis. Sci.*, 31, 452, 1990.
71. **Gussler, J. R., Ashton, P., Van Meter, W. S., and Smith, T. J.**, The effect of collagen shields on the topical delivery of trifluorothymidine into cornea and aqueous, *Invest. Ophthalmol. Vis. Sci.*, 31, 485, 1990.
72. **Jacob-La Barre, J. T. and Kaufman, H. E.**, Investigation of pilocarpine-loaded polybutylcyanoacrylate nanocapsules in collagen shields as a drug delivery system, *Invest. Ophthalmol. Vis. Sci.*, 31, 485, 1990.
73. **Loucas, S. P. and Haddad, H. M.**, Solid-state ophthalmic dosage systems in effecting prolonged release of pilocarpine in the cul-de-sac, *J. Pharm. Sci.*, 61, 985, 1972.
74. **Haddad, H. M. and Loucas, S. P.**, Les dérivés de l'acide polyuronique prolongeant le transport de la pilocarpine: evaluation clinique et expérimentale, *Bull. Mem. Soc. Fr. Opth.*, 1972, 621.
75. **Loucas, S. P. and Haddad, H. M.**, Solid state ophthalmic dosage systems. II. Use of polyuronic acid in effecting prolonged delivery of pilocarpine in the eye, *Metab. Ophthalmol.*, 1, 27, 1976.
76. **Capozza, R. C.**, Enzymatically decomposable bioerodable pharmaceutical carrier, German Patent 2,505, 305, 1975; *Chem. Abstr.*, 48, 35314s, 1976.
77. **Miyazaki, S., Ishii, K., and Takada, M.**, Use of fibrin film as a carrier for drug delivery: a long-acting delivery system for pilocarpine in the eye, *Chem. Pharm. Bull.*, 30, 3405, 1982.
78. **Hui, H.-W. and Robinson, J. R.**, Ocular delivery of progesterone using a bioadhesive polymers, *Int. J. Pharm.*, 26, 203, 1985.
79. **Gurny, R., Ibrahim, H., Aebi, A., Buri, P., Wilson, C. G., Washington, N., Edman, P., and Camber, O.**, Design and evaluation of controlled release systems for the eye, *J. Controlled Release*, 6, 367, 1987.
80. **Saettone, M. F., Chetoni, P., Torracca, M. T., Burgalassi, S., and Giannaccini, B.**, Evaluation of muco-adhesive properties and in vivo activity of ophthalmic vehicles based on hyaluronic acid, *Int. J. Pharm.*, 51, 203, 1989.
81. **Benedetti, L. M., Kyyrönen, K., Hume, L., Topp, E., and Stella, V.**, Steroid ester of hyaluronic acid in ophthalmic drug delivery, in *Proc. Int. Symp. Controlled Release Bioact. Mater.*, Controlled Release Society, 1991, 18.
82. **Bundgaard, H.**, *Design of Prodrugs*, Elsevier, Amsterdam, 1985.
83. **Sasaki, H., Bundgaard, H., and Lee, V. H. L.**, Design of prodrugs to selectively reduce systemic timolol absorption on the basis of the differential lipophilic characteristics of the cornea and the conjunctiva, *Invest. Ophthalmol. Vis. Sci.*, 21, 232, 1990.
84. **Lee, V. H. L., Li, S., Saettone, M. F., Chetoni, P., and Bundgaard, H.**, Systemic and ocular absorption of timolol prodrugs from erodible inserts, in *Proc. Int. Symp. Controlled Release Bioact. Mater.*, Controlled Release Society, 1991, 18.
85. **Lee, V. H. L.**, personal communication.
86. **Diepold, R., Kreuter, J., Himber, J., Gurny, R., Lee, V. H. L., Robinson, J. R., Saettone, M. F., and Schnaudigel, O. E.**, Comparison of different models for the testing of pilocarpine eyedrops using conventional eyedrops and a novel depot formulation (nanoparticles), *Albrecht von Graefes Arch. Klin. Exp. Ophthalmol.*, 227, 188, 1989.
87. **Casini, M.**, Structural properties of contact lens materials, in *Ophthalmic Drug Delivery — Biopharmaceutical, Technological and Clinical Aspects*, (Fidia Research Series), Vol. 11, Saettone, M. F., Bucci, G., and Speiser, P., Eds., Liviana Press, Padua, Italy, 1987.
88. **Baker, R. W. and Lonsdale, H. K.**, Controlled release: mechanism and rates, in *Controlled Release of Biologically Active Agents*, Tanquary, A. C. and Lacey, R. E., Eds., Plenum Press, New York, 1974, 15.
89. **Refojo, M. F.**, A critical review of properties and applications of soft hydrogel contact lenses, *Surv. Ophthalmol.*, 16, 233, 1972.
90. **Calabria, G. and Rathschuler, F.**, Contact lenses as therapeutic systems, in *Ophthalmic Drug Delivery — Biopharmaceutical, Technological and Clinical Aspects*, Vol. 11, (Fidia Research Series), Saettone, M. F., Bucci, G., and Speiser, P., Eds., Liviana Press, Padova, 1987.

91. **Sedlacek, J.,** Possibilities of application of ophthalmic drugs with the aid of gel contact lenses, *Cesk. Oftalmol.,* 21, 509, 1965.

92. **Waltman, S. R. and Kaufman, H. E.,** Use of hydrophilic contact lenses to increase ocular penetration of topical drugs, *Invest. Ophthalmol.,* 9, 250, 1970.

93. **Kaufman, H. E., Uotila, M. H., Gasset, A. R., Wood, T. O., and Ellison, E. D.,** The medical use of soft contact lenses, *Trans. Am. Acad. Ophthalmol. Otolaryngol.,* 75, 361, 1971.

94. **Podos, S. M., Becker, B., Asseff, C., and Hartstein, J.,** Pilocarpine therapy with soft contact lenses, *Am. J. Ophthalmol.,* 73, 336, 1972.

95. **Praus, R., Brettschneider, I., Krejci, L., and Kalodowá, D.,** Hydrophilic contact lenses as a new therapeutic approach for the topical use of chloramphenicol and tetracyline, *Ophthalmologica,* 165, 62, 1972.

96. **Matoba, A. Y. and McCulley, J. P.,** The effect of therapeutic soft contact lenses on antibiotic delivery to the cornea, *Ophthalmology,* 92, 97, 1985.

97. **Hull, D. S., Edelhauser, H. F., and Hyndiuk, R. A.,** Ocular penetration of prednisolone and the hydrophilic contact lens, *Arch. Ophthalmol.,* 92, 413, 1974.

98. **Hillman, J. S.,** Management of acute glaucoma with pilocarpine-soaked hydrophilic lens, *Br. J. Ophthalmol.,* 58, 674, 1974.

99. **Krohn, D. L. and Breitfeller, J. M.,** Quantitation of pilocarpine flux enhancement across isolated rabbit cornea by hydrogel polymer lenses, *Invest. Ophthalmol.,* 14, 152, 1975.

100. **Friedman, Z., Allen, R. C., and Raph, S. M.,** Topical acetazolamide and mathazolamide delivered by contact lenses, *Arch. Ophthalmol.,* 103, 963, 1985.

101. **Ozawa, H. Hosaka, S., Kunitomo, T., and Tanzawa, H.,** Ocular inserts for controlled release of antibiotics, *Biomaterials,* 4, 170, 1983.

102. **Hosaka, S., Ozawa, H., and Tanzawa, H.,** Controlled release of drug from hydrogel matrices, *J. Appl. Polym. Sci.,* 23, 2089, 1979.

103. **Lerman, S. and Reininger, B.,** Simulated sustained release pilocarpine therapy and aqueous humour dynamics, *Can. J. Ophthalmol.,* 6, 14, 1971.

104. **Heilmann, K.,** Therapeutic systems for local use, in *Therapeutic Systems. Rate-Controlled Drug Delivery: Concepts and Developments,* Thieme, G., Ed., Stuttgart, 1978, 66.

105. **Urquhart, J.,** Development of the Ocusert pilocarpine ocular therapeutic systems — a case history in ophthalmic product development, in *Ophthalmic Drug Delivery Systems,* Robinson, J. R., Ed., American Pharmaceutical Association, Washington, D.C., 1980, 105.

106. **Shell, J. W. and Baker, R. W.,** Diffusional systems for controlled release of drugs to the eye, *Ann. Ophthalmol.,* 6, 1037, 1974.

107. **Armaly, M. F. and Rao, K. R.,** The effect of pilocarpine Ocusert® with different release rates on ocular pressure, *Invest. Ophthalmol.,* 12, 491, 1973.

108. **Drance, S. M., Mitchell, D. W. A., and Schulzer, M.,** The duration of action of pilocarpine Ocusert® on intraocular pressure in man. *Can. J. Ophthalmol.,* 10, 450, 1975.

109. **Tomono, M. and Nanba, K.,** Long-term clinical trials of pilocarpine (second report) — a further follow-up study, *Folia Ophthalmol. Jpn.,* 32, 2095, 1985.

110. **Urtti, A., Pipkin, J. D, Rork, G. S., and Repta, A. J.,** Experimental surrogate devices for ocular biopharmaceutical studies: *in vitro* studies, *Proc. Int. Symp. Controlled Release Bioact. Mater.,* 14, 295, 1987.

111. **Urtti, A., Pipkin, J. D., Rork, G. S., and Repta, A. J.,** Controlled drug delivery devices for experimental ocular studies with timolol. 1. In vitro release studies, *Int. J. Pharm.,* 61, 235, 1990.

112. **Urtti, A., Sendo, T., Pipkin, J. D., Rork, G., and Repta, A. J.,** Application site dependent ocular absorption of timolol, *J. Ocular Pharmacol.,* 4, 335, 198.

113. **Urtti, A., Pipkin, J. D., Rork, G., Sendo, T., Finne, U., and Repta, A. J.,** Controlled drug delivery devices for experimental ocular studies with timolol. 2. Ocular systemic absorption in rabbits, *Int. J. Pharm.,* 61, 241, 1990.

114. **Gale, R. M., Ben-Dor, M., Keller, N.,** Ocular therapeutic system for dispensing a medication formulation, U.S. Patent 4,190,642, 1980.

115. **Birss, S. A., Longwell, A., Heckbert, S., and Keller, N.,** Ocular hypotensive efficacy of topical epi-nephrine in normotensive and hypertensive rabbits: continuous drug delivery vs. eyedrops, *Ann. Ophthalmol.,* 10, 1045, 1978.

116. **Gale, R., Chandrasekaran, S. K., Swanson, D., and Wright, J.,** Use of osmotically active therapeutic agents in monolythic systems, *J. Membr. Sci.,* 7, 319, 1980.

117. **Sutinen, R., Urtti, A., Miettunen, R., and Paronen, P.,** Water-activated and pH-controlled release of weak bases from silicone reservoir devices, *Int. J. Pharm.,* 62, 113, 1990.

118. **Hou, W.-M., Miyazaki, S., and Takada, M.,** Controlled release of pilocarpine hydrochloride from ethylene-vinyl alcohol copolymer matrices, *Chem. Pharm. Bull.*, 33, 1242, 1985.
119. **Salminen, L.,** Review: systemic absorption of topically applied ocular drugs in humans, *J. Ocular Pharm.*, 6, 243, 1990.
120. **Lee, V. H. L.,** Ophthalmic delivery of peptides and proteins, *Pharm. Technol.*, 12, 26, 1987.

Chapter 5

THE DEVELOPMENT AND USE OF *IN SITU* FORMED GELS, TRIGGERED BY pH

Robert Gurny, Houssam Ibrahim, and Pierre Buri

TABLE OF CONTENTS

I.   Introduction 82

II.   *In Situ* Gelling Systems 82

III.   pH-Triggered Systems 83

IV.   *In Vivo* Evaluation 85

References 89

0-8493-7296-8/93/$0.00 + $.50

I. INTRODUCTION

Ophthalmic dosage forms have been virtually limited to solutions, ointments, suspensions, and emulsions. Nevertheless, there have been a few successful efforts with ocular inserts. Such inserts have been known from pharmaceutical literature for more than 50 years. The excessively rapid drug exchange between the soluble insert and the tear fluid was overcome, however, only with the introduction of the Ocusert®, a diffusion-controlled system developed by Alza Corp. in the 1970s.[1] Inserts have a number of disadvantages such as compliance, especially by elderly people,[2] but are of considerable interest for controlled release to the eye.

In the early 1980s, researchers came up with a new concept, using polymeric dispersions in the nanometer size range.[3-5] A very careful selection of the polymeric material is essential. Most of these polymeric dispersions are prepared by well-known polymerization techniques. An alternative method for the preparation from already formed polymers (e.g., cellulose), is by mechanical dispersion using high-pressure homogenizers in conjunction with conventional emulsifiers and stabilizers.[6] Several new approaches for the preparation of these so-called ''latex-carriers'' from already existing polymers are possible, e.g., solution emulsification, phase inversion, self emulsification, or salting-out processes.[7-12] Nowadays, most of the latex formulations are still produced by the mechanism of emulsion polymerization. This technique requires that the initiator create radicals in the aqueous medium which are captured in the micelles formed by an emulsifier. These micelles are swollen by the diffusing monomer. The polymerization process takes place within the swollen micelles and as the monomer is consumed, it is replaced by diffusing additional amounts of monomer from the outer phase.[4] There are still some problems in using this type of pharmaceutical carrier,[13] such as the possibility of a toxic reaction (i.e., inflammation, carcinogenesis). To ensure the safety of these polymeric preparations for *in vivo* use, the final product must be free of residual products and the breakdown products must be nontoxic.

The disadvantages mentioned, and the impossibility of obtaining some latex systems by emulsion polymerization, led directly to a new technology, the so-called pseudolatices, currently used in the pharmaceutical industry for the film coating of solid dosage forms.[14] Figure 1 shows the main differences between two methods of preparing latex systems. One is a typical emulsion polymerization, the other, a dispersion of an already formed polymer in water, called pseudolatex.

For more than 10 years there have been numerous attempts to use colloidal carriers for different routes, such as nanocapsules,[15] macromolecular complexes,[16] and liposomes.[17] This chapter will only describe some recent applications of latex carriers to the eye.

Ticho and co-workers[18-23] worked on an aqueous polymer emulsion designed for use as pilocarpine-releasing eye drops for the treatment of glaucoma. In this particular example the active ingredient is chemically bound to the polymer.

In a large number of publications, Speiser,[24,27] Harmia,[24,25,27] and Kreuter[26-29] have described the use of nanoparticles to increase bioavailability. Rapidly biodegradable particles were produced using alkylcyanoacrylates. The authors investigated the sorption behavior of pilocarpine salts on hydrophilic polymethylmethacrylate (PMMA) and lipophilic butylcyanoacrylate (PBCA) or -hexylcyanoacrylate (PHCA). The method for producing these particles is relatively simple. Thus far, *in vivo* experiments seem promising, since they indicate good biocompatibility and prolonged duration of action.

II. *IN SITU* GELLING SYSTEMS

The new concept of producing a gel *in situ* (e.g., in the cul-de-sac of the eye) was suggested for the first time in the early 1980s. It is widely accepted that increasing the

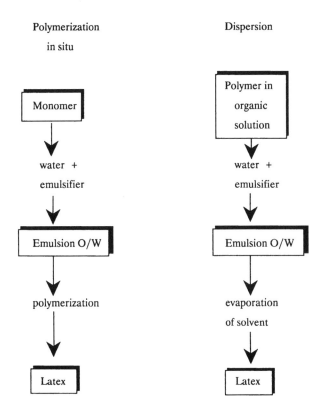

FIGURE 1. General methods of latex preparation of polymeric dispersions.

viscosity of a drug formulation in the precorneal region will lead to an increased bioavailability, due to slower drainage from the cornea.[30] Several concepts for *in situ* gelling systems have been investigated. These systems can be triggered by pH[31] or by temperature.[32] More recently, gellan gum (Gelrite®) has been suggested as a novel ophthalmic vehicle by Rozier et al.[33] and Greaves et al.[34] This material gels on contact with mono- and divalent cations.

III. pH-TRIGGERED SYSTEMS

The first method developed for the preparation of pilocarpine-containing nanoparticles was based on a solvent removal method (Figure 2). A second method, published recently, is based on a salting-out process (Figure 3).

In general, the latices produced by these methods can be defined as water-based systems characterized by low viscosities which are independent of the molecular weight of the dispersed polymer. A pH-triggered ophthalmic latex is a low-viscosity polymeric dispersion in water which undergoes spontaneous coagulation and gelation after instillation in the conjunctival cul-de-sac[35] (Figures 4 and 5). Any process which destabilizes a pseudolatex to such an extent that the particles agglomerate and coalesce in large numbers may be defined as coacervation.[36] Should the resulting coacervate assume a gel form, the process is described as gelation. In a gelation process, the polymeric dispersion gradually changes from a fluid system to a uniform gel. By incorporating a drug into such a formulation, the latter will form *in situ* (i.e., the cul-de-sac) a network of coacervated polymer particles, together with an entrapped amount of drug. These properties will be used to release a bioactive material from a soluble polymeric device onto the eye after instillation of a fluid polymeric dispersion.

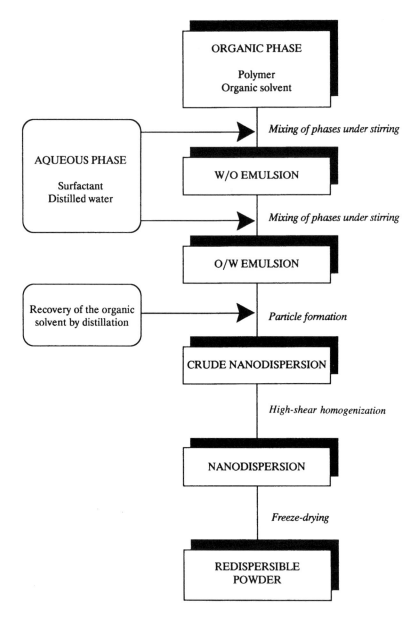

FIGURE 2.   Solvent evaporation process.

Destabilization of pseudolatex is effected by physical agents or by chemical coacervants. Physical destabilization can be induced by increasing the frequency or the energy of the collisions between nanoparticles.

The alkali-induced thickening phenomenon of anionic latices was considered most interesting for the concept of an ophthalmic drug delivery system, because of the presence of a carbonic buffer system regulating the pH of tears as described by Ibrahim.[37] Nanodispersions with a low viscosity and containing a large amount of polymeric material, exhibit an important increase in viscosity when neutralized with a base. Wesslau[38] described this effect as an "inner thickening" that is due to the swelling of the particles from the neutralization of the acid groups contained on the polymer chain and the absorption of water.

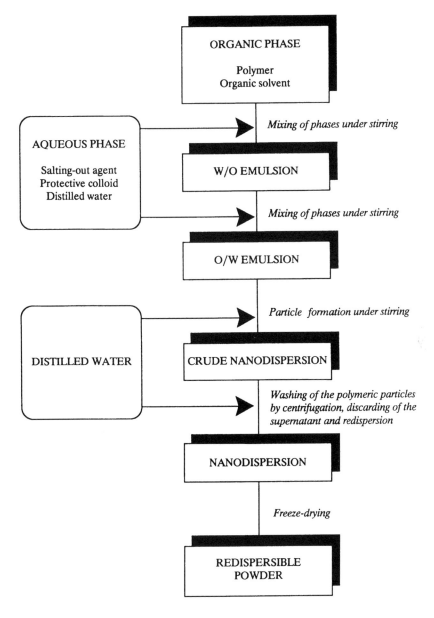

FIGURE 3. Salting-out process.

The pH of tears is normally about 7.2 to 7.4, but may rise up to pH 9, depending on the time between two blinks.[39] By selecting an anionic polymer, the dispersion typically shows a very low viscosity up to pH = 5, and will coacervate in contact with the tear fluid, forming a gel and releasing the active ingredients over a prolonged period of time.

IV. *IN VIVO* EVALUATION

Gamma-emitting radionuclides have been used for many years in nuclear medicine to image different regions of the body and to quantify organ functions. Developments have occurred in the field of radiopharmaceuticals and nuclides for diagnostic imaging, such as

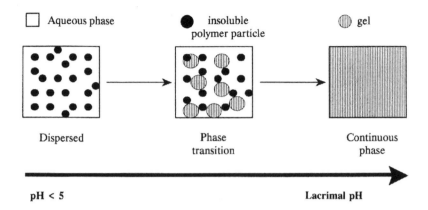

FIGURE 4. Schematic representation of the dispersion to gel transformation.

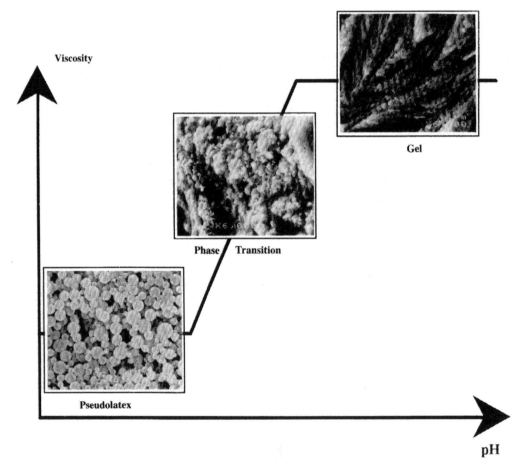

FIGURE 5. Scanning electron microscopic pictures of the transformation.

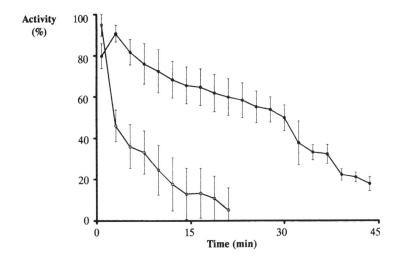

FIGURE 6. Corneal residence time of the pH-triggered 2% pilocarpine HCl preparation (●), compared to a 2% solution (○).

the use of radioiodide for the thyroid, and iodinated fatty acids for the myocardium.[40] With the introduction of lacrimal scintigraphy,[41] it became possible to study the dynamics of lacrimal drainage by visualizing the passage of a tracer through the lacrimal duct with the help of a gamma camera. Since then, lacrimal scintigraphy has been used to study the normal and pathological lacrimal drainage,[42,43] measure the flow rate of tears,[44] and determine the corneal contact time of ophthalmic vehicles.[45,46]

In recent studies the gamma scintigraphy technique was used to monitor the ocular residence time of a new drug delivery system to the eye.[47-50] This ophthalmic preparation is based on a cellulose acetate phthalate (CAP) dispersion which has a low viscosity and coagulates by a pH-induced phenomenon (as shown in Figures 4 and 5) when instilled into the conjunctival sac. The gelled system constitutes an *in situ* microreservoir of high viscosity. ^{99m}Technetium was chosen as tracer to monitor the elimination kinetics of a 25 μl instillation. ^{99m}Tc is easily available and has a short half-life (6 h).

To avoid the binding of technetium to eye tissue or its absorption into the eye, diethylenetriaminepentaacetic acid (DTPA) is added to the radionuclide (^{99m}Tc-DTPA) to form a hydrophilic complex. The radioactive drug-vehicle system was prepared by adding 25% (v/v) of the ^{99m}Tc-DTPA aqueous solution to 75% (v/v) of the polymeric dispersion with a CAP content of 30% (w/w).

In a recent study[47] on New Zealand albino rabbits, the clearance of polymeric dispersion was investigated. For measuring the elimination of the tracer the rabbit was positioned in a restraining box in a normal, upright posture. Twenty-five microliters of a saline solution of ^{99m}Tc-DTPA were first instilled into the eye of the rabbit to determine the clearance of the radionuclide without any viscosity enhancer. Afterwards, 25μl of liquid drug carrier were used. The progression of the radioactive tracer was followed through the lacrimal apparatus.

The clearance rate of the ^{99m}Tc-DTPA solution without polymer from the corneal surface was found to decrease very rapidly (Figure 6). In the majority of the cases, an initially rapid

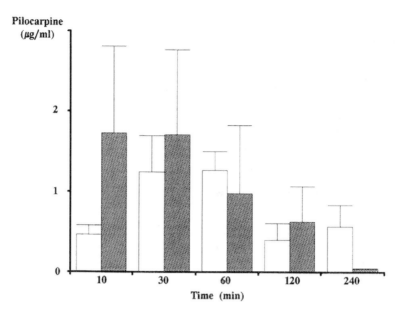

FIGURE 7. Mean concentration ($\pm$ s.e.m.) of pilocarpine in the aqueous humor of rabbits after a topical administration of 25 μl; ($\square$) 2% pilocarpine HCl in 0.58% HEC (n = 8); (▨) 3.4% pilocarpine base in a pH-triggered nanodispersion (n = 12).

loss was followed by a slower elimination. This can be explained as follows: after instillation of a known volume of tracer solution into the eye, the total volume (instilled preparation plus lacrimal fluid) drained out at a particular rate until the volume of the mixture was reduced to that of the initial lacrimal fluid. Subsequent clearance of the tracer was due to the normal turnover of the lacrimal fluid.

Therefore it is clear that the precorneal residence time can be significantly enhanced with pH-triggered systems, by comparison with simple solutions. Aqueous humor concentrations measured in rabbits after bilateral instillations of 50 μl of either 2% pilocarpine hydrochloride (1.7% base) in 0.58% hydroxyethylcellulose (HEC), or 3.4% pilocarpine base in a pH-triggered dispersion gave similar AUC (0 to 4 h) (Figure 7).[52]

Hence, the bioavailability of pilocarpine from a dispersion was approximately half that from hydroxyethylcellulose. In contrast, the peak concentration with the dispersion occurred at 60 min, compared to 10 min with the HEC preparations, and the 240 min levels in the aqueous humor obtained with the dispersion were higher.

For further details the reader is referred to a methodology for selecting solvents for the evaporation technique by Ibrahim.[53] The use of solubility parameters to find the optimal composition is demonstrated to be very efficient. Two successively published articles[54,55] explain in detail the technical options available for modifying nanodispersions when using the salting-out procedure. This technique offers new possibilities for the production of a large number of nanodispersed systems from a broad range of pH-sensitive polymers.

More work is needed to explore further applications of this most promising technology.

REFERENCES

1. **Shell, J. W.**, Diffusional systems for controlled release of drug to the eye, *Ann. Ophthalmol.*, 6, 1037, 1974.
2. **Hess, H.**, Arzneiformen und ihre Anwendung, *Ciba-Geigy*, Basel, 1974.
3. **Gurny, R. and Taylor, D.**, Development and evaluation of a prolonged acting drug delivery system for the treatment of glaucoma, in Proc. Int. Symp. Br. Pharm. Technol. Conf., London, (M. H. Rubinstein, Ed.), Solid Dosage Research Unit, Liverpool, 1980.
4. **Harmia, T. and Speiser, P.**, Polyalkylcyanoacrylate nanoparticles as drug carriers in ophthalmology, in *FIP 83 Abstr.*, Program of Short Communications, 43rd Int. Congr. Pharm. Sci., Montreux, 1983, 222.
5. **Blank, I. and Fertig, J.**, Pharmaceutical base salts, U.S. Patent 4,248,855, 1981.
6. **Vanderhoff, J. W., El-Aasser, M. S., and Ugelstad, J.**, Polymer emulsification process, U.S. Patent 4,177,177, 1979.
7. **Gurny, R.**, Latex systems, in *Topics in Pharmaceutical Sciences*, Breimer, D. D. and Speiser, P., Eds., Elsevier, Amsterdam, 1983, 277.
8. **Gurny, R.**, Preliminary study of prolonged acting drug delivery system for the treatment of glaucoma, *Pharm. Acta Halv.*, 56, 130, 1981.
9. **Gurny, R.**, Ocular therapy with nanoparticles, in *Polymeric Nanoparticles and Microspheres*, Guiot P. and Couvreur, P., Eds., CRC Press, Boca Raton, FL, 1985.
10. **Gurny, R.**, Controlled drug delivery with colloidal polymeric systems, in *Biopolymers*, Piskin, E., Ed., Nato-AST, 1985.
11. **Ibrahim, H., Gurny, R., Bindschaedler, C., Doelker, E., and Buri, P.**, A new technology for the preparation of dry nanodispersed systems for controlled release to the eye, *Proc. Int. Symp. Controlled Release Bioact. Mater.*, 17, 303, 1990.
12. **Bindschaedler, C., Gurny, R., and Doelker, E.**, Process for preparing a powder of water-insoluble polymer which can be redispersed in a liquid phase, the resulting powder and utilization thereof, U.S. Patent 4,968,350, 1990.
13. **Gesler, R. M., Garvin, P. J., Klamer, B., Robinson, R. U., Thompson, C. R., Gibson, W. R., Wheeler, F. C., and Carlson, R. G.**, The biologic effects of polystyrene latex particles administered intravenously to rats — a collaborative study, *Bull. Parenter. Drug Assoc.*, 27, 101, 1973.
14. **Gumowski, F., Doelker, E., and Gurny, R.**, The use of a new redispersible aqueous enteric coating material, *Pharm. Technol.*, 11, 26, 1987.
15. **Oppenheim, R. C.**, Nanoparticles in drug delivery systems, in *Drug Delivery Systems*, Juliano R. L., Ed., *Oxford University Press*, 177, 1980.
16. **Batz, J. H. G., Ringdorf, H., and Ritter, H.**, Pharmacologically active polymers, *Makromol. Chem.*, 175, 2229, 1974.
17. **Papahadjopoulos, P.**, Liposomes and their uses in biology and medicine, *Ann. N.Y. Acad. Sci.*, 308, 281, 1978.
18. **Ticho, U., Blumenthal, M. D., Zonis, S., Gal, A., Blank, I., and Azor, Z. W.**, A clinical trial with Piloplex — a new long-acting pilocarpine compound: preliminary report, *Ann. Ophthalmol.*, 11, 555, 1979.
19. **Mazor, Z., Ticho, U., Rehandy, U., and Rose, L.**, Piloplex, a new long-acting pilocarpine polymer salt. B: comparative study of the visual effects of pilocarpine and piloplex eye drops, *Br. J. Ophthalmol.*, 63, 48, 1979.
20. **Mazore, Z., Kazan, R., Kain, N., Ladkani, D., Ross, M., and Weiner, B.**, Glaubid® (piloplex 3,4) - a long-acting, antiglaucoma medication, in Proc. Int. Symp. Glaucoma, Jerusalem, 1983.
21. **Ticho, U., Blumenthal, M., Zonis, S., Gal, A., Blank, I., and Mazor, Z. W.**, Piloplex, a new long-acting pilocarpine polymer salt. A longterm study, *Br. J. Ophthalmol.*, 63, 45, 1979.
22. **Ticho, U., Lahav, M., Berkowitz, S., and Yoffe, P.**, Ocular changes in rabbits with corticosteroid-induced ocular hypertension, *Br. J. Ophthalmol.*, 63, 646, 1979.
23. **Robinson, J. R. and Li, V. H. K.**, Ocular disposition and bioavailability from Piloplex and other drug delivery systems, in Proc. Int. Symp. Glaucoma, Jerusalem, 1983.
24. **Harmia, T. and Speiser, P.**, Nanopartikel als Arzneistoffträger für Pilocarpin, in Proc. 30th Ann. Congr. Int. Pharm. Technol., Mainz, Germany, 1984, 62.
25. **Harmia, T.**, Nanopartikel als Trägersystem für Augenarzneien, Ph.D. thesis 7472, ETH, Zürich, Switzerland, 1976.
26. **Fitzgerald, P., Hadgraft, J., Kreuter, J., and Wilson, C. G.**, A gamma scintigraphic evaluation of microparticulate ophthalmic delivery systems: liposomes and nanoparticles, *Int. J. Pharmacol.*, 40, 81, 1987.
27. **Harmia, T., Kreuter, J., and Speiser, P.**, Optimization of pilocarpine loading on to nanoparticles by sorption procedures, *Int. J. Pharmacol.*, 33, 45, 1986.

28. **Kreuter, J., Mills, S. N., Davis, S. S., and Wilson, C. G.**, Polybutyl-cyanoacrylate nanoparticles for the delivery of [^{75}Se] norcholesterol, *Int. J. Pharmacol.*, 16, 105, 1983.

29. **Diepold, R., Kreuter, J., Himber, J., Gurny, R., Lee, V. H. L., Robinson, J. R., Saettone, M. F., and Schnaudigel, O. E.**, Comparison of different models for the testing of pilocarpine eyedrops using conventional eyedrops and a novel depot formulation (nanoparticles) *Albrecht von Graefes Arch. Klin. Exp. Ophthalmol.*, 227, 188, 1989.

30. **Patton, T. F. and Robinson, J. R.**, Ocular evaluation of polyvinyl alcohol vehicle in rabbits, *J. Pharm. Sci.*, 64, 1312, 1975.

31. **Gurny, R.**, Preliminary study of prolonged acting drug delivery system for the treatment of glaucoma, *Pharm. Acta Helv.*, 56, 130, 1981.

32. **Miller, S. C. and Donovan, M. D.**, Effect of poloxamer 407 gels on the miotic activity of pilocarpine nitrate in rabbits, *Int. J. Pharm.* 12, 147, 1982.

33. **Rozier, A., Mazuel, C., Grove, J., and Plazonnet, B.**, Gelrit®: a novel ion-activated, *in situ* gelling polymer for ophthalmic vehicles. Effect on bioavailability of timolol, *Int. J. Pharm.*, 57, 163, 1989.

34. **Greaves, J. L., Wilson, C. G., Rozier, A., Grove, J., and Plazonnet, B.**, Scintigraphic assessment of an ophthalmic gelling vehicle in man and rabbit, *Curr. Eye Res.*, 9, 415, 1990.

35. **Ibrahim, H.**, Concept et évaluation de systèmes polymériques dispersés (Pseudo-latex) à usage ophtalmique, Ph.D. thesis 2369, University of Geneva, 1989.

36. **Blachley, D. C.**, Fundamental principles, in *High Polymer Latices, Their Science and Technology*, Vol. 1, Maclaren & Sons, London, 1966.

37. **Ibrahim, H., Buri, P., and Gurny, R.**, Composition, structure et paramètres physiologiques du système lacrymal impliqués dans la conception de formes ophtalmiques, *Pharm. Acta Helv.*, 63, 146, 1988.

38. **Weslau, H.**, Zur Kenntnis von Acrylsäure enthaltenden Copolymer-dispersionen. II. Die Verdichbarkeit Acrylsäure enthaltender Dispersionen, *Makromol. Chem.*, 69, 220, 1963.

39. **Fischer, F. H. and Wiederholt**, Human precorneal tear film pH measured by microelectrodes, *Albrecht von Graefes Arch. Klin. Exp. Ophthalmol.*, 218, 168, 1982.

40. **Wilson, C. G., Hardy, J. G., Frier, M., and Davis, S. S.**, Radionuclide Imaging in Drug Research, *Croom Helm* , London, 1982.

41. **Rossomondo, R. M., Carlton, W. H., Trueblood, J. H., and Thomas, R. P.**, A new method of evaluating lacrimal drainage, *Arch. Ophthalmol.*, 88, 523, 1972.

42. **Amanat, L. A., Hilditch, T. E., and Kwok, C. S.**, Lacrimal scintigraphy. III. Physiological aspects of lacrimal drainage, *Br. J. Ophthalmol.*, 67, 729, 1983.

43. **Hurwitz, J. J., Maisey, M. N., and Welham, R. A. N.**, Quantitative lacrimal scintillography. I. Method and physiological application, *Br. J. Ophthalmol.*, 59, 308, 1975.

44. **Sorensen, T. and Jensen, F. T.**, Methodological aspects of tear flow determination by means of a radioactive tracer, *Acta Ophthalmol. (Kbh)*, 55, 726, 1977.

45. **Hardberger, R., Hanna, C., and Boyd, C. M.**, Effects of drug vehicles in ocular contact time, *Arch. Ophthalmol.*, 93, 42, 1975.

46. **Trueblood, J. H., Rossomondo, R. M., Carlton, W. H., and Wilson, L. A.**, Corneal contact times of ophthalmic vehicles, *Arch. Ophthalmol.*, 93, 127, 1975.

47. **Ibrahim, H., Gurny, R., Buri, P., Ryser, J.-E., and Donath, A.**, Evaluation of the precorneal residence time of a drug delivery system by gamma scintigraphy in rabbit, in Proc. 3rd Eur. Congr. Biopharm. Pharmacokinetics, Vol. I, 1987, 454.

48. **Gurny, R., Boye, T., Ibrahim, H., and Buri, P.**, Recent developments in controlled drug delivery to the eye, in *Proc. Int. Symp. Controlled Release Bioact. Mater.*, 12, 300, 1985.

49. **Gurny, R., Ibrahim, H., Aebi, A., Buri, P., Wilson, C. G., Washington, N., Edman, P., and Camber, O.**, Design and evaluation of controlled release systems for the eye, *J. Controlled Release*, 6, 367, 1987.

50. **Barendsen, H., Oosterhis, J. A., and van Haeringen, N. J.**, Concentration of fluorescein in tear fluid after instillation as eye-drops. I: isotonic eye-drops, *Ophthalmic Res.*, 11, 73, 1979.

51. **Chrai, S. S., Patton, T. F., Mehta, A., and Robinson, J. R.**, Lacrimal and instilled fluid dynamics in rabbit eyes, *J. Pharm. Sci.*, 62, 1112, 1973.

52. **Ibrahim, H., Gurny, R., Buri, P., Grove, J., Rozier, A., and Plazonnet, B.**, Ocular bioavailability of pilocarpine from a phase-transition latex system triggered by pH, *Eur. J. Drug. Metab. Pharmacokinet.*, Special Issue, 7, 1990.

53. **Ibrahim, H., Gurny, R., and Buri, P.**, Methodologie pour le choix de solvants dans la fabrication de pseudo-latex à base d'acétophtalate de cellulose, 4th Int. Conf. Pharm. Technol., Paris, 1986, 282.

54. **Ibrahim, H., Bindschaedler, C., Gurny, R., Doelker, E., and Buri, P.**, Concept and development of ophthalmic pseudo-latexes triggered by pH, *Int. J. Pharm.*, 77, 211, 1991.

55. **Ibrahim, H., Bindschaedler, C., Doelker, E., Buri, P., and Gurny, R.**, Aqueous nanodispersions prepared by a salting-out process, *Int. J. Pharm.*, accepted for publication, 1992.

Chapter 6

LIPOSOMES AND NANOPARTICLES AS OCULAR DRUG DELIVERY SYSTEMS

Michael Mezei and Dale Meisner

TABLE OF CONTENTS

I.   Introduction 92

II.   Liposomes as Drug Carriers 92

III. Liposome Constituents 92

IV.   Liposomes in Ocular Drug Delivery 93
      A.   Topical Instillation 93
      B.   Intravitreal Injection 96
      C.   Subconjunctival Injection 97

V.   Systemic Route of Administration 97

VI.   Nanoparticles as Drug Carriers 97

VII. Methods of Preparation 98

VIII. Drug Release from Nanoparticles 99

IX.   Nanoparticles for Ocular Drug Delivery 99

X.   Conclusion 100

References 101

I. INTRODUCTION

To achieve effective ophthalmic therapy, an adequate amount of ingredient must be delivered and maintained at its site of action within the eye. The anatomical structure and the protective physiological process of the eye (discussed in Chapter 1) exerts a formidable defense against ocular drug delivery. Often only 1% or less of the instilled dose of drug actually reaches the anterior segment tissues of the eye.[1-6] Subsequently, only a fraction of the absorbed dose partitions to posterior tissues. The most frequently used dosage forms, i.e., ophthalmic solutions and suspensions, are compromised in their effectiveness by several limitations. In solution form, many drugs display poor penetration through the lipophilic corneal barrier. Rapid nasolacrimal drainage of the instilled drug from tear fluid and non-productive absorption through the conjunctiva lead to a short duration of action and unwanted entrance into the systemic circulation. Tear turnover and drug binding to tear fluid proteins are additional precorneal factors that contribute to the poor ocular bioavailability of many drugs when instilled in the eye in the solution dosage form. Ophthalmic drops also rely on the pulse entry effect.[7] The rate of uptake of the drug from the tear fluid to ocular tissues is initially high, but rapidly declines. This rapid loading of drug results in a transient period of overdose and the associated risk of side effects, followed by an extended period of subtherapeutic levels before the next dose is administered. The need for an ocular drug delivery system that has the convenience of a drop, but will localize and prolong drug activity at its site of action is apparent. Other chapters in this book discuss some of the approaches to improve ophthalmic drug delivery. This chapter deals with liposomes and nanoparticles as novel dosage forms to prolong the residence time of the encapsulated drug within the eye, or used as drug carriers for targeting the drug to ocular tissues.

II. LIPOSOMES AS DRUG CARRIERS

Liposomes are microscopic vesicles composed of membrane-like lipid layers surrounding aqueous compartments. The lipid layers are comprised mainly of phospholipids. Phospholipids are amphiphilic, they have a hydrophilic head and a lipophilic tail. In aqueous solution they are arranged in bilayers, which form closed vesicles, like artificial cells. In the bilayer, the fatty acid tails, being nonpolar, are located in the interior of the membrane, and the polar head points outward. A single bilayer enclosing an aqueous compartment is referred to as a unilamellar lipid vesicle; according to their size they are known as small unilamellar vesicles (SUV) or large unilamellar vesicles (LUV). If more bilayers are present, they are referred to as multilamellar vesicles (MLV). Depending on the composition, liposomes can have positive, negative, or neutral surface charge. Depending on the lipid composition, methods of preparations, and the nature of the encapsulated agents, many types of liposomal products can be formulated.[8]

III. LIPOSOME CONSTITUENTS

The major components of liposomes are lipids, water, drug, and possibly electrolytes. The lipids are mainly phospholipids and cholesterol. Most liposomes are prepared by using lecithin of egg or vegetable (soy bean) origin. For investigative purposes, synthetic phospholipids, e.g., dipalmitoyl phosphatidylcholine, might be used, but for large-scale production, the price of synthetic lipids might be prohibitive. In our biocompatibility studies[9] the hydrogenated soy lecithin provided the best result. Since liposomes are made up of similar substances as cell membranes, it is expected that they are biocompatible and biodegradable preparations.[9]

Cholesterol is usually included in the formula to stabilize the liposomal membrane and to minimize leaching out of the encapsulated water soluble drug. Electrolytes are used to enhance the lipid bilayer formation and to provide isotonicity.

In cases of topically applied liposomes, it is desirable to use viscosity-inducing agents to produce a consistency which is easy to apply and has better cosmetic property and patient acceptability. Other auxiliary agents such as antioxidants and preservatives might also be included.[10]

Due to the biphasic nature of liposomes (lipid and water), both lipophilic and hydrophilic ingredients are accommodated depending on their solubility in the liposome components; consequently, almost any type of drug can be encapsulated. The ideal drug candidates for liposomal encapsulation are those that have potent pharmacological activity and are highly lipid or water soluble. If a drug is water soluble, it will be encapsulated within the aqueous compartment and its concentration in the liposomal product will depend on the volume of the entrapped water and the solubility of that drug in the encapsulated water. The lipophilic drug is usually bound to the lipid bilayer or "dissolved" in the lipid phase. A lipophilic drug is more likely to remain encapsulated during storage due to its partition coefficient. Since the lipophilic drug is associated with the lipid bilayers, it will not leach out as readily to the "external" water phase. Generally, the encapsulation efficiency is higher for lipophilic drugs than hydrophilic ones.

IV. LIPOSOMES IN OCULAR DRUG DELIVERY

Liposomes have been studied for ocular drug delivery by various ways of administration. Topical instillation is the most convenient and frequent means of administration for ophthalmic therapy, and most studies have administered liposomes by this route. Some investigators, however, have experimented with intravitreal and subconjunctival injection, while others have attempted to target ocular tissues by systemic route of administration.

A. TOPICAL INSTILLATION

The first use of liposomes in ocular therapy was reported by Smolin et al.[11] who described the advantages of liposome-associated idoxuridine over a solution of the drug in the treatment of herpes simplex keratitis in the rabbit eye. The procedure consisted of an "eye-drop"-like treatment three times a day. The liposomal idoxuridine proved to be more effective than the same therapy with the solution form of idoxuridine. Corneal penetration of idoxuridine was later shown to be significantly increased due to liposomal encapsulation.[12] The replication of herpes simplex virus has also been successfully inhibited by immunoliposomes.[13] Monoclonal antibody to herpes simplex virus glycoprotein D, incorporated into liposomes loaded with acyclovir, proved far more effective at inhibiting viral replication in the mouse cornea than free drug, or drug delivered in untargeted liposomes. *In vitro* experiments indicated that the immunoliposomes bound to intact mouse cornea infected with herpes simplex virus. The immunoliposomes could provide site-specific and sustained-release vehicles for ophthalmic therapy.[13]

Other attempts to target liposomes were reported by Megaw et al.[14] In their *in vitro* and *in vivo* studies, they concluded that lectin-mediated binding of liposomes to intraocular tissues may be useful as a specific drug delivery to ocular tissues. A slight nonspecific liposome binding to the lens can be potentiated by incorporating concanavalin A into the liposomal membranes. Schaeffer and Krohn[15] also investigated the lectin-mediated attachment of liposomes to freshly excised cornea and its influence on transcorneal drug flux. They tested uni- and multilamellar types of liposomes (SUV and MLV) with neutral, positive, or negative surface charge. *In vitro* liposome-corneal interaction studies showed that liposomes were taken up by cornea in the order of $MLV^+ > SUV^+ >> MLV^- > SUV^-$ $> MLV = SUV$. *In vitro* studies with various liposomal penicillin G preparations showed that the flux of the drug across the cornea was in the order of $SUV^+ > MLV^- > MLV^+$ $> SUV^- > SUV > MLV$ = free drug > free drug mixed with "empty" liposomes. These results indicated that liposomal encapsulation of the water soluble antibiotic enhanced the transcorneal flux *in vitro*, while the presence of "empty" liposomes did not alter the corneal drug penetration significantly. *In vivo* studies with a lipophilic anti-inflammatory agent, indoxole, revealed that the liposomal form provided 2.5 times higher drug levels in the aqueous humor than the indoxole solution.[15] The authors[15] proposed that the transfer of liposomal drug to the corneal surface could be the mechanism for delivery of the drug.

Stratford et al.[16] studied the ocular disposition of two model compounds, epinephrine and inulin, in rabbits. The liposomal drug was tested against free drug, free drug mixed with "empty" liposomes, and free drug administered 15 min after topical instillation of "empty" liposomes. As a result of liposomal encapsulation, epinephrine absorption was reduced by 50% whereas inulin absorption was increased 10 times.

Lee et al.[17] investigated the effects of some precorneal factors on the retention of liposomes in tears and their interaction with corneal and conjunctival surfaces. Also in this study, inulin, as a model compound, was encapsulated in multilamellar, neutral liposomes. They found that adsorption of liposomes on corneal and conjunctival surfaces was a requisite to the ocular absorption of inulin. Over a dose range of 10 to 50 µl, the availability of binding sites on these surfaces, rather than the size of the instilled volume, controlled the extent of liposomal adsorption, and consequently, the availability of inulin to the intraocular tissues. They concluded that liposomes can be suitable for ocular drug delivery provided they have affinity for, and are able to bind to the corneal surfaces, and release their contents at optimal rates.

Ahmed and Patton,[18,19] pursuing the investigations of ocular absorption of inulin, concluded that the increased inulin levels in the iris-ciliary body may be due to the adsorption of liposomes to the conjunctival surface. This provides higher inulin concentration and, therefore, higher drug flux across the conjunctival and scleral membranes. The liposomal dosage form can selectively promote noncorneal drug absorption which can provide enhanced drug levels in certain intraocular tissues, while minimizing high concentration of drug in the anterior chamber.[19]

Studies[20,21] in our laboratory also suggested that the alteration of drug disposition observed with liposomal encapsulation may be dependent on the type of liposome and on the physicochemical properties of the entrapped species. Liposomal triamcinolone acetonide, a model for lipophilic compounds, provided higher drug concentrations in ocular tissues when compared to the suspension dosage form.[20] However, liposome-encapsulated dihydrostreptomycin sulfate, a hydrophilic compound, produced lower drug levels in ocular tissues compared to its solution form.[21] Among the liposomal preparations, the large multi- and unilamellar vesicles provided higher drug concentration in all ocular tissue than the small unilamellar ones. Introduction of a positive charge on the liposome surface enhanced liposome-conjunctiva interactions.

The hypothesis suggested by Singh and Mezei[21] is that association between the drug molecules and the lipid vesicles can be a major factor influencing drug disposition. Liposomal drug delivery is probably more favorable for lipophilic drugs than for hydrophilic compounds. To confirm this hypothesis, we selected one drug that can be used both as a lipophilic (atropine base) and hydrophilic (atropine sulfate) model.[22] Another reason for selecting atropine was that in addition to biodisposition studies, we could conduct pharmacodynamic studies, since the biological pupil dilatory effect of atropine can be objectively and accurately measured.

In vivo drug disposition studies of [³H]-atropine base in liposomal and solution form, after topical instillation to rabbit eyes, demonstrated that liposomal encapsulation enhanced the pulse of drug to anterior ocular compartments such as cornea, aqueous humor, and iris/ciliary body. As a result, the duration of its pharmacological effect, pupil dilation, was prolonged in the order of positively charged MLV > neutral or negatively charged MLV > solution.[22]

Benita et al.[23] also conducted pharmacodynamic studies by encapsulating 0.2% pilocarpine into small MLV and testing it against 1 and 2% pilocarpine solution by measuring changes in the intraocular pressure of the rabbit. From their limited experiments, no clear conclusion could be drawn concerning the effect of liposome on the transcorneal transport. Preliminary results suggested that the liposome vehicle was probably unable to enhance corneal penetration of pilocarpine to reach satisfactory therapeutic levels when administered at lower concentrations (i.e., 0.2%) than commonly used. However, a more recent study,[24] examining the effects of pilocarpine hydrochloride on intraocular pressure and pupil contraction in rabbits with experimentally induced glaucoma, concluded that a liposomal formulation with lecithin:cholesterol:stearylamine (7:2:2 molar ratio) produced the greatest effect. The intraocular pressure decreased from 22.1 to 13.4 mmHg 120 min after administration. The maximum reduction of pupil area, 59.5%, occurred after 60 min.

Shek and Barber[25] successfully prevented the miotic effect of di-isofluorophosphate (DFP) by entrapping the cholinesterase enzyme. Pretreatment consisted of topical instillation of either acetylcholinesterase-containing liposomes, free enzyme, or empty liposomes. Miotic challenge by topical instillation of DFP was attempted 2 h later. While free enzyme and empty liposomes did not provide any protection against DFP, pretreatment with liposome-entrapped enzyme significantly reduced DFP-induced miosis. This was a unique strategy in that the effectiveness of enzyme-containing liposomes stemmed from the ability to bind the miotic agent, and thus, only the release of the entrapped enzyme was required to neutralize the toxic action of the agent. Ocular penetration of the entrapped enzyme was not a prerequisite for successful prophylaxis.

The biodisposition and efficacy of anti-inflammatory steroids were investigated by Taniguchi et al.[26,27] Dexamethasone and its esters were tested in liposomal and suspension forms. The liposome preparation containing dexamethasone valerate provided the highest ocular drug levels, but in the cases of dexamethasone and dexamethasone palmitate, the liposomal form provided a lower drug level than the suspension form. The corneal absorption of dexamethasone was increased by the incorporation of stearylamine which provided a positive surface charge to liposomes. Other reports also indicate that positive surface charge provides higher ocular drug concentration and prolonged activity.[21,22,24] *In vitro* studies have also demonstrated that binding of liposomes to cornea decreased in the order of positive, negative, and neutral liposomes.[15] In a gamma scintigraphic evaluation of the precorneal residency of liposomal formulations in rabbits, Fitzgerald et al.[28] came to the conclusion that the positive surface charge significantly decreased the drainage from the cornea; the positively charged multilamellar vesicles were retained longer in this region. Shek and Barber[25] suggested that liposomes with a positive surface charge can form a stable adsorption to the corneal surface because corneal epithelium is thinly coated with negatively charged mucin. It seems reasonable to consider that a closer and stronger association with the cornea provided greater resistance to removal from the tear fluid and ultimately augmented drug loading to anterior tissues. McCalden and Levy[29] also came to the same conclusion, ie., that liposomes composed of different types of phospholipids adhere to the surface of the cornea and the positively charged liposomes are retained longer.

The precorneal drainage of topically instilled liposomes has been demonstrated by Fitzgerald et al.[28] to be a multiphasic phenomenon. In their studies, three anatomical regions of interest were defined, the cornea, the inner canthus, and the lacrimal duct, to evaluate the precorneal residence of liposome formulations. It was reported that following instillation, an immediate distribution occurred in the corneal and inner canthral areas which was too rapid to be accurately measured. Greater than 70% of the initial dose was lost from the cornea within 15 s. A second, less rapid phase of drainage occurred from 15 to 150 s, followed by a much slower basal phase. Following the initial rapid appearance of drug in the inner canthus, preparations drained slowly and monophasically into the nasolacrimal duct.[28]

The binding of liposomes to bovine lens epithelial cells was enhanced by cytochalasin D *in vitro* experiments. The lipid transfer between plasma membranes and phosphatidyl-choline liposomes was also increased.[30] Lee et al.,[31] in their review, emphasized the importance of targeting liposomes to the corneal, as opposed to the conjunctival, surface and of retaining the liposomes at the corneal surface in order to provide and improve the ophthalmic drug delivery system.

Alvarado[32] utilized liposomal 5-fluoro-orotate for glaucoma surgery to enhance the wound healing process. In an experimental monkey model, the most effective chemotherapy was the use of liposomal 5-fluoro-orotate administered prior to surgery.

B. INTRAVITREAL INJECTION

Liposome encapsulation has the potential not only to increase the activity and prolong the duration of action of drugs administered to the eye, but also to reduce the toxicity of certain drugs. Liposome-encapsulated amphotericin B produced less toxicity than the commercial amphotericin B solution when injected intravitreally.[33,34] Although amphotericin B is the drug of choice for serious fungal infections of the eye, there are several problems with its ophthalmic use. First, even if it is injected subconjunctivally, it does not penetrate the ocular humors and often causes local tissue lesions. Liposomal encapsulation markedly reduced the ocular toxicity and provided active concentration of the drug in the vitreous humor of rabbis. A more recent study,[35] however, claimed that the reduced toxicity of intravitreally injected, liposome-bound drug was accompanied by reduced efficacy. Liu et al.[35] suggested increasing the dose of the liposomal amphotericin B above the dose of the free drug to achieve adequate antifungal activity. A substantial reduction of ocular toxicity can also be achieved by liposomal encapsulation of cytarabine.[36] Similar results were reported by Joondeph et al.[37] who studied the effect of liposomal encapsulation of 5-fluorouracil in the treatment of proliferative vitreoretinopathy. Liposomal encapsulation improved both the efficacy and safety of antiproliferative agents used for the treatment of ocular proliferative disorders.

Intravitreally injected, liposome-encapsulated clindamycin was found effective in the treatment of Staphylococcus aureus endophthalmitis in rabbits.[38] Intravitreal liposome-encapsulated antibiotics such as clindamycin, gentamycin, and antiviral drugs such as acyclovir, were used in patients with acute toxoplasmosis retinochoroiditis, presumed propionibacterium acne endophthalmitis after cataract surgery, and presumed cytomegalovirus retinitis associated with AIDS. A single intravitreal dose of clindamycin, gentamycin, or acyclovir was effective in the treatment of the above conditions.[39] Pharmacokinetic studies of gentamycin concluded that liposomal encapsulation resulted in decreased drug clearance and increased biological half-life in the vitreous compartment.[40] The pharmacokinetics of another intravitreally injected, liposome-encapsulated antibiotic was investigated by Kim and Kim.[41] Tobramycin was encapsulated into liposomes of phosphatidylcholine, phosphatidic acid, and α-tocopherol by the reverse phase evaporation method. One eye of the rabbit received an intravitreal injection of either liposome-encapsulated tobramycin (LET), tobramycin phosphate-buffered saline (TS), or a mixture of tobramycin and liposome-encapsulated saline (TEL). The results indicated that the concentrations of free tobramycin were significantly lower with LET than with TS or TEL at 1 h after intravitreal injection. The concentrations of free and total tobramycin were significantly higher with LET than TS or TEL at 5 and 8 d after intravitreal injection. Concentrations of free tobramycin with TS were lower than the minimal inhibitory concentration (MIC) of tobramycin for *Pseudomonas aeruginosa* at 8 d after intravitreal injection, while those with LET were higher than the MIC of tobramycin for *Pseudomonas aeruginosa* 18 d after injection.

Alghadyan et al.[42] reported that the retinal toxicity of intravitreally injected cyclosporine was reduced by liposomal encapsulation. Liposome encapsulation also increased the biological half-life of free cyclosporine, which is about 6 h to 3 d, indicating the possibility of prolongation of the duration of action.[42]

C. SUBCONJUNCTIVAL INJECTION

Barza et al.[43] studied the pharmacokinetics of liposome-encapsulated gentamycin by subconjunctival injection. Rabbits were given single injections of liposome-encapsulated gentamycin, free gentamycin, or a mixture of "empty" liposomes with free gentamycin. The liposomal form provided higher drug concentration in the sclera and cornea up to 24 h after injection. The differences were 5- to 20-fold in the cornea. The authors concluded that liposome encapsulation extended the effects of a subconjunctival injection of antibiotics. Simmons et al.[44] reported that the liposomal encapsulation prolonged the residence time of 5-fluorouracil in normal pigmented rabbit eye. A similar conclusion was reported by Assil et al.,[45] i.e., liposomes can provide a sustained-release vehicle for 5-fluorouridine monophosphate.

V. SYSTEMIC ROUTE OF ADMINISTRATION

The potential of targeting the delivery of dyes and drugs to specific sites in the eye was investigated using temperature-sensitive liposomes.[46] Carboxyfluorescein (CF) or an antineoplastic agent, cytosine arabinoside, were encapsulated into temperature-sensitive, large unilamellar vesicles and injected intravenously into rabbits. Increasing the temperature of the ciliary body with microwaves caused the dye or the drug to be selectively released from the liposomes. In the eyes receiving liposome-encapsulated dye or drug, the average concentration in the anterior chamber of the heated eyes was 40 and 8 times higher, respectively, than in the contralateral unheated control eyes. In another study,[47] to visualize the retinal microvasculature, liposome-encapsulated fluorescein was injected intravenously into rhesus monkeys. The release of CF in a retinal artery was induced by a short heat pulse from a laser. The comparison of the results with conventional fluorescein angiography illustrated the advantage of the liposomal delivery.

The heat-sensitive, liposomal, selective delivery of cytosine arabinoside and 5-fluorouridine by systemic injection was also investigated, and the results confirmed the potential advantages of this novel delivery system.[46,48]

VI. NANOPARTICLES AS DRUG CARRIERS

Nanoparticles are solid particles of polymeric nature ranging in size from 10 to 1000 nm. Biologically active materials can be incorporated into the carrier or adsorbed on the surface of the nanoparticle.[49] Several recent reviews discuss, in detail, nanoparticles and their application in drug delivery.[50-53] The versatility of polymer chemistry provides unique opportunities to impart specific and desirable properties required for the biological use of nanoparticles as drug carriers. In the area of ocular drug delivery, the slow release and mucoadhesive properties of nanoparticles represent a potential means to provide selective and prolonged therapeutic activity in the eye.

VII. METHODS OF PREPARATION

Biodegradable nanoparticles can be prepared by emulsion polymerization of polyalkyl-cyanoacrylates.[54] Water soluble monomers are emulsified in an aqueous phase which often contains dextran as a protectant to prevent aggregation and glucose for isotonicity.[51] Polymerization occurs spontaneously at room temperature, with stirring to form nanoparticles approximately 200 nm in size. To prevent excessively rapid polymerization and promote the formation of nanoparticles, emulsion polymerization is carried out at acidic pH. Drugs can be incorporated by addition to the media prior to polymerization or adsorbed by addition to the nanoparticle suspension after polymerization is complete.[49] Once polymerization is complete, the suspension is filtered to remove the large particles and neutralized to ensure the disappearance of residual monomers. The nanoparticle suspension is ready to use or can be lyophilized, and later suspended when needed.

Other methods used to prepare nanoparticles include interfacial polymerization and denaturation, or desolvation of natural proteins or carbohydrates.[50-53] The interfacial polymerization technique involves dissolving the polyalkylcyanoacrylate monomers and lipophilic drug in an oil and slowly injecting this mixture into a well-stirred solution of 0.5% poloxamer 338 in water at pH 6.[55] At the oil-water interface, nanoparticles with a shell-like wall are formed spontaneously by hydroxyl-ion-induced polymerization. Macromolecules such as albumin or gelatin can form nanoparticles through desolvation and denaturation processes. In the first process, desolvation of macromolecules in solution can be induced by changes in pH, charge, or the addition of a desolvating agent such as ethanol.[49,56] Normally a coacervate is produced by desolvation; however, prior to formation of the coacervate, the desolvation process induces swollen macromolecules to coil tightly. At this point, tightly coiled macromolecules can be fixed and hardened by crosslinking with glutaraldehyde to form nanoparticles rather than microcapsules. Nanoparticles are then purified by gel filtration. The denaturation process involves preparing an emulsion from an aqueous phase containing the drug, magnetite particles, and the macromolecule and an oil (e.g., cottonseed oil).[57-60] Polymerization is carried out by heat denaturization at temperatures above 120°C, or by chemical crosslinking. Nanoparticles are precipitated out and washed with ether, or in the case of gelatin,[61] acetone, and stored in dry form.

The size of nanoparticles produced can be influenced by several physicochemical factors. The pH of the solution during polymerization and, to some extent, the monomer concentration have been shown to effect the size of nanoparticles in the range of 100 to 200 nm.[62] Stabilizers (e.g., dextran) and nonionic surfactants can affect the diameter in the 20 to 770 nm size range depending on the molecular weight of the stabilizer used; the use of B-cyclodextrin can produce particles up to 3000 nm in diameter.[63] The carrier capacity of nanoparticles is dependent on the method of loading.[51] For example, the incorporation process provided an eightfold increase in the maximum loading capacity of rose bengal into nanoparticles, as compared to the adsorption process.[64] The amount of drug that is incorporated or adsorbed can also be influenced by the polymeric composition of the nanoparticles, pH of the solution, the temperature at which nanoparticles were produced, presence of stabilizers and surfactants, electrolyte concentration, and the drug itself.[64-68] The porous nature of nanoparticles provides a high surface area for drug binding.

VIII. DRUG RELEASE FROM NANOPARTICLES

Some studies have demonstrated that the release of compound from nanoparticles can be correlated to nanoparticle degradation.[69,70] Considering that the rate of degradation of cyanoacrylate polymers is dependent on their alkyl chain length,[71] it is theoretically possible to select a monomer whose polymerized form has the desired release characteristics. However, in some cases, the release of drug cannot be attributed to degradation of the polymer alone. Drug desorption from the polymer surface and diffusion through the polymeric matrix are other mechanisms by which drug can be released from nanoparticles.[72] As observed with liposomes, drug release from nanoparticles has sometimes displayed a biphasic pattern. For example, release of ampicillin from polyisohexylcyanoacrylate nanoparticles was initially fast, followed by a period of zero-order release.[73] The period of rapid release was likely due to loss of adsorbed drug, while the slower phase may represent release due to nanoparticle degradation. This is supported by the observation that, with rose bengal as model compound, initial release *in vitro* was faster when the marker was adsorbed to nanoparticle surfaces rather than incorporated into the polymeric matrix.[64] Whether nanoparticles with specific release characteristics *in vivo* can be designed is a major issue which needs to be addressed for ocular drug delivery, as well as for other routes of administration.

IX. NANOPARTICLES FOR OCULAR DRUG DELIVERY

Studies that have investigated the potential of nanoparticles for ocular drug delivery have been limited and have yet to demonstrate conclusively if they are superior to the conventional eye drop; however, there have been some promising results. Using a radiotracer technique, the ocular disposition of nanoparticles following topical instillation to the rabbit eye was investigated by Wood et al.[74] It was found that although nanoparticles composed of poly-hexyl-2-cyanoacrylate were rapidly cleared from the precorneal site, approximately 1% of the instilled dose was able to adhere to corneal and conjunctival surfaces. Predosing with a mucolytic agent did not significantly alter levels of radioactivity in the cornea and the aqueous humor suggesting that nanoparticles or their degradation products adhered directly to the corneal tissue, and that the mucin layer did not appear to represent a barrier to corneal permeation. Radioactivity detected in the aqueous humor was assumed to be a product of polymer degradation rather than intact nanoparticles. The same pretreatment increased the concentration of nanoparticles in the conjunctiva, which possibly contributed to the formation of a gel-like substance in the cul-de-sac. There was also a relatively rapid rate of degradation of the nanoparticles in tear fluid during the first hour, but the rate declined over the remaining time course. In terms of drug delivery, this would be advantageous since the degradation of the nanoparticles would facilitate drug release from the polymer matrix.

The elimination of ^{111}In-labeled nanoparticles from tear fluid was compared to liposomes and control solutions by gamma-ray scintigraphy.[75] All three preparations were cleared from the cornea much faster than from the inner canthus. Clearance half-life of the solution from the cornea and inner canthus were 1.3 and 5 min, respectively. Positively charged liposomes displayed the longest corneal half-life at 3.7 min, while nanoparticles had the longest inner canthal half-life at 17.3 min and an intermediate value of 2.2 min in the cornea. In comparison, radiotracer technique indicated that polyalkylcyanoacrylate nanoparticles had a half-life in tears of about 20 min.[74] The residence time of these same nanoparticles in inflamed eye tissues was about 4 times higher than that observed in healthy tissues.[76] Under inflamed conditions, relatively constant concentrations of nanoparticles were maintained in the cornea and conjunctiva for up to 4 h, while aqueous humor concentrations displayed a fivefold increase up to 1 h. Increased retention of nanoparticles in the inflamed eye was possibly attributed to specific and nonspecific protein binding, partial blockage of the nasolacrimal duct, and enhanced bioadhesiveness of the inflamed tissue to the polymer. If the latter explanation is valid, it suggests that nanoparticles may be particularly useful in the delivery of anti-inflammatory and anti-allergic drugs.

The main objective of employing nanoparticles as a carrier for ophthalmic drug delivery is to provide sustained drug release and prolonged therapeutic activity. Using pilocarpine as a model drug, Harmia et al.[77] were able to demonstrate prolonged miosis in rabbits following topical administration of drug adsorbed to polybutylcyanoacrylate nanoparticles. A commercial pilocarpine solution was used as a control. Interestingly, when pilocarpine was incorporated into nanoparticle matrix, no significant prolongation of the miotic was observed. It was suggested that an insufficient amount of drug was released from the nanoparticles prior to their removal from the precorneal site; thus, there was also a limited quantity of drug available for absorption. Conversely, when drug was adsorbed to the surface of the nanoparticles, drug release did not restrict the amount of drug available for absorption and may have facilitated a direct interaction with epithelial surfaces of tissues in the precorneal site. In another study, the use of polyalkylcyanoacrylate nanoparticles prolonged the intraocular pressure-reducing effect of pilocarpine for more than 9 h in a rabbit model.[78]

The use of polybutylcyanoacrylate nanoparticles to improve the ocular delivery of progesterone following topical administration proved unsuccessful.[79] Comparison of drug disposition in ocular tissues following topical instillation as a solution or a nanoparticle suspension indicated that progesterone levels in the cornea and aqueous humor was 4 to 5 times less for the encapsulated drug. As observed with pilocarpine, the release of drug from nanoparticles was too slow to provide adequate absorption during its residence time in the precorneal area. The high affinity of the compound for nanoparticles may have significantly contributed to the diminished availability of free drug at the absorptive site. A similar result was reported for betaxolol chlorhydrate adsorbed to isobutylcyanoacrylate nanoparticles.[80] Modification of surface charge allowed different levels of adsorption; however, none of these provided any increase or prolongation of therapeutic activity.

X. CONCLUSION

Most of the reports, as reviewed above, concluded that liposome-mediated drug delivery to ocular tissues is a promising means to improve selective drug treatment. In some cases liposomes can provide increased efficacy, reduced toxicity, prolonged activity, and even site-specific activity. In other cases, however, no advantage is gained by liposome encapsulation. The differences in this conclusion are mainly due to the different types of lipid vesicles, the physicochemical properties of the encapsulated active ingredient, and the physiological processes at the site of administration. The type of liposome, particularly the surface charge, has a major effect on the biodisposition and activity of the encapsulated drug. The binding of the liposomes to the cornea and, consequently, the residence time extent of absorption is decreasing in the order of positive, negative, and neutral liposomes. Although the mechanism involved has not been clearly elucidated, it remains apparent that the physicochemical properties of the entrapped species also have an important effect on the ocular absorption of topically instilled, liposome-encapsulated compounds. If encapsulated compounds are released from liposomes prior to absorption, then upon release the extent to which a drug will be absorbed will be dictated by its physicochemical properties. Corneal epithelium provides a greater barrier to hydrophilic compounds as compared to lipophilic ones.[3] Compounds that did not significantly benefit from liposome encapsulation were either hydrophilic salts or highly ionized in aqueous mediums. Of the liposome-encapsulated compounds that improved ocular bioavailability, idoxuridine, indoxole, triamcinolone acetonide, and atropine base were all lipophilic. Although inulin and penicillin G are not lipophilic, they may be secondarily associated with liposomal membranes[15] and thus may similarly associate with corneal epithelium.

Nanoparticles appear to offer several advantages in the area of ophthalmic drug delivery. Particularly attractive are their bioadhesive properties which, if optimized, may overcome a major shortcoming of most ophthalmic products, i.e., inadequate retention time in the precorneal site. Another important feature is the versatility of nanoparticles as a drug carrier. Many different types of compounds can be incorporated or adsorbed to nanoparticles, and depending on the composition, nanoparticles with different release characteristics can be designed. Furthermore, nanoparticles are easy to manufacture and form a stable, yet biodegradable product. Biodegradability suggests that nanoparticles will have low toxicity.

Although most of the investigations provided results that promised an advantage of the liposomal or nanoparticle ophthalmic drug delivery, there is a need for further studies to elucidate the pharmacodynamic and pharmacokinetic fate of the liposome and nanoparticle ophthalmic products, the safety of long-term use of this new type of ophthalmic dosage form, and also the aspects of the industrial product development.

REFERENCES

1. **Makoid, M. C. and Robinson, J. R.,** Pharmacokinetics of topically applied pilocarpine in the albino rabbit eye, *J. Pharm. Sci.*, 68, 435, 1979.
2. **Schoenwald, R. D. and Huang, H. S.,** Corneal penetration behaviour of β-blocking agents. I. Physicochemical factors, *J. Pharm. Sci.*, 72, 1266, 1983.
3. **Huange, H. S., Schoenwald, R. D., and Lach, J. L.,** Corneal penetration behaviour of β-blocking agents. II. Assessment of barrier contributions, *J. Pharm. Sci.*, 72, 1271, 1983.
4. **Lee, V. H. L. and Robinson, J. R.,** Review: topical ocular drug delivery: recent development and future challenges, *J. Ocular Pharmacol.*, 2, 67, 1986.
5. **Tang-Hui, D., Lui, S., Neft, J., and Sandri, R.,** Disposition of levobunolol after an ophthalmic dose to rabbits, *J. Pharm. Sci.*, 76, 780, 1987.
6. **Ling, T. and Combs, D.,** Ocular bioavailability and tissue distribution of [14C]-ketorolac trimethamine in rabbits, *J. Pharm. Sci.*, 76, 280, 1987.
7. **Shell, J. W.,** Ophthalmic drug delivery systems, *Surv. Ophthalmol.*, 29, 117, 1984.
8. **Gregoriadis, G., Ed.,** *Liposome Technology*, Vol 1–3, CRC Press, Boca Raton, FL, 1983.
9. **Foong, W. C., Harsanyi, B. B., and Mezei, M.,** Effect of liposome on hamster mucosa, *J. Biomed. Mater. Res.*, 23, 1213, 1989.
10. **Mezei, M.,** Liposomes in topical application of drugs, in *Liposomes as Drug Carriers: Trends and Progress*, Gregoriadis, G., Ed., John Wiley & Sons, Toronto, 1988, 663.
11. **Smolin, G., Okumoto, M., Feiler, S., and Condon, D.,** Idoxuridine-liposome therapy for herpes simplex keratitis, *Am. J. Ophthalmol.*, 91, 220, 1981.
12. **Dharma, S. K., Fishman, P. H., and Peyman, G. A.,** A preliminary study of corneal penetration of ^{125}I-labelled idoxuridine liposomes, *Acta Ophthalmol.*, 64, 298, 1986.
13. **Norley, S. G., Sendele, D., Huang, L., and Rouse, B. T.,** Inhibition of herpes simplex virus replication in the mouse cornea by drug containing immunoliposomes, *Invest. Ophthalmol. Vis. Sic.* 28, 591, 1987.
14. **Megaw, J. M., Takei, Y., and Lerman, S.,** Lectin-mediated binding of liposomes to the ocular lens, *Exp. Eye Res.*, 32, 395, 1981.
15. **Schaeffer, H. E. and Krohn, D. K.,** Liposomes in topical drug delivery, *Invest. Ophthalmol. Vis. Sci.*, 22, 220, 1982.

16. **Stratford, R. E., Yang, D. C., Redell, M., and Lee, V. H. L.,** Effects of topically applied liposomes on disposition of epinephrine and inulin in the rabbit eye, *Int. J. Pharm.,* 13, 263, 1983.

17. **Lee, V. H. L., Takemoto, K. A., and Limoto, D. S.,** Precorneal factors influencing the ocular distribution of topically applied liposomal inulin, *Curr. Eye Res.,* 3, 585, 1984.

18. **Ahmed, I. and Patton, T. F.,** Importance of the non-corneal absorption route in topical ophthalmic drug delivery, *Invest. Ophthalmol.,* 26, 584, 1985.

19. **Ahmed, I. and Patton, T. F.,** Selective intraocular delivery of liposome encapsulated inulin via the non-corneal absorption route, *Int. J. Pharm.,* 34, 163, 1986.

20. **Singh, K. and Mezei, M.,** Liposomal ophthalmic drug delivery system. I. Triamcinalone acetonide, *Int. J. Pharm.,* 16, 339, 1983.

21. **Singh, K. and Mezei, M.,** Liposomal ophthalmic drug delivery system. II. Dihydrostreptomycin sulphate, *Int. J. Pharm.,* 19, 263, 1984.

22. **Meisner, D., Pringle, J., and Mezei, M.,** Liposomal ophthalmic drug delivery. III. Pharmacodynamic and biodisposition studies of atropine, *Int. J. Pharm.,* 55, 105, 1989.

23. **Benita, S., Plenecassagne, J. D., Cave, G., Drouin, D., Dong, P. H. L., and Sincholle, D.,** Pilocarpine hydrochloride liposomes: characterization *in vitro* and preliminary evaluation *in vivo* in rabbit, *J. Microencaps.,* 1, 203, 1984.

24. **Szulc, J., Woyczikowski, B., and De Laval, W.,** Influence of pilocarpine hydrochloride liposomes on the intraocular pressure and the rabbit eye pupil, *Farm. Pol.,* 44, 462, 1988.

25. **Shek, P. N. and Barber, R. F.,** Liposomes are effective carriers for the ocular delivery of prophylactics, *Biochim. Biophys. Acta,* 902, 229, 1987.

26. **Taniguchi, K., Yamazawa, N., Itakura, K., Morisaki, K., and Hayashi, S.,** Partition characteristics and retention of anti-inflammatory steroids in liposomal ophthalmic preparations, *Chem. Pharm. Bull.,* 35, 1214, 1987.

27. **Taniguchi, K., Itakura, K., Yamazawa, N., Morisaki, K., Hayashi, S., and Yamada, Y.,** Efficacy of a liposome preparation of anti-inflammatory steroids as an ocular drug-delivery system *J. Pharmacobiodyn.,* 11(1), 39, 1988.

28. **Fitzgerald, P., Hadgrast, J., and Wilson, C. G.,** A gamma scintigraphic evaluation of the precorneal residence of liposomal formulations in the rabbit, *J. Pharm. Pharmacol.,* 39, 487, 1987.

29. **McCalden, T. A. and Levy, M.,** Retention of topical liposomal formulations on the cornea, *Experientia,* 46(7), 713, 1990.

30. **Baibakov, B. A., Iwig, M., Glaesser, D., and Margolis, L. B.,** Influence of cytochalasin D on the lipid transfer between cells and liposomes, *Biomed. Biochim. Acta,* 49(1), 129, 1990.

31. **Lee, V. H. L., Urrea, P. T., Smith, R. E., and Schanzlin, D. J.,** Ocular drug bioavailability from topically applied liposomes, *Surv. Ophthalmol.,* 29, 335, 1985.

32. **Alvarado, J. A.,** The use of a liposome-encapsulated 5-fluoroorotate for glaucoma surgery. I. Animal studies, *Trans. Am. Ophthalmol. Soc.,* 87, 489, 1990.

33. **Tremblay, C., Barza, M., Szoka, F., Lahav, M., and Baum, J.,** Reduced toxicity of lioposome-associated amphotericin B injected intravitreally in rabbits, *Invest. Ophthalmol. Vis. Sci.,* 26, 711, 1985.

34. **Barza, M., Baum, J., Tremblay, C., and Szoka, F.,** Ocular toxicity of intravitreally injected liposomal amphotericin B in rhesus monkeys, *Am. J. Ophthalmol.,* 100, 259, 1985.

35. **Liu, K. R., Peyman, G. A., and Khoobehi, B.,** Efficacy of liposome-bound amphotericin B for the treatment of experimental fungal endophthalmitis in rabbits, *Invest. Ophthalmol. Vis. Sci.,* 30(7), 1527, 1989.

36. **Liu, K. R., Peyman, G. A., She, S. C., Niesman, M. R., and Khoobehi, B.,** Reduced toxicity of intravitreally injected liposome-encapsulated cytarabine, *Ophthalmic Surg.,* 20(5), 358, 1989.

37. **Joondeph, B. C., Peyman, G. A., Khoobehi, B., and Yue, B. Y.,** Liposome-encapsulated 5-fluorouracil in the treatment of proliferative vitreoretinopathy, *Ophthalmic Surg.,* 19(4), 252, 1988.

38. **Rao, V. S., Peyman, G. A., Khoobehi, B., and Vangipuram, S.,** Evaluation of liposome-encapsulated clindamycin in Staphylococcus aureus endophthalmitis, *Int. Ophthalmol.,* 13(3), 181, 1989.

39. **Peyman, G. A., Charles, H. C., Liu, K. R., Khoobehi, B., and Niesman, M.,** Intravitreal liposome-encapsulated drugs: a preliminary human report, *Int. Ophthalmol.,* 12(3), 175, 1988.

40. **Fishman, P. H., Peyman, G. A., and Lesar, T.,** Intravitreal liposome-encapsulated gentamicin in a rabbit model, *Invest. Ophthalmol. Vis. Sci.,* 27, 1103, 1986.

41. **Kim, E. K. and Kim, H. B.,** Pharmacokinetics of intravitreally injected liposome-encapsulated tobramycin in normal rabbits, *Yonsei Med. J.,* 31(4), 308, 1990.

42. **Alghadyan, A. A., Peyman, G. A., Khoobehi, B., Milner, S., and Liu, K. R.,** Liposome-bound cyclosporine: clearance after intravitreal injection, *Int. Ophthalmol.,* 12(2), 109, 1988.

43. **Barza, M., Baum, J., and Szoka, F.,** Pharmacokinetics of subconjunctival liposome-encapsulated gentamicin in normal rabbit eyes, *Invest. Ophthalmol. Vis. Sci.,* 25, 486, 1984.

44. **Simmons, S. T., Sherwood, M. B., Nichols, D. A., Penne, R. B., Sery, T., and Spaeth, G. L.,** Pharmacokinetics of a 5-fluorouracil liposomal delivery system, *Br. J. Ophthalmol.,* 72(9), 688, 1988.
45. **Assil, K. K., Lane, J., and Weinreb, R. N.,** Sustained release of the antimetabolite 5-fluorouridine-5'-monophosphate by multivesicular liposomes, *Ophthalmic Surg.,* 19(6), 408, 1988.
46. **Khoobehi, B., Peyman, G. A., McTurnan, W. G., Niesman, M. R., and Magin, R. L.,** Externally triggered release of dye and drugs from liposomes into the eye: an *in vitro* and *in vivo* study, *Ophthalmology,* 95(7), 950, 1988.
47. **Zeimer, R. C., Guran, T., Shahidi, M., and Mori, M. T.,** Visualization of the retinal microvasculature by targeted dye delivery, *Invest. Ophthalmol. Vis. Sci.,* 31(8), 1459, 1988.
48. **Khoobehi, B., Peyman, G. A., Niesman, M. R., and Oncel, M.,** Hyperthermia and temperature-sensitive liposomes: selective delivery of drugs into the eye, *Jpn. J. Ophthalmol.,* 33(4), 405, 1989.
49. **Kreuter, J.,** Evaluation of nanoparticles as drug-delivery systems. I. Preparation methods, *Pharm. Acta Helv.,* 58, 196, 1983.
50. **Douglas, S. J., Davis, S. S., and Illum, L.,** Nanoparticles in drug delivery, *Crit. Rev. Ther. Drug Carrier Syst.,* 3, 233, 1987.
51. **Couvreur, P.,** Polyalkylcyanoacrylates as colloidal drug carriers, *Crit. Rev. Ther. Drug Carrier Syst.,* 5, 1, 1988.
52. **Kreuter, J.,** Nanoparticle-based drug delivery systems, *J. Controlled Release,* 16, 169, 1991.
53. **Kreuter, J.,** Possibilities of using nanoparticles as carriers for drugs and vaccines, *J. Microencap.,* 5, 115, 1988.
54. **Couvreur, P., Kante, B., Roland, M., Guiot, P., Bauduin, P., and Speiser, P.,** Polycyanoacrylate nanocapsules as potential lysosomotropic carriers: preparation morphological and sorptive properties, *J. Pharm. Pharmacol.,* 31, 331, 1979.
55. **Al Khouri Fallouh, N., Roblot-Treupel, L., Fess, H., Devissaguet, J.Ph., and Puisieux, F.,** Development of a new process for the manufacture of polyisobutyl-cyanoacrylate nanoparticles, *Int. J. Pharm.,* 28, 125, 1986.
56. **Marty, J. J., Oppenheim, R. C., and Speiser, P.,** Nanoparticles — a new colloidal drug delivery system, *Pharm. Acta Helv.,* 53, 17, 1978.
57. **Scheffel, U., Rhodes, B. A., Natarajan, T. K., and Wagner, H. N., Jr.,** Albumin microspheres for the study of the reticuloendothelial system *J. Nucl. Med.,* 13, 498, 1972.
58. **Kramer, P. A.,** Albumin microspheres as vehicles for achieving specificity in drug delivery, *J. Pharm. Sci.,* 63, 1646, 1974.
59. **Widder, K., Flouret, G., and Senyei, A.,** Magnetic microspheres: synthesis of a novel parenteral drug carrier, *J. Pharm. Sci.,* 68, 79, 1979.
60. **Gallo, J. M., Hung, C. T., and Perrier, D. G.,** Analysis of albumin microsphere preparation, *Int. J. Pharm.,* 22, 63, 1984.
61. **Yoshioka, T., Hashida, M., Muranishi, S., and Sekazi, H.,** Specific delivery to the liver, spleen and lung: nano- or microspherical capsules of gelatin, *Int. J. Pharm.,* 8, 131, 1981.
62. **Douglas, S. J., Illum, L., Davis, S. S., and Kreuter, J.,** Particle size and size distribution of poly(butyl-2-cyanoacrylate) nanoparticles. I. Influence of physicochemical factors, *J. Colloid Interface Sci.,* 101, 149, 1983.
63. **Douglas, S. J., Illum, L., and David, S. S.,** Particle size and size distribution of poly(butyl-2-cyanoacrylate) nanoparticles. II. Influence of stabilizers, *J. Colloid Interface Sci.,* 103, 154, 1985.
64. **Illum, L., Khan, M. A., Mak, E., and Davis, S. S.,** Evaluation of the carrier capacity and release characteristics for poly(butyl-2-cyanoacrylate) nanoparticles, *Int. J. Pharm.,* 30, 17, 1986.
65. **El Egakey, M. A. and Speiser, P.,** Drug loading studies on ultrafine solid carriers by sorption procedures, *Pharm. Acta Helv.,* 57, 236, 1982.
66. **Douglas, S. J., Illum, L., and Davis, S. S.,** Poly(butyl 2-cyanoacrylate) nanoparticles with differing surface charges, *J. Controlled Release,* 3, 15, 1986.
67. **Harmia, T., Speiser, P., and Kreuter, J.,** A solid colloidal drug delivery system for the eye: encapsulation of pilocarpine in nanoparticles, *J. Microencaps.,* 3, 3, 1986.
68. **Harmia-Pulkkinen, T., Tuomi, A., and Kristoffersson, E.,** Manufacture of polyalkylcyanoacrylate nanoparticles with pilocarpine and timolol by micelle polymerization: factors influencing particle formation, *J. Microencapsulation,* 6, 87, 1989.
69. **Lenaerts, V., Couvreur, P., Christiaens-Leyh, D., Joiris, E., Roland, M., Rollman, B., and Speiser, P.,** Degradation of poly-Isobutylcyanoacrylate) nanoparticles, *Biomaterials,* 5, 65, 1984.
70. **Couvreur, P., Kante, B., Roland, M., and Speiser, P.,** Adsorption of antineoplastic drugs to polyalkylcyanoacrylate nanoparticles and their release characteristics in calf serum, *J. Pharm. Sci.,* 68, 1521, 1979.
71. **Vezin, W. and Florence, A.,** *In vitro* degradation rates of biodegradable poly-N-alkylcyanoacrylates, *J. Pharm. Pharmacol.,* 30, 5P, 1978.

72. **El-Samaligy, M. and Rohdewald, P.,** Triamcinolone diacetate nanoparticles, a sustained release drug system available for parenteral administration, *Pharm. Acta Helv.,* 57, 201, 1983.

73. **Henry-Michelland, S., Alonso, M. J., Andremont, A., Maincen, P., Sauzieres, J., and Couvreur, P.,** Attachment of antibiotics to nanoparticles: preparation, drug release and antimicrobial activity in vitro, *Int. J. Pharm.,* 35, 121, 1987.

74. **Wood, R. W., Li, V. H. K., Kreuter, J., and Robinson, J. R.,** Ocular disposition of polyhexyl-2-cyano[3-^{14}C] acrylate nanoparticles in the albino rabbit, *Int. J. Pharm.,* 23, 175, 1985.

75. **Kreuter, J.,** Nanoparticles and liposomes in ophthalmic drug delivery, in *Ophthalmic Drug Delivery. Biopharmaceutical, Technological and Clinical Aspects,* Saettone, M. S., Bucci, G., and Speiser, P., Eds., Liviana Press, Padua, Italy, 1987, 101.

76. **Diepold, R., Kreuter, J., Guggenbuhl, P., and Robinson, J. R.,** Distribution of polyhexyl-2-cyano-[3–14C]acrylate nanoparticles in healthy and chronically inflamed rabbits eyes, *Int. J. Pharm.,* 54, 149, 1989.

77. **Harmia, T., Kreuter, J., Speiser, P., Boye, T., Gurny, R., and Kubis, A.,** Enhancement of the myotic response of rabbits with pilocarpine-loaded polybutylcyanoacrylate nanoparticles, *Int. J. Pharm.,* 33, 187, 1986.

78. **Diepold, R., Kreuter, J., Himber, J., Gurny, R., Lee, V. H. L., Robinson, J. R., Saettone, M. F., and Schnaudigel, O. E.,** Comparison of different models for the testing of pilocarpine eyedrops using conventional eyedrops and a novel depot formulation (nanoparticles), *Albrecht von Graefes Arch. Klin. Exp. Ophthalmol.,* 227, 188, 1989.

79. **Li, V. H. K., Wood, R. W., Kreuter, J., Harmia, T., and Robinson, J. R.,** Ocular drug delivery of progesterone using nanoparticles, *J. Microencaps.,* 3, 213, 1986.

80. **Marchal-Heussler, L., Maincent, P., Hoffman, M., Spittler, J., and Couvreur, P.,** Antiglaucomatous activity of betaxolol chlorhydrate sorbed onto different isobutylcyanoacrylate nanoparticle preparations, *Int. J. Pharm.,* 58, 115, 1990.

Chapter 7

USE OF HYALURONIC ACID IN OCULAR THERAPY

Stéphanie F. Bernatchez, Ola Camber, Cyrus Tabatabay, and Robert Gurny

TABLE OF CONTENTS

I.   Introduction 106

II. Hyaluronic Acid: Biological Properties 107
     A.   Source 107
     B.   Molecular Structure 107
     C.   Viscosity and Other Physicochemical Properties......................... 108
     D.   Use in Eye Surgery... 109

III. Use of Hyaluronic Acid in Ocular Drug Delivery............................. 109
     A.   Effect on the Precorneal Residence Time 109
     B.   Treatment of Dry Eye 113
     C.   Use as a Vehicle for Controlled Drug Delivery......................... 115

References... 118

0-8493-7296-8/93/$0.00 + $.50

I. INTRODUCTION

The sodium salt of hyaluronic acid (SH) is a high-molecular-weight biological polymer, made of repeating disaccharide units of glucuronic acid and N-acetyl-β-glucosamine. Figure 1 shows the structure of the molecule. This glycosaminoglycan is a ubiquitous component of the extracellular matrix of tissues such as connective tissue, vitreous body, skin, tendons, muscles, and cartilage.[1]

In the eye, SH is present in the vitreous body and, in lower concentrations, the aqueous humor. Its use for the replacement of human vitreous and aqueous humor was suggested by Balazs, who developed a test in the monkey eye to establish the noninflammatory nature of this product, and who patented a specific fraction of SH under the name of Healon®.[2] Further studies established that repeated implantations of SH in the monkey eye did not increase the inflammatory reaction.[3]

The behavior of endogenous SH in different states of disease has been investigated, and various uses for exogenous SH have been developed. Examples of such investigations include the following: serum SH levels correlated with the development of arthritic lesions and with the arthritic score in a rat model of experimentally induced arthritis, suggesting that SH can be used as a marker to follow the progression of this disease.[4,5] SH increased chemoattraction and replication of fibroblasts, and collagen deposition in an *in vivo* wound-healing model. The combination of SH and fibronectin was synergistic in this model.[6] SH was also found to increase the nasal absorption of vasopressin in a rat model.[7] Drug release devices based on SH derivatives have also been studied: films prepared from ester derivatives of SH showed a high permeability and a high degree of hydration, leading to a rapid release (200 min) of the physically incorporated chlorpromazine used as a tracer.[8] SH esters have also been used to prepare microspheres, in which the release of physically incorporated hydrocortisone was compared to the release of the covalently bound drug. The physically incorporated hydrocortisone was released within 10 min, whereas the covalently bound drug showed a zero-order release rate over 100 h.[9] These results suggest that esters of SH can be used to form polymeric prodrug devices for prolonged drug delivery.

SH is currently widely used in intraocular surgery, and many researchers are now working to understand the interactions between SH and ocular tissues, and to explore innovative uses for this product, making use of its particular physicochemical characteristics. The purpose of this chapter is to review the recent advances in the use of sodium hyaluronate in ophthalmic therapy, giving the general principles, working hypotheses, and experimental results obtained so far.

Ocular drug delivery faces important constraints due to the physiology of the eye. Topical instillation, for instance, induces blinking and lacrimation, which in turn increase tear turnover and decrease precorneal residence time. Moreover, the corneal permeability is very low for most substances. The combination of a low permeability and a short residence time, therefore, leads to a poor bioavailability for topically administered ophthalmic drugs.[10,11]

Various ways of improving bioavailability can be thought of, such as: (1) increasing the precorneal residence time by the use of viscous vehicles,[12-16] (2) using penetration enhancers which modify the integrity of the corneal epithelium,[17-19] and (3) using ion pair formation or prodrugs.[19] The potential advantage of SH-containing formulations for topical ocular drug delivery is their ability to form viscous hydrogels with excellent tolerance and increased precorneal residence time.

Other routes of drug delivery to the eye include subconjunctival and intraocular injections during eye surgery. Recently, SH has been experimentally used in rabbits as a vehicle to deliver bleomycin through subconjunctival injection to investigate a potential adjunct to

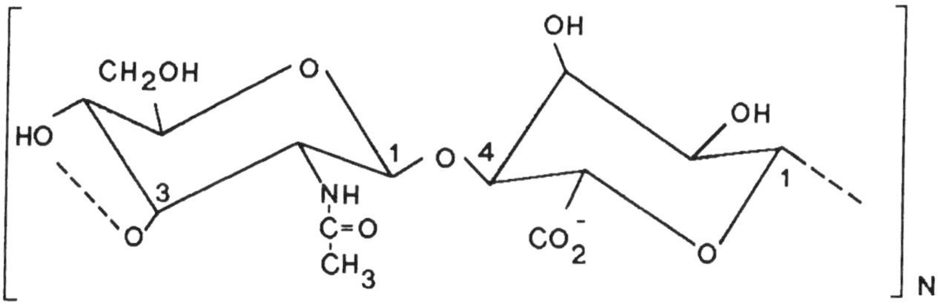

FIGURE 1. Structure of hyaluronate.

glaucoma filtering surgery. SH prolonged drug delivery when compared with an injection of the same drug in saline solution, but it was less efficient than a collagen implant.[20]

Finally, vehicles intended for ocular use must fulfill a large number of requirements regarding pH, osmolality, stability, tolerance, safety, and compatibility with a preservative for multiple-dose formulations. Additionally, if a topically applied viscous vehicle is used to increase the residence time, its viscosity must be sufficiently low not to cause blurred vision in order to insure the comfort and compliance of patients.

II. HYALURONIC ACID: BIOLOGICAL PROPERTIES

A. SOURCE

SH was discovered in the bovine vitreous body by Meyer and Palmer.[21] Since then, this large polysaccharide molecule was found to be present in nearly all connective tissue matrices of vertebrate organisms. The concentrations (expressed as percent of total weight) of SH in some representative tissues and fluids are: human vitreous body 0.02%, human adult skin 0.03 to 0.09%, normal human urine 0.002%, streptococcal cultures 0.01 to 0.1%, and rooster comb 0.75%.[22] The concentration of SH in human and animal vitreous body varies considerably according to topography, species, and age. It is the highest in the vitreous cortical gel close to the ciliary body and the retina in the several species tested.[23] Among various species, the highest concentration of SH in the vitreous has been found in cattle and owls, whereas the lowest has been found in rabbits, dogs, and cats. The human vitreous body has an intermediate concentration. Adult vitreous levels of SH are about 20 to 100 times lower than at birth.[24]

Increased pathological levels of SH have been found in patients with rheumatoid arthritis, due to an increased production, and in patients with liver cirrhosis, due to a decreased catabolism of the polysaccharide.[25]

The normal metabolism of SH in the body has not yet been described in detail. SH is synthesized in the cell membranes, and the polysaccharide is directly extruded into the extracellular space.[26] In recent years, the interest in SH for medical use and skin care has tremendously increased; therefore, there is a growing need to find a good source for this polysaccharide. Various biological sources containing a large amount of SH such as umbilical cord, bovine vitreous, or rooster comb are being considered. Production of SH may also be achieved by bacterial synthesis. However, there is a problem in achieving SH of high molecular weight with this latter technique.

B. MOLECULAR STRUCTURE

SH consists of repeating disaccharide units (Figure 1) of N-acetyl-D-glucosamine and glucuronate linked by β (1,3) and β (1,4) glycoside bonds.[27] Balazs reported that SH is a linear unbranched polysaccharide with a random coil conformation.[24] SH of various molecular weights (M.W.) have been identified. Bothner-Wik analyzed in detail the molecular structure of this polysaccharide. She reported that SH having a molecular weight of 4×10^6 Da consists of approximately 10,000 disaccharide units and shows an average chain diameter of 10 nm.[28]

SH contains one carboxyl group per disaccharide unit. At physiological pH, this group is dissociated, thus conferring a polyanionic character to the compound. The ionic strength and pH of the medium will affect size and shape of the molecule, and therefore influence physicochemical factors such as viscosity.

The chemical structure is independent of the origin, but the molecular weight varies dramatically depending on the source.[22] A low-molecular-weight polymer is produced by streptococcal cultures, whereas very large molecules have been found in synovial fluid. Products containing SH for use in ophthalmic surgery vary considerably with respect to molecular weight. Bothner and Wik (1989)[29] investigated the molecular weight of the following products: Viscoat® (Alcon), IAL® (Fidia), Amvisc® (Med-Chem Products), and Healon® (Kabi Pharmacia), and found that the molecular weight ranged from 5×10^5 to 4×10^6 Da.

C. VISCOSITY AND OTHER PHYSICOCHEMICAL PROPERTIES

The use of SH as an aid in medicine is due to a combination of the good biocompatibility and the physicochemical properties of this polysaccharide.[30] These properties are dependent upon the concentration and the molecular weight. SH has a very large hydrodynamic volume, and due to the expanded coil structure the molecules will come in contact with each other even at very low concentrations. At higher concentrations, the coils will start to entangle and form a continuous, flexible, three dimensional network.[22] Physicochemical properties such as flow resistance, osmotic pressure, sieve effect, exclusion effect, and rheological behavior are affected. From a physiological point of view, the above-mentioned properties retard the bulk flow of solvent, and sterically exclude large-size molecules thereby affecting their distribution and chemical activity. SH also works as a sieve or filter for macromolecules and exhibits a nonideal colloid osmotic pressure, thereby acting as an osmotic buffer.[29] The physical properties such as shear viscosity, viscoelasticity, and lubrication of SH are of major importance when the latter is used as a medical aid in eye surgery. This kind of surgery is called viscosurgery. This term, first introduced by Balazs,[31] is used to describe procedures in which viscoelastic solutions or gels are used to protect cells from mechanical trauma, to maintain or create tissue spaces, and to insure separation and lubrication of tissue surfaces.

The viscosity of SH solutions is shear-dependent: they exhibit a typical pseudoplastic behavior with a low viscosity at high shear rates and a constant viscosity at low shear rates (zero shear viscosity).[29] It can be noted that both concentration and molecular weight of SH have a great influence on the rheological properties. At high shear rates, the viscosity is mainly dependent on concentration. However, the zero shear viscosity is greatly influenced by both the molecular weight and the concentration. An increase in the zero shear viscosity of a SH solution also leads to an increase in the elastic properties. The elastic properties of a solution can be studied by oscillating motion.[32] It was found that at low strain frequencies, the solutions were viscous, whereas at high frequencies they show an elastic behavior. High-molecular-weight SH solutions are mainly elastic at high frequencies. On the other hand, at low molecular weights the viscous character is predominant. In surgery, the elasticity of SH is of great importance since SH prevents the cells from coming in contact with the surgical instruments.

D. USE IN EYE SURGERY

Various commercial formulations of sodium hyaluronate are available for ocular surgery: Healon® and Hylorin® (Kabi Pharmacia, Sweden); Hyalectin;®, Hyalistil®, and IAL (Fidia, Italy); Viscoat® (Alcon), which is a mixture of SH and sodium chondroitin sulfate; Amvisc® (Med-Chem Products); Vitrax® (Edward Weck); and Hylumed® (Genzyme, England). Products based on SH are mostly used during cataract surgery to maintain the shape of the anterior chamber and to protect the corneal endothelium during phakoemulsification and lens implantation. This protective role of SH was established by replacing rabbit aqueous humor with SH and by subsequently examining the corneal endothelium with scanning electron microscopy.[33] SH also showed a topical protective effect for the cornea and conjunctiva during cataract extraction in humans.[34] It has been suggested that this protective mechanism may be due to the ability of SH to retain water.[35] In fact, specific cellular binding sites for SH have been found on the corneal endothelium, which is covered with SH in the normal eye in the rat, rabbit, and monkey.[36] The amount of SH in the cornea seems to increase during the healing of the corneal stroma.[37] The effect of SH on the healing of corneal epithelium has also been studied in rabbits, using three different models of corneal epithelial defect. When the epithelium was removed with iodine vapor, leaving the basement membrane essentially intact, neither 0.1 nor 0.25% SH had an effect on the healing. When the epithelium was removed with n-heptanol, denaturing the basement membrane, 0.1% SH did not affect healing, but 0.25% SH did. When the epithelium, the basement membrane, and a part of the stroma were surgically removed, both 0.1 and 0.25% SH improved healing. These authors established a correlation between the type of defect and: (1) the corneal production of fibronectin, and (2) the retention of SH on the cornea. Their results suggest that SH may accelerate corneal epithelial healing when the fibronectin production of the cornea is induced, or when the retention of SH is increased.[38]

SH has been evaluated in different types of human anterior segment surgeries. Pape and Balazs found it safe and efficient for intracapsular cataract extraction, extracapsular cataract extraction glaucoma filtration, and corneal transplantation. They reported an enhancement in the quality of the filtering bleb in glaucoma filtration surgery.[39] However, Liebmann and co-workers reported an increased risk of an early rise in intraocular pressure (IOP) after the use of SH to reform the anterior chamber in trabeculectomy. They therefore recommend caution when using SH during surgery on eyes with severe glaucomatous optic nerve damage or visual field loss.[40] Conflicting studies have been published reporting either a transient increase in IOP after anterior segment surgery using SH,[41,42] no difference in IOP in a SH-treated group compared to a control group,[43,44] or even an improvement in IOP in a SH-treated group compared to a control group.[45,46] However, the measurement of IOP values has not been performed at the same time points by the various authors. Overall, it is agreed that a transient increase in IOP occurs shortly after surgery, followed by a subsequent satisfactory control of IOP. In a rabbit model, the use of hyaluronidase to increase outflow facility has been suggested to counterbalance the early IOP rise described above.[47]

III. USE OF HYALURONIC ACID IN OCULAR DRUG DELIVERY

A. EFFECT ON THE PRECORNEAL RESIDENCE TIME

The effect of SH on precorneal residence time has been evaluated on the basis of its potential muco-adhesive properties, and several methods have been used. Table 1a summarizes these methods and the results obtained in humans, whereas Table 1b presents the results obtained with rabbit models.

Two forms of SH have been used for ocular administration, i.e., solutions and inserts. Ludwig and Van Ooteghem[14] found that SH increases the precorneal residence time of

TABLE 1a
Effect of Sodium Hyaluronate on the Precorneal Residence Time of a Topically Applied Solution in Humans

Tracer (volume instilled)	n^a	SH (%)	Viscosity parameters^b	M_r^b (kDa)	Half-life^c (s)	C_{max}^b	Ref.
Fluorescein 0.5%	4	0	—	—	96	27^d	14
(10 μl)		0.1	10 mPa·s	>4000	144	43^d	
		0.19	21 mPa·s	>4000	138	51^d	
		0.25	247 mPa·s	>4000	>240	78^d	
^{99m}Tc	7	0	—	—	96	—	16
(25 μl)		0.125	—	—	168^e	—	
		0.250	—	—	$>1200^f$	—	
^{99m}Tc	6	0	—	—	36	—	15
(25 μl)		0.2	—	—	279^e	—	
		0.3	—	—	437^e	—	
^{99m}Tc	12 KCS^g	0	—	—	40	—	
(25 μl)		0.2	—	—	468^f	—	
		0.3	—	—	909^f	—	

^{a} Number of healthy individuals unless mentioned otherwise.
^{b} When available.
^{c} Half-life values estimated from the available data.
^{d} Concentration in units of fluorescence.
^{e} Not significantly different from control.
^{f} Significantly different from control.
^{g} KCS = Keratoconjunctivitis sicca.

TABLE 1b
Effect of Sodium Hyaluronate on the Precorneal Residence Time of a Topically Applied Solution in Rabbits

Tracer (volume instilled)	n^a	SH (%)	Viscosity parameters^b	M_r^b (kDa)	Half-life^c (s)	Residence time^d (min)	Ref.
Fluorescein 1%	≥5	5	$[\eta] = 10.8$ dl/g	620		45	49
(50 μl, or 1 insert)		15	$[\eta] = 3.2–4$ dl/g	134		10	
		dry film (casting)	$[\eta] = 10.8$ dl/g	620		60	
		idem	$[\eta] = 3.2–4$ dl/g	134		45	
		dry film (compression)	$[\eta] = 10.8$ dl/g	620		60	
		idem	$[\eta] = 3.2–4$ dl/g	134		15	
		ethyl ester of hyaluronic acid (compression)	—	160		no uniform corneal film	
^{99m}Tc	5	0	—	—	40		46
(25 μl)							
		0.125	—	—	$>600^e$		

^{a} Number of healthy animals.
^{b} When available.
^{c} Half-life values estimated from the available data.
^{d} Persistence of detectable corneal film fluorescence.
^{e} Significantly different from control.

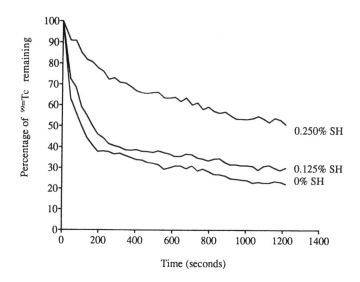

FIGURE 2. Percentage of sodium pertechnetate ^{99m}Tc remaining in the human precorneal area (n = 7). Linear regression analysis for a period of <195 s gives the following elimination rate constants: 0.250% SH, k = −0.11% s^{-1}; 0.125% SH, k = −0.25% s^{-1}; 0% SH, k = −0.28% s^{-1}. Linear regression analysis for a period of >195 s gives the following elimination rate constants: 0.250% SH, k = −0.018% s^{-1}; 0.125% SH, k = −0.009% s^{-1}; 0% SH, k = −0.013% s^{-1}. (Reprinted from Gurny, R. et al., *Albrecht von Graefes Arch. Klin. Exp. Ophthalmol.*, 228, 510, 1990. With permission.)

fluorescein in humans, the optimal SH concentration being 0.25% (for a preparation with a molecular weight higher than 4 × 10⁶ Da). No strong binding exists between fluorescein and SH; this tracer diffuses freely in the solution. Higher concentrations of SH may not mix easily with tears and may be irritative, causing an increase in lacrimation.

Radioactive labeling has also been used to evaluate the precorneal residence time of ophthalmic solutions. Gurny and co-workers[16] incorporated technetium (^{99m}Tc) into 0.125 and 0.250% SH solutions (M$_r$ of 3 × 10⁶ Da), and measured, by gamma scintigraphy, the precorneal residence time of these solutions compared to a phosphate buffer solution (PBS) in healthy humans.

As shown by Figure 2, the 0.250% solution significantly increased residence time of the tracer, whereas the 0.125% solution gave results similar to those obtained with PBS.[16] In a rabbit experiment using the same technique, 0.125% SH remained longer on the cornea,[48] suggesting an interspecies difference such as that reported by Saettone.[49] Figure 3 shows the results obtained with rabbits. These results may suggest a viscosity effect, where a more viscous vehicle would be more slowly drained out of the eye. They may also suggest a bioadhesion effect, where a more concentrated solution would establish a greater number of molecular interactions with the lacrimal fluid through the mucin layer in contact with the microvilli of superficial corneal epithelial cells. Either of the two phenomena, or a combination of both, would lead to an increased residence time of SH.

Comparisons of equiviscous solutions of different polymers on ocular retention time have been performed to investigate the above-mentioned viscosity effect. Saettone and co-workers compared five viscous polymeric vehicles for their retention time and for their effect on the bioavailability of tropicamide in humans and in rabbits: carboxymethylcellulose (CMC), low-molecular-weight hydroxypropylcellulose (HPCL), medium-molecular-weight hydroxypropylcellulose (HPCM), polyvinylpyrrolidone (PVP), and polyvinylalcohol (PVA). Their concentrations were adjusted to give equiviscous solutions. All of these vehicles

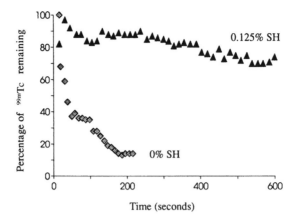

FIGURE 3. Percentage of sodium pertechnetate ^{99m}Tc remaining in the rabbit precorneal area (n = 5). (Reprinted from Gurny, R. et al., *J. Controlled Release*, 6, 367, 1987. With permission.)

increased the bioavailability of the drug, with PVP and PVA being significantly more efficient than the others in humans, but not in rabbits.[49] The increase in bioavailability, therefore, would not be solely due to a viscosity effect, but also to molecular properties of the vehicles, and possibly to physiological parameters, which would explain the interspecies differences in sensitivity to vehicle effect. However, these vehicles have never been compared to SH. Ludwig and Van Ooteghem[14] compared the effect of equiviscous SH and hydroxyethylcellulose (HEC) solutions on the retention of fluorescein in healthy volunteers, and found comparable results with both polymers. However, the experiment was done on only 4 subjects and over a period of 4 min, with an important variability between the subjects. The relative contributions of viscosity and bioadhesion effects to the increased precorneal residence time of SH remains to be established.

Snibson and co-workers[15] used ^{99m}Tc to label SH solutions. Gamma scintigraphy was used to quantify the residence time of 0.2 and 0.3% SH solutions in a group of healthy humans and in a group of patients with keratoconjunctivitis sicca (KCS). Interestingly, the results were different for the two groups: no statistical difference between PBS, 0.2, and 0.3% SH was observed for normal subjects, although SH showed a tendency to increase the precorneal residence time of the tracer. In KCS patients, the residence time was significantly increased by 0.2 and 0.3% SH, with the 0.3% solution remaining longer on the cornea than the 0.2% SH. Figure 4 illustrates these findings. These authors hypothesized that an alteration of tear mucin in dry eyes might modify the interaction of SH with the ocular surface and explain the difference between the two groups.

The effect of SH on precorneal residence time has been investigated for an insert formulation. A matrix of SH was prepared either by casting or by compression and was then applied on rabbit eyes. Fluorescein was incorporated to describe the corneal film obtained. This type of insert formed what the author described as a long-lasting corneal film compared to SH solutions and polyacrylic acid gels.[50] Here, again, an interaction between SH and the tear film can be hypothesized. The existence of a real bioadhesion phenomenon remains to be established.

An indirect way of following the drainage of SH from the ocular surface is to incorporate a drug, such as pilocarpine[51] in a rabbit model, and to monitor the biological response (in this case, miosis). The fact that a vehicle has an increased precorneal residence time does not necessarily imply that an incorporated drug will also have a correspondingly increased biological response. In fact, the rate of diffusion of the drug out of the matrix can be faster

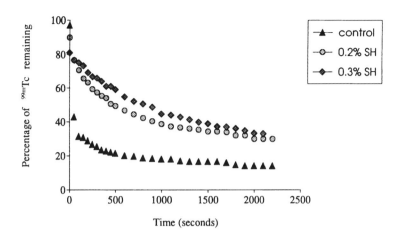

FIGURE 4. Clearance of the test formulations from the ocular surface in dry-eye patients (mean data, n = 12). (Adapted from Snibson, G. R. et al., *Eye* 4, 594, 1990. With permission.)

than the rate of erosion of this matrix. Factors such as the solubility of the drug in water, its diffusion characteristics in the vehicle, and its molecular interactions with the matrix determine its release kinetics. Results for a given drug, therefore, cannot be extrapolated from results obtained with another drug tested in the same matrix. The incorporation of a bioactive tracer to test precorneal residence time will be further discussed in Section III.C.

B. TREATMENT OF DRY EYE

The dry-eye syndrome is associated with a variety of symptoms, from mild ocular discomfort to severe pain, depending on the gravity of the case. In the most severe cases, decreased vision and photophobia can occur. Ultimately, corneal ulceration can occur, threatening the integrity of the eye. Conventional treatment of this condition with artificial tears is not always satisfactory, and the use of SH seems to provide a better and a longer-lasting lubrication of the ocular surface. Many groups have investigated the effect of SH on dry eye, and Table 2 summarizes these studies.

The precorneal tear film is made of a mucin layer, in direct contact with the corneal epithelium. This layer is covered with a watery film, which is externally overlayed with a lipid layer facing the atmosphere. The total structure provides a protection 6.5 μm thick for the corneal epithelium.[52] The dry-eye syndrome occurs when one of the two first components of the tear film is abnormal. Artificial tears can treat this condition by providing a substitution for tears, lubrication, and by preventing the corneal epithelium from drying. However, the question of precorneal residence time is also important in dry-eye therapy. In severe cases, instillation must be performed as frequently as every 10 to 15 min in order to relieve the symptoms when a balanced salt solution is used as medication.[53] Two problems arise from this situation: patient discomfort and side effects due to preservatives which are known to be potentially toxic to the corneal epithelium after repeated instillations. Various tear substitutes having viscous properties are then introduced as they are supposed to increase the corneal residence time: methylcellulose (and other substituted cellulose ethers), polyvinylalcohol, polyvinylpyrrolidone, polyethylene oxide, polysorbate, gelatin, dextran, and SH.[52] The particular feature that distinguishes SH from many of the polymers used in commercial preparations is its non-Newtonian behavior. In fact, SH has a pseudoplastic behavior, and resembles tear mucus glycoprotein in that it has a high viscosity between blinks; it undergoes shear-thinning during each blink.[54] This property provides an increased residence time

TABLE 2
Summary of the Results Obtained with Sodium Hyaluronate
on Dry-Eye Patients

Criteria	References reporting an improvement	References reporting no improvement
Subjective		
Pain	52, 57, 61	
Itching and burning	54, 59, 60	
Foreign body sensation	54, 59	60
Photophobia	59	
Objective		
Vision	52	
Inflammation	52	
Keratitis	60	
Tear meniscus		54, 60
Tear production (Schirmer's test)		54, 59, 60, 61
Tear break-up time	54, 61, 62	59, 60
Tear-film osmolality	61	
Filaments		60
Mucus strand formation	54, 60	
Rose-bengal or fluorescein staining of conjunctiva and/or cornea	54, 57, 59, 61, 62	
Impression cytology of conjunctiva	59	61

combined with an acceptable comfort.[52] As a consequence of these properties, a number of clinical studies have been performed to evaluate the efficacy of SH to relieve patients suffering from dry eye.

Polack[53] reported a decrease of pain and ocular redness, and an improvement of vision in a group of 20 patients (uncontrolled study) after instillation of a 0.1% solution of SH. In this study, SH was found to coat the corneal surface for at least 1 h in most patients. De Luise and Peterson[55] recorded subjective and objective improvement in 26 of 28 patients treated with 0.1% SH in an uncontrolled study. Tabatabay[56,57] has reported that cases of severe xerophthalmy greatly improved by either 0.1 or 0.9% SH after failure of conventional therapy. Stuart and Linn[58] treated 14 dry-eye patients with 0.1% SH and recorded subjective improvement in 13 of them. No adverse effects were seen in 6 patients using SH continuously for over 1 year, and for 1 patient using it for over 2 years. Limberg and co-workers[59] performed a crossover study on 20 KCS patients to compare 4 solutions, including 0.1% SH. The four solutions were effective in the treatment of dry eye, and none of them were preferred over the others by the majority of the patients. However, moderate KCS patients tended to prefer SH or polyvinylalcohol solutions, whereas severe KCS patients preferred a chondroitin sulfate solution or a mixture of chondroitin sulfate and SH. Orsoni and co-workers[60] treated 11 dry-eye patients with SH and performed impression cytology of the conjunctiva. They found an improvement in the morphology of conjunctival cells after 30 d of treatment. Laflamme and Swieca[61] found a significant reduction in keratitis and mucus strands, as well as in burning and irritation in 12 severe dry-eye patients treated with preservative-free 0.1% SH and 1.4% PVA in a crossover study. Nelson and Farris[62] treated 35 patients with moderate KCS with either preservative-free 0.1% SH or 1.4% PVA with 0.5% chlorobutanol in a randomized study. The following parameters were studied: pain/ discomfort, tear film osmolality, Schirmer's test values, tear breakup time, rose bengal staining scores, and bulbar and palpebral cytology grades. They found no intergroup differences for all those parameters, but a significant mean percentage of change from baseline, except for cytology grades. Both preparations were effective. A double-blind clinical trial was performed by Sand and co-workers[63] on 20 KCS patients who received 0.1 and 0.2% SH, and placebo in a crossover design. Rose bengal staining of the cornea was lower and tear breakup time was longer for the 0.2% SH solution compared with the placebo. No significant difference was observed between the 0.1% SH solution and the placebo. Scanning electron microscopy studies were performed to understand the interaction between corneal epithelium and hyaluronic acid. Hazlett and Barrett[64] applied 0.1% SH on eyes of adult and pup mice, and they observed the corneal epithelium up to 60 min after application. Adult mice present a preocular mucus coat, whereas pup mice lack morphologically detectable mucus on the corneal surface. The latter may facilitate the study of the mucus-deficient eye. The eyes of both adult and pup mice revealed, at all observation times (up to 60 min), a 0.5 mm thick filamentous material covering the cornea and regionally associated with epithelial cell microvilli, the distribution becoming patchy with time. Their study shows that SH remains on the ocular surface of both adult and pup mice for at least 60 min. Another study using chick embryo corneal epithelium showed that SH (0.1 and 1%) has no toxic effects on these cells, and that the architecture of the cells and the morphology of the microvilli are well preserved. Moreover, SH had a protective effect against the damage caused by benzalkonium chloride.[65]

The interest in using SH in dry-eye therapy has been well established. A large majority of patients experience a subjective improvement of their condition from this therapy, and no side effects have been observed up to now. Good compliance can therefore be expected. Further studies need to be done to investigate the stability of SH in the presence of the usual preservatives used in ocular drug formulations. The studies on precorneal residence time and the use of SH in dry eye therapy showed that solutions of this product remain on the corneal surface longer than balanced salt solutions. It was then hypothesized that SH could be used as a vehicle for ocular drugs in order to increase the duration of their effect. This topic is discussed in the following section.

C. USE AS A VEHICLE FOR CONTROLLED DRUG DELIVERY

The potential benefit of new vehicles for controlled ocular drug administration can be evaluated by incorporating a drug into the tested vehicle and directly measuring the biological effect obtained. The capacity of SH to prolong the release of a drug by increasing its precorneal residence time has been investigated, mostly in rabbits, for some of the most commonly used ophthalmic drugs. Many ophthalmic drugs affect the iris. The resulting miosis or mydriasis have, in several studies, been used to evaluate the drug bioavailability from various ophthalmic preparations.[51,66,67]

Camber and Edman[13] reported a miotic response study in rabbits using 2% pilocarpine-HCl in solutions of SH at different concentrations (M.W. 4.6×10^6). Table 3 shows their results. A significant increase in the miotic response (t-test on independent observations, $p < 0.05$) is seen when comparing solutions with and without SH. The same statement holds for preparations with 0.075 and 0.1% SH. Similar results have been reported by Gurny and co-workers,[48] supporting the assumption that the SH concentration is critical for the effect of SH on the duration of the miotic response induced by pilocarpine. Above 0.1% and up to 0.25% SH, the influence on the miotic response is rather constant. Higher concentrations of SH increase the drug bioavailability even more. However, these vehicles, owing to their high viscosity, would probably interfere with vision, which would render them unfavorable for use during waking hours. The effect of the molecular weight of SH on the miotic response induced by pilocarpine-HCl is presented in Table 4.[13] The miotic response observed with

TABLE 3

**Analysis of Miotic Response Curves for 2%
Pilocarpine-HCl Formulations**

Formulations	I_{max}[a]	Duration[b] > 10%	AUC[c] S.D.[d]	Relative AUC	N
H_2O	25	120	2538 (441)	1	6
0.075% SH	27	160	3400 (686)	1.34	6
0.100% SH	32	194	4628 (955)	1.82	6
0.125% SH	31	194	4492 (1004)	1.77	6
0.250% SH	33	200	5072 (1230)	2.00	6

[a] Maximal change in pupil diameter, in percent of the initial pupil diameter.
[b] Time when the pupil size differs more than 10% from its normal size (min).
[c] Area under miosis-time curve (%·min^{-1}).
[d] Standard deviation of the mean.

TABLE 4

**Influence of Molecular Weight of Solution Hyaluronate on
Miotic Effect of 2% Pilocarpine-HCl**

Molecular weight	Concentration of sodium hyaluronate			
	0.125%	0.25%	0.50%	0.75%
0.6×10^6	2640[a] (404)[b]	3539 (750)	3900 (906)	3990 (857)
1.6×10^6	3246 (612)	4182 (955)	4304 (963)	4460 (882)
4.6×10^6	4492 (1004)	5072 (1230)	—	—

[a] Area under the miosis-time curve (%·min^{-1}).
[b] Standard deviation of the mean.

the pilocarpine solution containing sodium hyaluronate (0.125%) with a M_r of 0.6×10^6 Da was similar to that observed with an aqueous solution.

Statistical analysis (t-test for independent observations) indicates that the influence of molecular weight of SH on the miotic effect of pilocarpine may be seen at lower concentrations of SH. At 0.125% SH, a significant increase ($p < 0.05$) was observed for samples of M_r of 4.6×10^6 Da over those of a M_r of 1.6×10^6 Da. No difference was seen between SH of M_r 0.6×10^6 Da and 1.6×10^6 Da. A possible explanation for the observed increase in bioavailability may be the differences in the rheological properties influencing the persistence of the SH vehicle in the eye.

The decreased drainage and the increased miotic response seen in the presence of SH would thus suggest that SH may raise the pilocarpine concentrations in the ocular tissues. This was investigated in a study where 25 µl of 1% ^{3}H-pilocarpine-HCl in 0.125% SH or buffer were administered to rabbit eyes. The amount of drug in the cornea and in the aqueous humor was nearly doubled, 30 min and 1 h post instillation, when the SH vehicle was used.[13]

The above-mentioned studies on rabbits show that the addition of SH (0.125%, $M_r > 3 \times 10^6$ Da) to an aqueous pilocarpine solution gives: (1) a twofold increase of pilocarpine concentration in cornea and aqueous humor, and (2) an increase in the miotic response as can be inferred from the area under the miosis time curve (AUC) and the duration of the effect.

The viscosity of a SH solution is a function of concentration and molecular weight. The effective SH concentrations leading to a prolonged miotic effect of pilocarpine are in the range of 0.075 to 0.1%. Although the bioavailability increases with increasing viscosity of the hyaluronate solution, there is an additional effect of the molecular weight. This suggests that other physicochemical properties of sodium hyaluronate are presumably of importance for the ocular bioavailability.[13]

The effect of SH on the mydriatic activity of tropicamide has also been investigated. Since tropicamide is less watersoluble than pilocarpine, it was hypothesized that less diffusion out of the vehicle would occur. Saettone and co-workers[50] found that SH solutions and compressed matrices had a bioavailability-enhancing effect for both pilocarpine and tropicamide, this effect being more important for tropicamide. Drugs of selected optimal physicochemical properties, i.e., reduced solubility and/or diffusivity, may therefore benefit most from the prolonged residence time offered by viscous vehicles.

The capacity of SH to increase the precorneal residence time of gentamicin sulfate (GS) in male volunteers has recently been under investigation (Bernatchez, Tabatabay, and Gurny, unpublished results). GS (0.5%) was incorporated into a 0.25% SH solution (GS-SH), and this preparation was compared to the same concentration of GS in a phosphate buffer solution (GS-PBS). Each volunteer received 25 μl of GS-PBS in the left eye and 25 μl of GS-SH in the right eye. Lacrimal fluid was sampled using a 1-μl capillary before instillation, and at 5, 10, 20, and 40 min after instillation. The concentration of GS was determined by radioimmunoassay. We observed a significantly higher concentration of GS in SH-treated eyes at 5 min ($p <0.01$) and 10 min ($p <0.05$), and a similar, but not statistically significant trend at 20 min (n = 9). At 40 min, similar concentrations of GS remained in both eyes, except for one subject who still benefited from the SH treatment (n = 8). Figure 5 illustrates these findings. These results suggest that SH increased GS bioavailability on the ocular surface, resulting in higher concentrations for at least 10 min after instillation. Severe cases of bacterial corneal ulcers requiring frequent instillations could benefit from such a treatment. Frequent instillation would probably still be necessary, but a higher concentration of GS could induce a faster healing of the infection. This hypothesis remains to be tested in a corneal bacterial ulcer model, and in patients suffering from infected corneal ulcers. It is also possible that an increased concentration may lead to a deeper corneal penetration of GS, with more GS eventually reaching the aqueous humor. This will also have to be tested on corneal bacterial ulcers, since topically applied GS seldom reaches the aqueous humor in the healthy eye.[68]

In summary, SH is a nonimmunogenic glycosaminoglycan having a broad spectrum of applications in wound healing and drug delivery. SH has several uses in ophthalmic therapy, such as protecting corneal endothelial cells during intraocular surgery, replacing vitreous humor, acting as a tear substitute in the treatment of dry eye, and increasing the precorneal residence time of various drugs. This latter use is still the subject of experimentation, and it is worth noting that the use of vehicles that increase residence time in ocular drug delivery and subsequently the drug bioavailability has so far been investigated mainly in rabbits. However, this species proved to be less sensitive than humans to increases in vehicle viscosity.[12,69] Care should therefore be taken when a rabbit model is used to test the effect of SH on the precorneal residence time of a drug, since concentrations which may be efficient in humans could have no pronounced effect in rabbits. Another point to be mentioned is the lack of data concerning the molecular weight and viscosity of the SH that has been used in most of the published work. It is hoped that a more complete characterization of the innovative formulations will be available in the near future.

Methods for the preparation of purified SH from bacterial cultures have been reported. For example, SH isolated from streptococci has been used in the routine determination of antistreptococcal hyaluronidase in human serum samples.[70] SH can also be prepared from uridine 5'-diphosphoglucuronic acid and uridine 5'-diphospho N-acetyl glucosamine, the

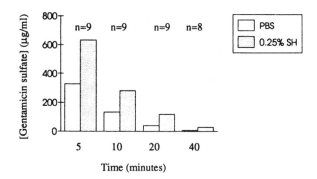

FIGURE 5.   Concentration of gentamicin sulfate (GS) in human tear samples. Instillation of 25 μl of 0.5% GS in a phosphate buffer solution (PBS) or in a 0.25% SH solution (unpublished data).

polymerization reaction being initiated by the addition of a streptococcal membrane suspension.[71] Therefore, it will be worthwhile to extensively characterize the hyaluronic acid from such sources to determine if it can be used safely in human therapy, and if the same advantageous physicochemical characteristics are retained (molecular weight and viscosity). The cost of SH may then be lowered. Further research on bacterial sources, genetic engineering, and laboratory synthesis of SH, although these sources until now lead to a low molecular weight product, should be strongly encouraged, given the high interest in this product for ocular therapy, as well as in many fields of biomedical therapy.

REFERENCES

1. **Balazs, E. A. and Band, P.,** Hyaluronic acid: its structure and use, *Cosmet. Toiletries,* 99, 65, 1984.
2. **Balazs, E. A.,** Ultrapure hyaluronic acid and the use thereof, U.S. Patent 4,141,973, 1979.
3. **Denlinger, J. L. and Balazs, E. A.,** Replacement of the liquid vitreous with sodium hyaluronate in monkeys. I. Short-term evaluation, *Exp. Eye Res.,* 31, 81, 1980.
4. **Goldberg, R. L. and Rubin, A. S.,** Serum hyaluronate as a marker for disease severity in the Lactobacillus casei model of arthritis in the rat, *J. Rheumatol.,* 16, 92, 1989.
5. **Smedegard, G., Björk, J., Kleinau, S., and Tengblad, A.,** Serum hyaluronate levels reflect disease activity in experimental arthritis models, *Agents Actions,* 27, 356, 1989.
6. **Doillon, C. J. and Silver, F. H.,** Collagen-based wound dressing: effects of hyaluronic acid and fibronectin on wound healing, *Biomaterials,* 7, 3, 1986.
7. **Morimoto, K., Yamaguchi, H., Iwakura, Y., Morisaka, K., Ohashi, Y., and Nakai, Y.,** Effects of viscous hyaluronate-sodium solutions on the nasal absorption of vasopressin and an analogue, *Pharm. Res.,* 8, 471, 1991.
8. **Hunt, J. A., Joshi, H. N., Stella, V. J., and Topp, E. M.,** Diffusion and drug release in polymer films prepared from ester derivatives of hyaluronic acid, *J. Controlled Release,* 12, 159, 1990.
9. **Benedetti, L. M., Topp, E. M., and Stella, V. J.,** Microspheres of hyaluronic acid esters — fabrication methods and in vitro hydrocortisone release, *J. Controlled Release,* 13, 33, 1990.
10. **Benson, H. and Alto, P.,** Permeability of the cornea to topically applied drugs, *Arch. Ophthalmol.,* 91, 313, 1974.
11. **Lee, V. H. L. and Robinson, J. R.,** Review: topical ocular drug delivery: recent developments and future challenges, *J. Ocular Pharmacol.,* 2, 67, 1986.
12. **Saettone, M. F., Giannaccini, B., Barattini, F., and Tellini, N.,** The validity of rabbits for investigations on ophthalmic vehicles: a comparison of four different vehicles containing tropicamide in humans and rabbits, *Pharm. Acta Helv.,* 57, 47, 1982.
13. **Camber, O. and Edman, P.,** Sodium hyaluronate as an ophthalmic vehicle: some factors governing the effect of pilocarpine in rabbits, *Curr. Eye Res.,* 8, 563, 1989.

14. **Ludwig, A. and Van Ooteghem, M.,** Evaluation of sodium hyaluronate as viscous vehicle for eye drops, *J. Pharm. Belg.,* 44, 391, 1989.
15. **Snibson, G. R., Greaves, J. L., Soper, N. D. W., Prydal, J. I., Wilson, C. G., and Bron, A. J.,** Precorneal residence times of sodium hyaluronate solutions studied by quantitative gamma scintigraphy, *Eye,* 4, 594, 1990.
16. **Gurny, R., Ryser, J. E., Tabatabay, C., Martenet, M., Edman, P., and Camber, O.,** Precorneal residence time in humans of sodium hyaluronate as measured by gamma scintigraphy, *Albrecht von Graefes Arch. Klin. Exp. Ophthalmol.,* 228, 510, 1990.
17. **Keller, N., More, D., Carper, D., and Longwell, A.,** Increased corneal permeability induced by the dual effects of transient tear film acidification and exposure to benzalkonium chloride, *Exp. Eye Res.,* 30, 203, 1980.
18. **Burstein, N. L.,** Preservative alteration of corneal permeability in humans and rabbits, *Invest. Ophthalmol. Vis. Sci.,* 25, 1453, 1984.
19. **Lee, V. H. L.,** Mechanisms and facilitation of corneal drug penetration, *J. Controlled Release,* 11, 79, 1990.
20. **Kay, J. S., Litin, B. S., Woolfenden, J. M., Chvapil, M., and Herschler, J.,** Delivery of antifibroblast agents as adjuncts to filtration surgery. Part I — Periocular clearance of cobalt-57 bleomycin in experimental drug delivery: pilot study in the rabbit, *Ophthalmic Surg.,* 17, 626, 1986.
21. **Meyer, K. and Palmer, J. W.,** The polysaccharide of the vitreous humor, *J. Biol. Chem.,* 107, 629, 1934.
22. **Laurent, T. C.,** Structure of hyaluronic acid, in *Chemistry and Molecular Biology of the Intercellular Matrix,* Vol. 2, Balazs, E. A., Ed., Academic Press, London, 1970.
23. **Balazs, E. A.,** Amino sugar-containing macromolecules in the tissues of the eye and the ear, in *The Amino Sugars: The Chemistry and Biology of Compounds Containing Amino Sugars. II A. Distribution and Biological Role,* Balazs, E. A. and Jeanloz, R. W., Eds., Academic Press, New York, 1965.
24. **Balazs, E. A.,** Sodium hyaluronate and viscosurgery, in *Healon (Sodium Hyaluronate),* Miller, D. and Stegmann, R., Eds., John Wiley & Sons, New York, 1983.
25. **Laurent, U. B. G. and Laurent, T. C.,** Catabolic fate of hyaluronan in the organism, in *Viscoelastic Materials, Basic Science and Clinical Applications,* Rosen, E. S., Ed., Pergamon Press, New York, 1989.
26. **Prehm, P.,** Hyaluronate is synthesized at plasma membranes, *Biochem. J.,* 220, 597, 1984.
27. **Weissmann, B. and Meyer, K.,** The structure of hyalubiuronic acid and of hyaluronic acid from umbilical cord, *J. Am. Chem. Soc.,* 76, 1753, 1954.
28. **Bothner-Wik, H.,** Rheological studies of sodium hyaluronate in pharmaceutical preparations, Ph.D. thesis, University of Uppsala, Sweden, 1991.
29. **Bothner, H. and Wik, O.,** Rheology of intraocular solutions, in *Viscoelastic Materials, Basic Science and Clinical Applications,* Rosen, E .S., Ed., Pergamon Press, New York, 1989.
30. **Balazs, E. A. and Denlinger, J. L.,** Clinical uses of hyaluronan, in *The Biology of Hyaluronan,* Evered, D. and Whelan, J., Eds., Wiley, Chichester, 1989.
31. **Balazs, E. A., Miller, D., and Stegmann, R.,** Viscosurgery and the use of Na-hyaluronate in intraocular lens implantation, paper presented at the Int. Congr. Intraocular Implantation, Cannes, France, 1979.
32. **Gibbs, D. A., Merrill, E. W., Smith, K. A., and Balazs, E. A.,** Rheology of hyaluronic acid, *Biopolymers,* 6, 777, 1968.
33. **Graue, E. L., Polack, F. M., and Balazs, E. A.,** The protective effect of Na-hyaluronate to corneal endothelium, *Exp. Eye Res.,* 31, 119, 1980.
34. **Norn, M. S.,** Peroperative protection of cornea and conjunctiva, *Acta Ophthalmol.,* 59, 587, 1981.
35. **Polack, F. M.,** Healon®(Na Hyaluronate). A review of the literature, *Cornea,* 5, 81, 1986.
36. **Madsen, K., Schenholm, M., Jahnke, G., and Tengblad, A.,** Hyaluronate binding to intact corneas and cultured endothelial cells, *Invest. Ophthalmol. Vis. Sci.,* 30, 2132, 1989.
37. **Fitzsimmons, T., Fagerholm, P., Schenholm, M., and Härfstrand, A.,** Hyaluronic acid in the rabbit cornea after superficial keratectomy with the excimer laser, *Invest. Ophthalmol. Vis. Sci. Suppl.,* 32, 1247, 1991.
38. **Sugiyama, T., Miyauchi, S., Machida, A., Miyazaki, K., Tokuyasu, K., and Nakazawa, K.,** The effect of sodium hyaluronate on the migration of rabbit corneal epithelium. II. The effect of topical administration, *J. Ocular Pharmacol.,* 7, 53, 1991.
39. **Pape, L. G. and Balazs, E. A.,** The use of sodium hyaluronate (Healon®) in human anterior segment surgery, *Opthalmology,* 87, 699, 1980.
40. **Liebmann, J. M., Ritch, R., DiSclafani, M., and Stock, L.,** Early intraocular pressure rise after trabeculectomy, *Arch. Ophthalmol.,* 108, 1549, 1990.
41. **Percival, S. P. B.,** Complications from use of sodium hyaluronate (Healonid) in anterior segment surgery, *Br. J. Ophthalmol.,* 66, 714, 1982.
42. **Alpar, J. J.,** Sodium hyaluronate (Healon®) in glaucoma filtering procedures, *Ophthalmic Surg.,* 17, 724, 1986.

43. **Hung, S. O.,** Role of sodium hyaluronate (Healonid) in triangular flap trabeculectomy, *Br. J. Ophthalmol.,* 69, 46, 1985.
44. **Wilson, R. P. and Lloyd, J.,** The place of sodium hyaluronate in glaucoma surgery, *Ophthalmic Surg.,* 17, 30, 1986.
45. **Blondeau, P.,** Sodium hyaluronate in trabeculectomy: a retrospective study, *Can. J. Ophthalmol.,* 19, 306, 1984.
46. **Raitta, C. and Setälä, K.,** Trabeculectomy with the use of sodium hyaluronate. A prospective study, *Acta Ophthalmol.,* 64, 407, 1986.
47. **Hein, S. R., Keates, R. H., and Weber, P. A.,** Elimination of sodium hyaluronate-induced decrease in outflow facility with hyaluronidase, *Opthalmic Surg.,* 17, 731, 1986.
48. **Gurny, R., Ibrahim, H., Aebi, A., Buri, P., Wilson, C. G., and Washington, N.,** Design and evaluation of controlled release systems for the eye, *J. Controlled Release,* 6, 367, 1987.
49. **Saettone, M. F., Giannaccini, B., Ravecca, S., La Marca, F., and Tota, G.,** Polymer effects on ocular bioavailability — the influence of different liquid vehicles on the mydriatic response of tropicamide in humans and in rabbits, *Int. J. Pharm.,* 20, 187, 1984.
50. **Saettone, M. F., Chetoni, P., Torracca, M. T., Burgalassi, S., and Giannaccini, B.,** Evaluation of muco-adhesive properties and in vivo activity of ophthalmic vehicles based on hyaluronic acid, *Int. J. Pharm.,* 51, 203, 1989.
51. **Camber, O., Edman, P., and Gurny, R.,** Influence of sodium hyaluronate on the miotic effect of pilocarpine in rabbits, *Curr. Eye Res.,* 6, 779, 1987.
52. **Bron, A. J.,** Prospects for the dry eye, *Trans. Ophthalmol. Soc. U.K.,* 104, 801, 1985.
53. **Polack, F. M. and McNiece, M. T.,** The treatment of dry eyes with Na hyaluronate (Healon), *Cornea,* 1, 133, 1982.
54. **Camber, O. and Lundgren, P.,** Diffusion of some low molecular weight compounds in sodium hyaluronate, *Acta Pharm. Suec.,* 22, 315, 1985.
55. **De Luise, V. P. and Peterson, W. S.,** The use of topical Healon tears in the management of refractory dry-eye syndrome, *Ann. Ophthalmol.,* 16, 823, 1984.
56. **Tabatabay, C.,** Utilisation du Healon lors d'épithélialisation cornéenne défectueuse, *J. Fr. Ophthalmol.,* 7, 755, 1984.
57. **Tabatabay, C.** Instillation d'acide hyaluronique à 0.1% lors de kératite sèche sévère, *J. Fr. Ophthalmol.,* 8, 513, 1985.
58. **Stuart, J. C. and Linn, J. G.,** Dilute sodium hyaluronate (Healon) in the treatment of ocular surface disorders, *Ann. Ophthalmol.,* 17, 190, 1985.
59. **Limberg, M. B., McCaa, C., Kissling, G. E., and Kaufman, H. E.,** Topical application of hyaluronic acid and chondroitin sulfate in the treatment of dry eyes, *Am. J. Ophthalmol.,* 103, 194, 1987.
60. **Orsoni, J. G., Chiari, M., Guazzi, A., De Carli, M., and Guidolin, D.,** Efficacité de l'acide hyaluronique en collyre dans le traitment de l'oeil sec, *Ophtalmologie,* 2, 355, 1988.
61. **Laflamme, M. Y. and Swieca, R.** A comparative study of two preservative-free tear substitutes in the management of severe dry eye, *Can. J. Ophthalmol.,* 23, 174, 1988.
62. **Nelson, J. D. and Farris, R. L.,** Sodium hyaluronate and polyvinyl alcohol artificial tear preparations, *Arch. Ophthalmol.,* 106, 484, 1988.
63. **Sand, B. B., Marner, K., and Norn, M. S.,** Sodium hyaluronate in the treatment of keratoconjunctivitis sicca, *Acta Ophthalmol.,* 67, 181, 1989.
64. **Hazlett, L. D. and Barrett, R.,** Sodium hyaluronate eye drop. A scanning and transmission electron microscopy study of the corneal surface, *Ophthalmic Res.,* 19, 277, 1987.
65. **Wysenbeek, Y. S., Loya, N., and Ben Sira, I.,** The effect of sodium hyaluronate on the corneal epithelium. An ultrastructural study, *Invest. Ophthalmol. Vis. Sci.,* 29, 194, 1988.
66. **Chrai, S. and Robinson, J. R.,** Ocular evaluation of methyl-cellulose vehicle in albino rabbits, *J. Pharm. Sci.,* 63, 1218, 1974.
67. **Gurny, R.,** Preliminary study of prolonged acting drug delivery for the treatment or glaucoma, *Pharm. Acta Helv.,* 56, 130, 1981.
68. **Ellerhorst, B., Golden, B., and Jarudi, N.,** Ocular penetration of topically applied gentamicin, *Arch. Ophthalmol.,* 93, 371, 1975.
69. **Zaki, I., Fitzgerald, P., Hardy, J. G., and Wilson, C. G.,** A comparison of the effect of viscosity on the precorneal residence time of solutions in rabbit and man, *J. Pharm. Pharmacol.,* 38, 463, 1986.
70. **Kjems, E. and Lebech, K.,** Isolation of hyaluronic acid from cultures of Streptococci in a chemically defined medium, *Acta Pathol. Microbiol. Scand.,* B84, 162, 1976.
71. **Simon, E. S., Toone, E. J., Ostroff, G., Bednarski, M. D., and Whitesides, G. M.,** Preparation of cytidine 5'-monophospho-N-acetylneuraminic acid and uridine 5'-diphosphoglucuronic acid; syntheses of alpha-2,6-sialyllactosamine, alpha-2, 6-sialyllactose, and hyaluronic acid, in *Methods in Enzymology, Complex Carbohydrates,* Part F, Ginsburg, V., Ed., Academic Press, New York, 1989, 275.

Chapter 8

IMPROVED OCULAR DRUG DELIVERY BY USE OF CHEMICAL MODIFICATION (PRODRUGS)

Vincent H. L. Lee

TABLE OF CONTENTS

I.   Introduction 122

II.   Applications of Prodrugs in Ophthalmic Drug Delivery 122
      A.   Improvement of Corneal Drug Penetration 122
      B.   Prolongation of Duration of Action 125
      C.   Reduction of Systemic Absorption 125
      D.   Reduction of Ocular Side Effects 128

III. Functional Groups Amenable to Prodrug Derivatization 129

IV.   Enzymes Involved in the Activation of Prodrugs 130

V.   Physicochemical Considerations in the Design of Prodrugs 131
      A.   Lipophilicity 132
      B.   Aqueous Solubility 133
      C.   Chemical Stability 134

VI.   Formulation Considerations 136

VII. Toxicity Considerations 136

VIII. Conclusions 137

Acknowledgments 137

References 137

0-8493-7296-8/93/$0.00 + $.50
© 1993 by CRC Press, Inc.

I. INTRODUCTION

Prodrugs are bioreversible derivatives of drugs with the potential to alter absorption, decrease side effects, or prolong duration of action.[1] Inactive as such, prodrugs must be converted either enzymatically or nonenzymatically to their parent drugs in the body for expression of pharmacological activity (Scheme 1). Steroids were perhaps the first class of ophthalmic drugs to which the prodrug principle was applied. The aim then was to enhance corneal absorption or aqueous solubility.[2] The concept of prodrugs was not formalized in ophthalmology until the introduction of dipivefrin for improvement of corneal penetration of epinephrine in the late 1970s.[3] Since then, several other ophthalmic drugs have been investigated for prodrug derivatization; they are timolol,[4-10] nadolol,[11] pilocarpine,[12-15] $PGF_{2\alpha}$,[16-20] phenylephrine,[21-24] terbutaline,[25,26] L-643,799 (a carbonic anhydrase inhibitor),[27,28] acyclovir,[29] vidarabine,[30] and idoxuridine.[31,32] So far, this approach has been investigated both preclinically and clinically with nadolol only.

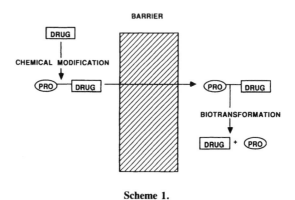

Scheme 1.

The purpose of this chapter is to review the following aspects of prodrugs in ophthalmic drug delivery: (1) applications, (2) functional groups amenable to prodrug derivatization, (3) enzymes involved in the activation of prodrugs, (4) physicochemical considerations, (5) formulation considerations, and (6) toxicity considerations.

II. APPLICATIONS OF PRODRUGS IN OPHTHALMIC DRUG DELIVERY

Prodrugs may improve ophthalmic drug delivery in several ways: (1) by enhancing corneal drug penetration, (2) by prolonging duration of action, (3) by reducing systemic side effects, or (4) by reducing ocular side effects.

A. IMPROVEMENT OF CORNEAL DRUG PENETRATION

The main application of prodrugs in ophthalmology is to enhance corneal drug penetration. Corneal drug penetration is usually poor due to a mismatch of the physicochemical properties of the drug with those of the cornea. The difficulty is largely due to the fact that all of the existing ophthalmic drugs, which were originally developed for systemic use, lack the physicochemical properties to overcome the resistance to penetration offered by the top two layers of the corneal epithelium.[33]

Because of its important role in limiting corneal drug penetration, compromising the integrity of the corneal epithelium should lead to improved corneal drug penetration. Except for very lipophilic drugs, e.g., prednisolone acetate,[34] fluorometholone,[34] and betaxolol,[33] there is usually a minimum of a twofold increase in the extent of corneal penetration when the corneal epithelial barrier is absent. The degree of penetration enhancement can be as high as 10- to 30-fold, as is the case for 5-fluorouracil, which penetrates the cornea poorly because of its hydrophilicity [log partition coefficient (PC) = −0.96];[35] 14-fold, as is the case for methionine enkephalin,[36] which penetrates the cornea poorly mainly because of susceptibility to aminopeptidase-mediated hydrolysis;[37] and 60-fold, as is the case for inulin, which penetrates the cornea poorly because of its size (M.W. 5000) and hydrophilicity (PC = 0.00127).[38] The above extent of improvement in drug penetration upon de-epithelializing the cornea is theoretically the upper limit to which corneal drug penetration can be improved by prodrug derivatization.

Two examples will be cited to illustrate the usefulness of prodrugs in enhancing corneal drug penetration: idoxuridine and phenylephrine.

Idoxuridine (5-iodo-2′-deoxyuridine) (1), a halogenated pyrimidine derivative currently indicated in the topical treatment of herpes simplex keratitis, is poorly absorbed into the cornea, resulting in a high incidence of treatment failure unrelated to resistant viral strains.[39] Promising results in corneal penetration were obtained when the 5′-propionyl, butyryl, isobutyryl, valeryl, and pivaloyl ester prodrugs of idoxuridine were administered. Of the 5 prodrugs tested, the 5′-butyryl ester (2) was the best, improving the ocular absorption of idoxuridine about 4 times.[32] Whether improved ocular absorption will increase the therapeutic efficacy of idoxuridine remains to be seen.

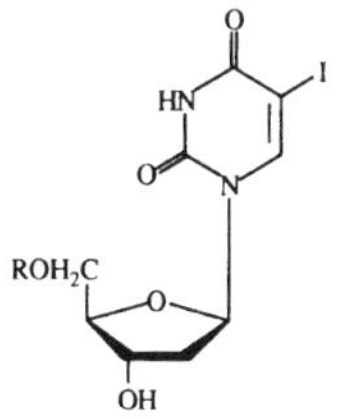

(1) R = H

(2) R = -C- $CH_2CH_2CH_3$
     ‖
     O

Phenylephrine (3) is another drug with poor corneal penetration characteristics that would benefit from prodrug derivatization.[40,41] The therapeutic goal here is to reduce the incidence of systemic side effects of phenylephrine, made possible by reduction in the instilled dose in proportion to the extent in corneal penetration enhancement. The two prodrugs that have been investigated, the pivalate ester (4) and oxazolidine (5) prodrugs, are about ten times more potent than phenylephrine.[21-24]

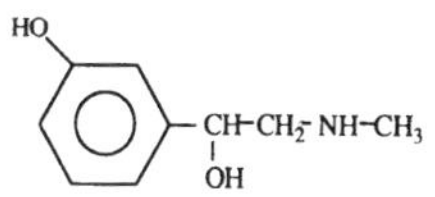

(3) 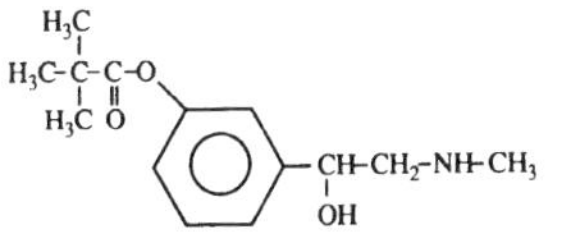   (4) 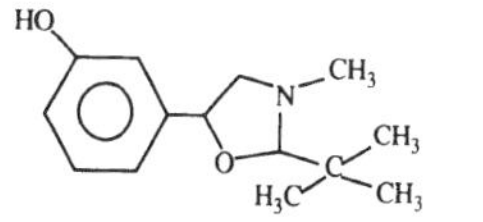   (5)

The increase in potency afforded by the oxazolidine prodrug is consistent with the 1000-fold increase in its partition coefficient.[24] As a result, a ten times lower dose of the oxazolidine prodrug can be used, leading to a 3.5-fold reduction in the systemic absorption of phenylephrine following topical instillation.[42] A similar degree in corneal penetration enhancement was observed *in vitro* when phenylephrine was used in combination with flurbiprofen in a molar ratio of 1:16 (Figure 1).[43] This was attributed partly to the increase in lipophilicity

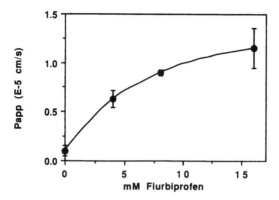

FIGURE 1. Influence of varying concentrations of flurbiprofen on the corneal penetration of 1 mM phenylephrine. Error bars represent the standard deviation for n = 4. (From Ashton, P., Clark, D. S., and Lee, V. H. L., *Curr. Eye Res.*, 11, 85, 1992. With permission.)

of phenylephrine due to ion-pair formation with flurbiprofen, and partly to lowering in the barrier function of the corneal epithelium by flurbiprofen.[43]

The new drugs on the therapeutic horizon that may benefit immensely from prodrug derivatization are the peptide drugs. A major obstacle to their clinical utility is their poor membrane penetration and rapid proteolytic degradation. Theoretically, both problems may be solved by derivatization of peptides to yield lipophilic prodrugs that are capable of protecting the parent peptides against proteolytic degradation. The potential usefulness of such an approach has been reviewed by Bundgaard.[44] The modifications that have been investigated thus far include (1) N-acylation and N-aminomethylation of the N-terminal pyroglutamyl residue in peptides such as thyrotropin-releasing hormone, luteinizing hormone-releasing hormone, and neurotensin (Scheme 2);[45-47] (2) condensation of α-aminoamide moiety with aldehydes or ketones to form 4-imidazolidones (Scheme 3);[48] and (3) condensation of an α-amino acid or an N-acylated amino acid with an aldehyde (N-α-hydroxy-alkylation) to form 5-oxazolidinones (Scheme 4).[49,50] At this early stage of development, only the bioreversibility of the peptide prodrugs and their ability to protect their parent peptides against proteolytic degradation have been investigated. Their effectiveness in enhancing corneal peptide penetration remains to be determined.

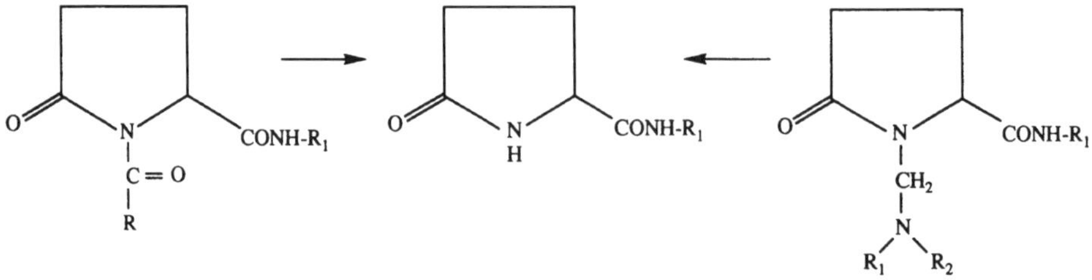

Scheme 2.

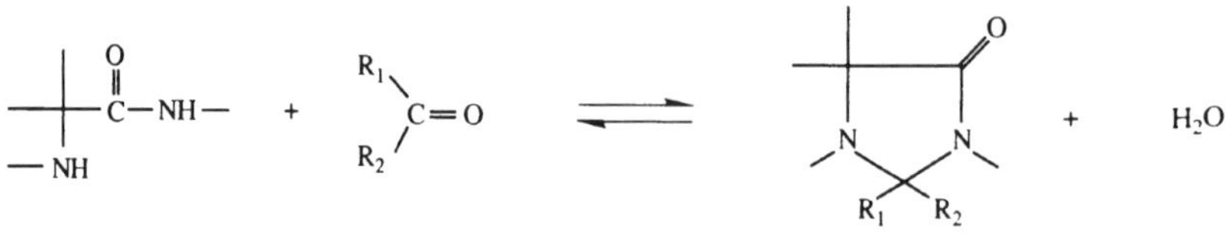

Scheme 3.

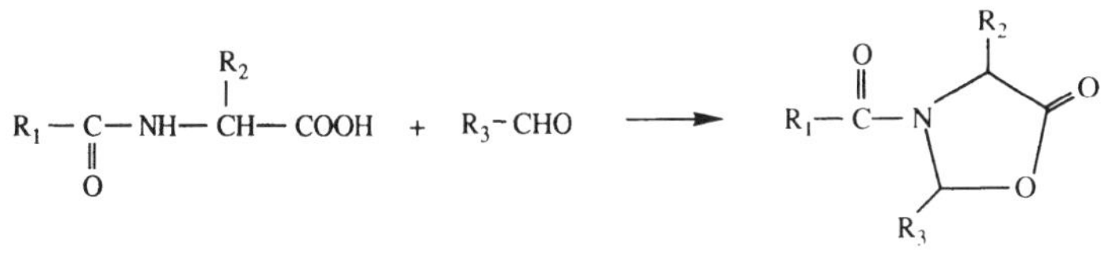

$$R_1 - \underset{\underset{O}{\|}}{C} - NH - \underset{\underset{|}{R_2}}{CH} - COOH \; + \; R_3 - CHO \; \longrightarrow \; R_1 - \underset{\underset{O}{\|}}{C} - N\underset{R_3}{\overset{R_2}{\diagdown}}O$$

Scheme 4.

B. PROLONGATION OF DURATION OF ACTION

Theoretically, the greater lipophilicity of prodrugs probably would result in their enhanced deposit in ocular tissues serving as a depot from which the active parent drug is slowly released. This has been shown to be the case for timolol and pilocarpine prodrugs. For timolol, there is a two- to fourfold increase in its duration of β-adrenergic antagonistic activity in the pigmented rabbit eye following prodrug derivatization.[51] For pilocapine, the factor of increase in its duration of miotic activity in the albino rabbit eye following prodrug administration is 4.5[15] These pilocarpine prodrugs appear to be comparable in effectiveness as the vehicle approaches based on viscous solutions,[52,53] mucoadhesives,[54,55] latices,[56] emulsions,[57-59] and presoaked soft contact lenses.[60]

C. REDUCTION OF SYSTEMIC ABSORPTION

A very powerful application of prodrugs is reduction of systemic side effects of ophthalmic drugs. Systemic absorption of the topically applied dose that has reached the nasal mucosa following solution drainage is an often neglected aspect of ocular drug therapy. This is partly due to the fact that the majority of ophthalmic drugs in use prior to 1978 had wide therapeutic indices, or that the patient population who had suffered from systemic side effects elicited by topically applied ophthalmic drugs was small. This situation changed dramatically when timolol, a potent mixed β_1 and β_2 antagonist, was introduced into glaucoma therapy in 1978. Van Buskirk was the first to caution about the systemic risk associated with its use.[61] In 1986, Nelson et al.[62] reported 450 cases of serious systemic side effects elicited by timolol, of which 32 resulted in patient deaths. As many as 23% of the patients experienced their adverse event on the first day of timolol therapy, and 33% did so within the first week.[62] The incidence of side effects is not as well documented for the other β-blockers in clinical use, namely, betaxolol, levobunolol, and carteolol. A recent study by Phan et al.[63] revealed that, following twice a day dosing of these three β-blockers for 10 d in albino rabbits, 3 to 29 times and at least 6 times the drug concentrations required for β_1 blockade were achieved in the plasma at 1 and 12 h after the last dose, respectively (Table 1). Other drugs known to be absorbed systemically from topical dosing, thereby eliciting systemic side effects, include epinephrine,[64] dipivalyl epinephrine,[64] terbutaline,[25] phenylephrine,[65] oxymetazoline,[66] clonidine,[67] pilocarpine,[68] hydrocortisone,[69] flurbiprofen,[70] tetrahydrocannabinol,[71] and cyclosporine,[72]

Restricting entry of a topically applied ophthalmic dose into the nasal cavity is an obvious approach to reduce the extent of systemic absorption of topically applied ophthalmic drugs. This objective can be achieved by (1) nasolacrimal occlusion for 5 min, with or without eyelid closure;[73,74] (2) making changes in vehicle composition, e.g., incorporation of polymers,[75,76] alteration in solution pH and tonicity,[75] and adjustment of preservative concentration (Figure 2);[75] (3) changing vehicle type;[77,78] and (4) reducing instilled volume.[75] Other means of reducing systemic drug absorption include coadminstration with low doses of vasoconstrictors, e.g., phenylephrine and epinephrine,[76,77,79] and selecting a dosing time that minimizes systemic absorption while maximizing ocular drug absorption (Figure 3).[80-83] The effectiveness of the above approaches has been reviewed.[84] Because the majority of the above approaches aim primarily at the nasal mucosa (the main site of systemic drug

TABLE 1
Peak (1 h) and Trough (12 h) Drug Concentrations
Following Topical Drop Instillation of Various
β-Adrenergic Antagonists

Drug	Plasma drug concentrations (ng/ml)			
	1 h		**12 h**	
Levobunolol	1.60 ± 0.16	(14.10)[a]	0.66 ± 0.19	(5.82)
Carteolol	8.00 ± 0.60	(29.22)	1.61 ± 0.54	(5.88)
Timolol	9.89 ± 2.42	(12.00)	0.94 ± 0.12	(1.11)
Betaxolol	22.28 ± 1.54	(3.08)	9.43 ± 1.68	(1.30)

[a] Mean ± s.e.m. Figure in parentheses denotes drug concentration ratio
     relative to β₁-adrenergic blockade.

From Phan, T.-M. M., Nguyen, K. P. V., Giacomini, J. C., and Lee,
D. A., *J. Ocular Pharmacol.*, 7, 243, 1991. With permission.

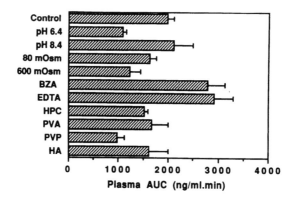

FIGURE 2.   Formulation influence on the extent of systemic timolol absorption following the topical instillation
of 25 µl of various 15 m*M* timolol maleate solutions in pigmented rabbits. The area under plasma concentration-
time curve serves as an index for the extent of systemic absorption. Error bars represent standard error of the mean.
About 4 to 6 rabbits were used per condition. Key: BZA, benzalkonium chloride; EDTA, ethylenediaminetetraacetic
acid; HPC, hydroxypropylcellulose; PVA, polyvinylalcohol; PVP, polyvinylpyrrolidone; HA, hyaluronic acid.
(From Podder, K., Moy, K. C., and Lee, V. H. L., *Exp. Eye Res.*, 54, 747, 1992. With permission.)

absorption) rather than at the conjunctival sac, reduction in systemic drug absorption may
not necessarily lead to enhanced corneal drug absorption. This has been found to be the
case when epinephrine was coadministered with timolol to reduce the systemic absorption
of timolol.[77]

Designing ophthalmic drugs that are poorly absorbed into the bloodstream[85] using the
prodrug approach is yet another approach that may be considered. The first hint that prodrugs
may be effective in this regard was indicated by dipivefrin, an epinephrine prodrug.[86] Recent
work with timolol prodrugs has provided additional evidence supporting this new application
of prodrugs. Except for the short chain alkyl esters, all other alkyl, cycloalkyl, and aryl
ester prodrugs were less readily absorbed systemically, yet they were ocularly absorbed
either equally well or better than timolol[87] (Figure 4). As a result, the therapeutic index,
defined as the ratio of aqueous humor to plasma timolol concentrations, was improved as
much as 16 times. The basis for this approach is the differential lipophilic characteristics
of the cornea, the conjunctiva, and, presumably, the nasal mucosa.[88]

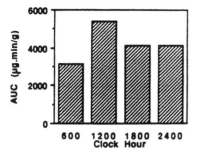

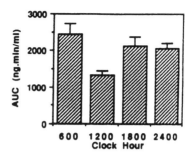

FIGURE 3. Influence of dosing time on the area under the concentration-time curves (AUC) of timolol in the iris-ciliary body (left plot) and plasma (right plot) of the pigmented rabbit following the topical instillation of 25 µl of 0.65% timolol maleate solutions. Error bars represent standard deviation for n = 4. No error bars were shown for the iris-ciliary body since pooled data were used. (From Ohdo, S., Grass, G. M., and Lee, V. H. L., *Invest. Ophthalmol. Vis. Sci.*, 32, 2790, 1991. With permission.)

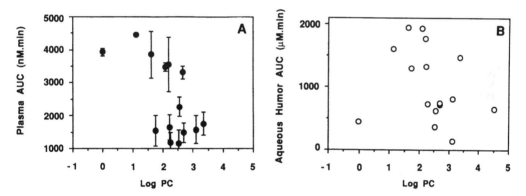

FIGURE 4. Influence of prodrug lipophilicity on the systemic (plasma AUC, plot A) and ocular absorption (aqueous humor AUC, plot B) of topically applied timolol ester prodrugs in the pigmented rabbit. Error bars represent standard error of the mean for n = 4–6. No error bars are shown for the aqueous humor since pooled data are used.

Traditionally, drug candidates are selected on the basis of potency: only the very potent ones are selected for preclinical evaluation. They are, therefore, prone to induce systemic side effects. Consequently, it seems logical to consider a new approach that selects the less potent candidate for evaluation and then offsets the loss in potency through prodrug derivatization. Hopefully, the prodrugs are also poorly absorbed by the conjunctival and nasal mucosa because of enhanced lipophilicity, rendering them less likely to be absorbed systemically. Such an approach has been described by Sugrue et al.[89] These investigators reported that L-653,328 (7), an acetate ester of the β-blocker L-652,698 (6), was as potent as timolol in lowering the intraocular pressure in the α-chymotrypsinized albino rabbit, but was at least 100 times less potent than timolol against the heart. This lack of systemic potency was consistent with the modest affinity of L-652,698, the active moiety of L-653,328, for the extraocular β-receptors.

$$R-OCH_2CH_2-\langle\bigcirc\rangle-OCH_2-\underset{OH}{\underset{|}{CH}}-CH_2-NH-\underset{CH_3}{\overset{CH_3}{\underset{|}{\overset{|}{C}}}}-CH_3$$

(6) R = H

(7) R = $-\underset{\underset{O}{\parallel}}{C}-CH_3$

The approach just described is akin to the soft drug approach. Soft drugs can be defined as biologically active drugs that may structurally resemble known active drugs or may be entirely new structures, but which are all characterized by predictable *in vivo* destruction (metabolism) to nontoxic moieties after they have achieved their therapeutic role.[90] Such a concept has been applied to β-blockers[91-94] as well as to antimicrobials,[95] anticholinergics,[96] and steroids.[97] Of the eight lipophilic esters of the acidic metabolite (8) of metoprolol tested in albino rabbits, the adamantylethyl ester (9) was the best in terms of intraocular pressure lowering potency[98] and possible low incidence of systemic side effects associated with a very fast rate of hydrolysis ($t_{1/2}$ = 7 min) to the inactive metabolite (8) in human blood.

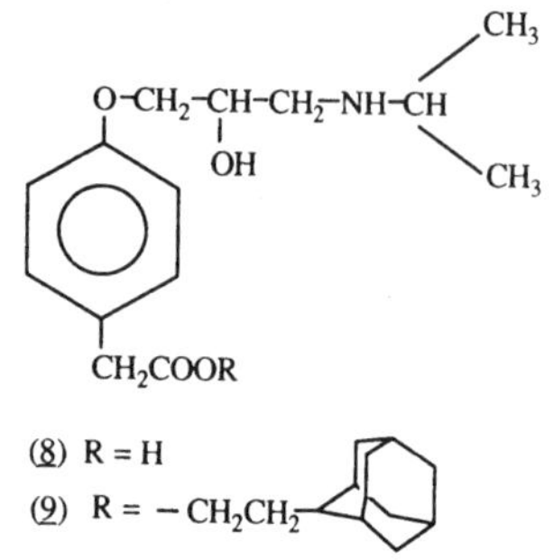

(8) R = H
(9) R = – CH₂CH₂–

D. REDUCTION OF OCULAR SIDE EFFECTS

The ability of prodrugs to reduce ocular side effects has not been well established. Thus far, this potential application of prodrugs has been suggested only for dipivefrin, an epinephrine prodrug.[86] Because 0.1% dipivefrin solution was as effective as a 2% epinephrine solution in lowering intraocular pressure,[99] it was anticipated that the incidence of extraocular side effects (e.g., conjunctival hyperemia, foreign body sensation, and follicular conjunctivitis) would be lowered. While this expectation was fulfilled when the prodrug was used on a short-term basis,[100,101] its incidence of side effects was no different from that of its parent compound when used for an extended period of time (1 to 2 years).[102,103] This outcome is not surprising since the prodrug itself can presumably be absorbed by the conjunctiva.

A class of drugs that can benefit from reduction in extraocular side effects is the prostaglandins, which are being investigated for their ocular hypotensive effect.[16] Local eye irritations have been reported for $PGF_{2\alpha}$ (10).[104] Interestingly, its methyl (11), ethyl (12), and isopropyl (13) ester prodrugs, which were designed to improve its corneal penetration, have been reported to be less irritating with the additional advantage of a 10 to 30 times gain in intraocular pressure that lowers potency.[17,105] The lower incidence of eye irritation is possibly due to the 25 to 50 times lower dose of ester prodrugs required.[106] Nevertheless, in a randomized, double-masked, placebo-controlled study, some glaucoma patients on 0.25 or 0.5 μg of prostaglandin $F_{2\alpha}$-1-isopropyl ester experienced mild irritation lasting for several minutes and conjunctival hyperemia that reached a maximum at 30 to 60 min after drop instillation.[107] As was the case with $PGF_{2\alpha}$, the isopropyl ester of PGA_2 also improved the intraocular pressure lowering potency of the parent drug, the factor of improvement being about 15.[108,109]

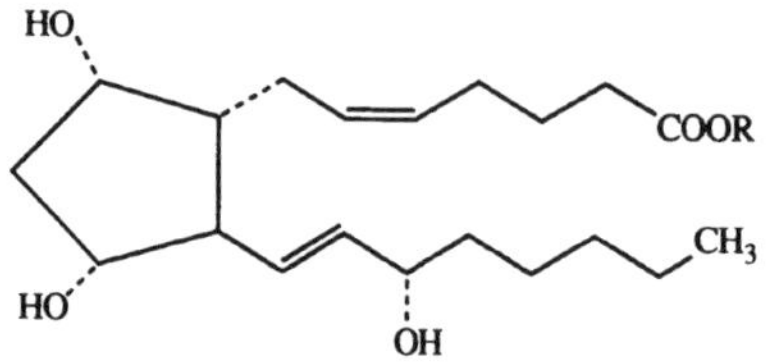

(10) R = H
(11) R = -CH₃
(12) R = -CH₂CH₃
(13) R = -CH(CH₃)CH₃

III. FUNCTIONAL GROUPS AMENABLE TO PRODRUG DERIVATIZATION

The majority of ophthalmic prodrugs developed thus far are esters derived from hydroxyl or carboxylic acid groups present in the parent molecules. In a number of cases, however, other strategies are required since the drug to be modified does not contain functional groups amenable to esterification. These strategies include dealkylation, reduction, and N-acylation.

Even though amines can be readily acylated, amide prodrugs have rarely been used. The main reason is their relative stability *in vivo*.[110] This problem can, however, be circumvented by preparing (acyloxy)alkyl carbamate derivatives. Such derivatives may be promising biolabile prodrugs for amino functional drugs, since they are neutral compounds that combine high stability in aqueous solution[111] with high susceptibility to undergo enzymatic regeneration of the parent amine by ester hydrolysis.[35,111,112] For instance, the N-acylated derivative (14) of timolol shows a half-life of degradation of 1410 min in a pH 7.4 phosphate buffer at 37°C and 10 min in dog plasma.[112] This prodrug approach has been applied to pindolol, propranolol, and betaxolol besides timolol[112] and has been found to improve *in vitro* corneal permeation.

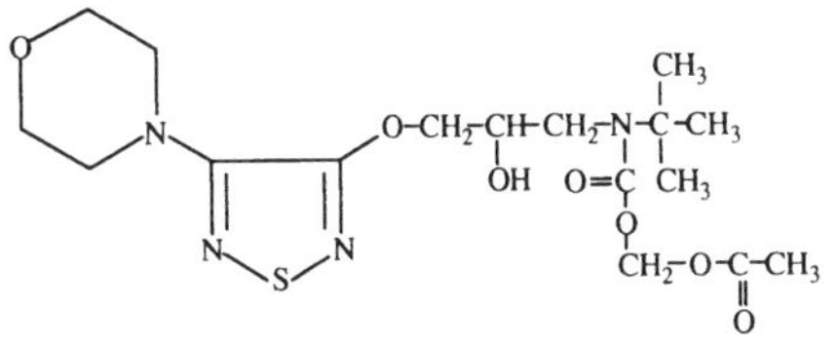

(14)

An alternative to the approach just described is to synthesize highly chemically reactive hydroxyamides of amines, which rapidly lactonize with a half-life of approximately 1 min at near-physiological pH and temperature to liberate the amines.[113] Two approaches have been attempted to retard this rapid rate of conversion: (1) esterification of the hydroxyamide[114] and (2) oxidation of the hydroxyl group to a quinone.[114] Regeneration of the amine from these double prodrugs depends on esterase-mediated hydrolysis and reduction of the quinone to hydroquinone, respectively (Scheme 5).

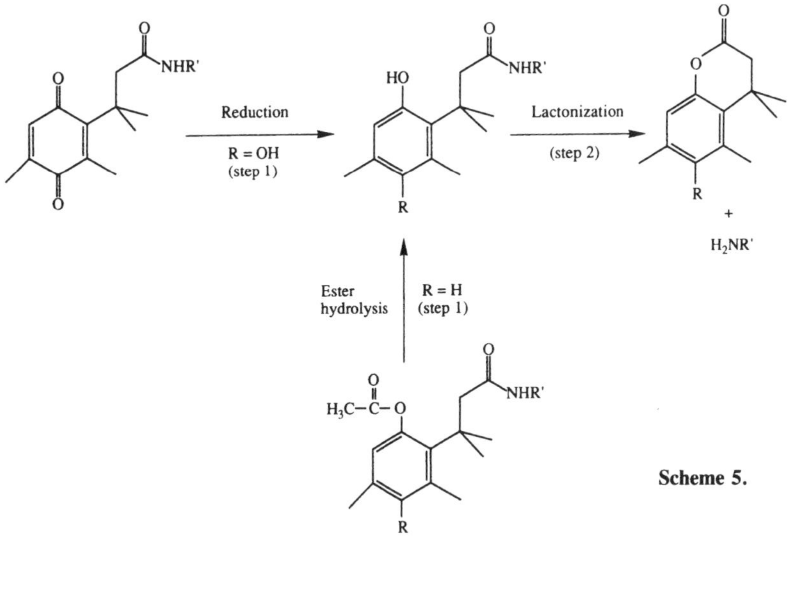

Scheme 5.

The prodrug approach is not applicable to all drugs, especially those with functional groups that are not amenable to prodrug derivatization. A case in point is carbonic anhydrase inhibitors. The most prominent functional moiety in these drugs is the primary sulfonamide group, so attempts to develop useful prodrug derivatives have been focused on this group.[115-119] Unfortunately, N-acyl derivatives of the primary sulfonamides of these carbonic anhydrase inhibitors are very resistant to chemical or enzymatic hydrolysis, although secondary sulfonamide derivatives are more reactive and easily hydrolyzed enzymatically.[116]

IV. ENZYMES INVOLVED IN THE ACTIVATION OF PRODRUGS

Of all the enzymes participating in the activation of prodrugs, esterases have received the most attention. This is because ester prodrugs are the most widely investigated in ophthalmology. Esterases are present in all anterior segment tissues[120] except tears.[121] Their activity is highest in the iris-ciliary body, being twice that in the cornea, where about 70% of the activity resides in the epithelium.[122] Except in the corneal epithelium, butyrylcholinesterase contributes to over 75% of the esterase activity in anterior segment tissues.[123] The substrate specificities of ocular esterases and their kinetic properties have been reviewed.[124]

Ketone reductase, which plays a role in the activation of ketoximes of various β-adrenergic blocking agents,[93] is not as ubiquitous as the esterases.[125] This enzyme is present primarily in the corneal epithelium and the iris-ciliary body, but not in the corneal stroma, aqueous humor, or conjunctiva.[125] Activation of the ketoximes proceeds via an initial hydrolysis of the oxime functionality to yield a ketone, which subsequently is enzymatically reduced to yield the parent β-blocker, principally in the iris-ciliary body,[93,125] as depicted in Scheme 6 for the ketoxime derivative (15) of propanolol (16).

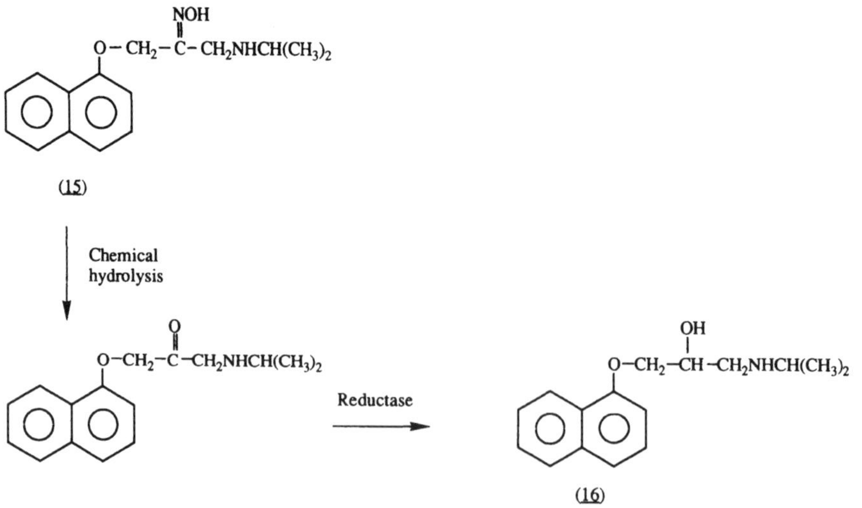

Scheme 6.

An enzyme that has received some attention recently is the N-dealkylating enzyme. The existence of this enzyme in ocular tissues is implicated by the purported ability of rabbit ocular tissues to metabolize *N*-methylacetazolamide to acetazolamide,[126] a process that was not observed subsequently by Lee and Bundgaard.[126a] This, perhaps, is a partial explanation for the inactivity of topically applied N-methylated ethoxzolamide.[127]

Theoretically, the marked differences in the ratio of two or more enzymes can be exploited for activating a sequentially labile prodrug so as to achieve site-specific release of the parent compound. Such an approach has been investigated by Bodor and Visor.[128] These investigators exploited the marked differences in the ratio of ketone reductase[125] to esterase levels[129] among the anterior segment tissues to achieve site-specific delivery of di-isovaleryl adrenalone (17), a bioreversible derivative of epinephrine (19), in the ciliary body, where epinephrine is regenerated and where this drug acts. Epinephrine is regenerated only when the diester is reduced before hydrolysis occurs; no epinephrine is regenerated from adrenalone (20) formed from diester hydrolysis (Scheme 7). The proportion of the diester undergoing only hydrolysis vs. the reduction-hydrolysis sequence, hence its duration of action, is a function of susceptibility of the ester linkage to hydrolysis.[128] Thus, di(ethylsuccinyl) adrenalone (18), with a plasma half-life of 1 min, is anticipated to have a shorter duration of action than its di-isovaleryl counterpart, which has a plasma half-life of 19 min. It is reasonable to expect that a better understanding of the enzymatic systems in the various anterior segments would enhance the usefulness of this approach to achieve drug targeting in the eye.

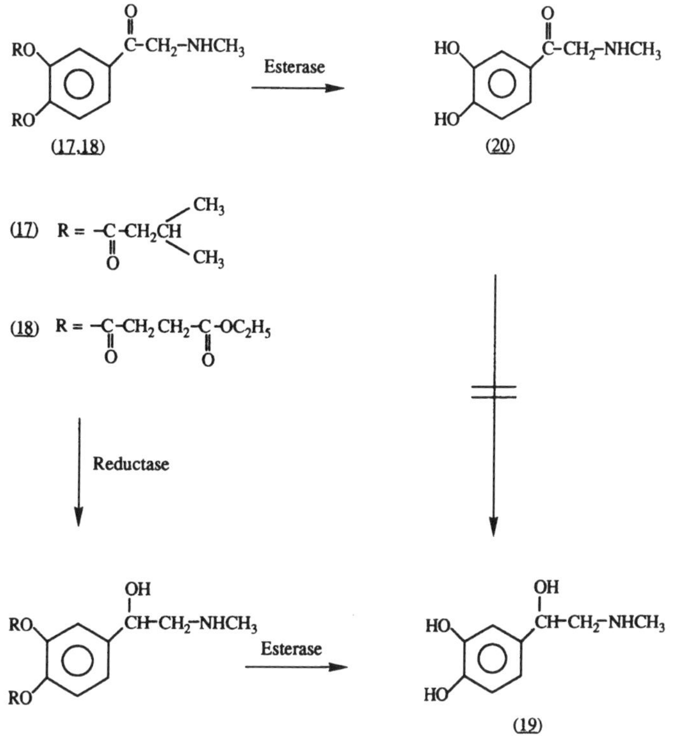

Scheme 7.

V. PHYSICOCHEMICAL CONSIDERATIONS IN THE DESIGN OF PRODRUGS

To be successful, an ocular prodrug should (1) possess the correct lipophilicity that balances ocular against systemic drug absorption, (2) possess sufficient aqueous solubility and stability for formulation as eye drops, and (3) be converted to the active parent drug within the eye quantitatively and at a rate consistent with the therapeutic need.

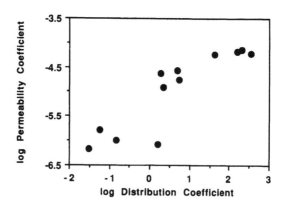

FIGURE 5.   Influence of drug lipophilicity (log Distribution Coefficient) on the corneal permeability (log Permeability Coefficient) of various β-blockers. (From Schoenwald, R. D. and Huang, H. S., *J. Pharm. Sci.*, 72, 1266, 1983. With permission.)

TABLE 2
Model Parameter Estimates (l, m, and n) and
Goodness-Of-Fit Indices (r and s) on the
Relationship Between the Corneal
Permeability Coefficient (Papp) and the
Partition Coefficient (PC) of β-Blockers

Parameter	Sigmoidal model[a]	Parabolic model[a]
l	-0.050 (0.49)[b]	0.28 (0.74)
m	7.26 (0.74)	0.40 (0.19)
n	354.0 (151.9)	-0.17 (0.75)
r[c]	0.9579	0.9040
s[d]	7.20	15.97

[a]   The model equations are Papp $= 1 + $ m·PC/(n + PC) for
       the sigmoidal model and Papp $= 1 + $ m log PC $+ $ n (log
       PC)^2 for the parabolic model
[b]   Asymptotic standard deviation.
[c]   Correlation coefficient.
[d]   Residual sum of squares.

Based on data from Schoenwald, R. D. and Huang, H. S., *J. Pharm. Sci.*, 72, 1266, 1983.

A. LIPOPHILICITY

The design of prodrugs for improved corneal penetration has been guided by the parabolic relationship between corneal penetration and log partition coefficient.[130] Such parabolic relationships have been reported for steroids,[131] *n*-alkyl *p*-aminobenzoate esters,[132] substituted anilines,[133] β-blockers,[134] and prodrugs of timolol.[135] It must be cautioned that the parabolic relationship reported from β-blockers is based on heavy weighting on one or two lipophilic compounds beyond the purported maximum in the parabola (Figure 5). As shown by Wang et al.,[136] a sigmoidal relationship statistically described the influence of lipophilicity on the corneal penetration of β-blockers better than the parabolic relationship reported by Schoenwald and Huang[134] (Table 2). The same argument probably holds for steroids.[134] Deviation from the parabolic relationship has also been reported by Grass and Robinson,[137] when compounds of diverse chemical structure and molecular size are considered. Such deviations are to be expected, because not all the compounds selected for study utilize the usual transcellular pathway for penetration. Compounds that penetrate via the less common paracellular pathway include low-molecular-weight alcohols and the ionized form of such drugs as pilocarpine,[138,139] sulfonamides,[140] and cromolyn Na.[141]

In addition to lipophilicity, enzymatic lability is another factor that may influence the extent of improvement in corneal drug penetration by prodrugs. Thus, the penetration of aliphatic timolol esters across the isolated rabbit cornea was found to depend on both lipophilicity and enzymatic lability.[6,10] The rates of penetration increased with increased susceptibility of the esters to undergo hydrolysis in the cornea (Figure 6). Thus, the enzymatically more labile straight-chain alkyl esters penetrated the cornea more readily than the more stable branched-chain esters of comparable lipophilicity. This finding may be ascribed to the possibility that facile prodrug cleavage increases the concentration gradient governing prodrug absorption. It is, therefore, not surprising that, 1 mM eserine sulfate, an esterase inhibitor, reduced the corneal permeation of O-butyryltimolol, 1'-methylcyclopropanolytimolol, and O-pivaloyltimolol by 30, 50, and 80%, respectively.[6] The above inverse relationship between corneal permeability and rate of prodrug hydrolysis has also been observed in the lipophilic O,O'-(1,4-xylylene)bispilocarpic acid ester prodrugs of pilocarpine (log PC $\geq$ 3) (21).[142] It was proposed that the corneal permeability of these prodrugs was controlled by the formation of pilocarpine in the corneal epithelium rather than by their absorption into the corneal epithelium or their diffusion across the stroma-endothelium.

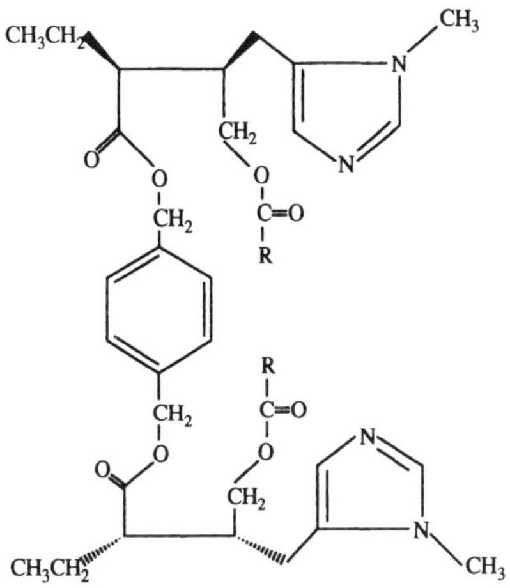

(21) R = –CH₃
    = –CH₂CH₃
    = –CH₂CH₂CH₃
    = –CH₂CH₂CH₂CH₃
    = ◁

B. AQUEOUS SOLUBILITY

In addition to possessing the correct lipophilicity, drugs must also possess adequate aqueous solubility, since they must diffuse across a water-filled corneal stroma to gain access to the intraocular tissues, and since it is the initial concentration in the tear film that determines the driving force for corneal drug penetration. The role of drug solubility in determining ocular drug bioavailability is best exemplified by the recent findings of Usayapant et al.[143] that solubilizing dexamethasone and its acetate ester prodrug in 5 and 8% solutions of hydroxypropyl-β-cyclodextrin, respectively, enhanced their ocular absorption about 2 times.

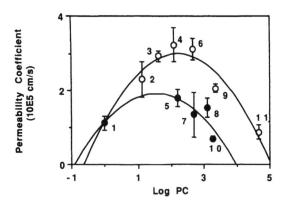

FIGURE 6. Influence of prodrug lipophilicity (log PC) on the corneal penetration of alkyl esters of timolol in the pigmented rabbit. The symbol ○ refers to straight chain alkyl esters and the symbol ● refers to branched chain alkyl esters. Error bars represent standard deviation (n = 4–6). Where not shown, the error bars are smaller than the size of the symbols. Key: 1, timolol; 2, *O*-acetyl timolol; 3, *O*-propionyl timolol; 4, *O*-butyryl timolol; 5, *O*-isobutyryl timolol; 6, *O*-valeryl timolol; 7, *O*-pivaloyl timolol; 8, *O*-neopentanoyl timolol; 9, *O*-hexanoyl timolol; 10, *O*-2-ethylbutyryl timolol; and 11, *O*-octanoyl timolol. (From Chien, D. S., Sasaki, H., Bundgaard, H., Buur, A., and Lee, V. H. L., *Pharm. Res.*, 8, 728, 1991. With permission.)

The most commonly used esters for increasing the aqueous solubility of hydroxyl-containing agents are esters containing an ionizable group, namely, dicarboxylic acid hemiesters, phosphate esters, and α-amino acid esters.[110] Various α-amino acid esters of the antiviral acyclovir have been prepared to improve its corneal penetration via more water-soluble prodrugs.[144] Whereas acyclovir itself (<u>22</u>) is not effective against stromal keratitis and iritis[39,145,146] — probably due to its low aqueous solubility (<0.02% at 25°C) and poor corneal penetration — its glycine ester (<u>23</u>) was effective.[29] Because of the enhanced solubility of the glycine ester, as high as a 6% aqueous solution at pH 4 to 5 can be formulated. Presumably, the ester is rapidly hydrolyzed by corneal enzymes, but like other α-amino acid esters, it suffers from instability in aqueous formulations.

(<u>22</u>) R = H

(<u>23</u>) R = $-\overset{\text{O}}{\underset{\|}{\text{C}}}-\text{CH}_2\text{NH}_2$

C. CHEMICAL STABILITY

A major challenge in prodrug design is to obtain derivatives that are chemically stable in solution (the preferred dosage form) and yet enzymatically labile. A case in point is most of the sterically unhindered straight-chain aliphatic esters of timolol, which are rapidly hydrolyzed chemically. This problem has been solved by utilizing sterically hindered esters, e.g., the 2-ethylbutyryl, 3,3-dimethylbutyryl, cyclopropanoyl, and 1′-methylcyclopropanoyl derivatives. For these compounds, it is feasible to obtain aqueous solutions with shelf-lives greater than 2 years when stored at 10 to 15°C.[5]

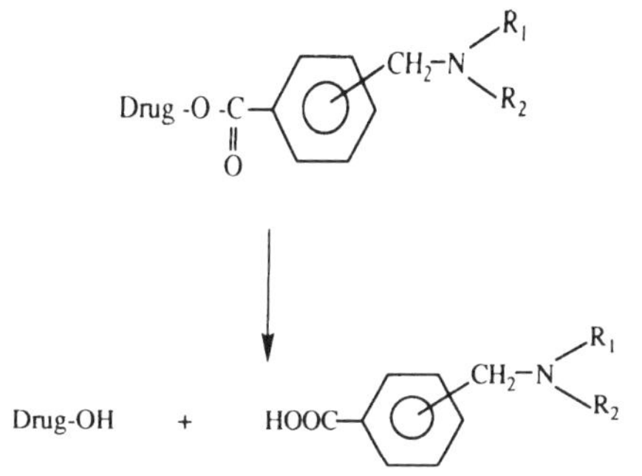

Scheme 8.

α-Amino and short chain aliphatic amino acid esters of various corticosteroids,[147] acyclovir,[29,144] ganciclovir,[148] and other hydroxyl-containing drugs[147] are additional examples of chemically unstable esters. There are two major reasons for their high instability in aqueous solution at pH values (pH 3 to 5) where they are most water soluble: (1) the strongly electron-withdrawing effect of the protonated amino group, thereby activating the ester linkage toward hydroxide ion attack, and (2) intramolecular catalysis or assistance by the neighboring amino group of ester hydrolysis.[149] An effective and simple means to completely block the hydrolysis-facilitating effect of the amino group described above, while retaining a rapid rate of enzymatic ester hydrolysis, is to incorporate a phenyl group, via a methylene spacer, between the ester moiety and the solubilizing amino group (Scheme 8).[147,150] In this way, the intramolecular catalytic reactions of the amino group are no longer possible for sterical reasons. Moreover, the ester-labilizing effect of the protonated amino group due to its polar character is greatly diminished. Such N-substituted 3- or 4-aminomethylbenzoate esters have been found to be readily soluble in water at weakly acidic pH values (10% at pH 5.1) and to possess very high aqueous solution stability ($t_{0.9}$ of 26 years at pH 3 to 4), while remaining highly susceptible to enzymatic hydrolysis in plasma ($t_{0.5}$ of 10 min or less).[147,150] In the case of ganciclovir, the solution instability problem of dipropionate ester has been solved by using the diadamantoate ester,[148] which remains susceptible to esterase-mediated hydrolysis. A drawback of this ester is its extremely low aqueous solubility (24 μg/ml vs. 2.1 mg/ml for the dipropionate ester and 3.7 mg/ml for the parent drug).

Carboxylic acid monester prodrugs of pilocarpine are a third example of unstable ester prodrugs. This stability problem has been solved by cascade latentiation or double prodrug formation (pro-prodrugs),[151,152] whereby an enzymatic release mechanism is required prior to the spontaneous release of the parent drug. This goal is achieved by esterifying the free hydroxy group in the carboxylic monoesters. The double esters (24) thus obtained are highly stable in aqueous solutions, even at pH 6 to 7 (shelf-lives exceeding 5 years at 25°C), and yet are enzymatically labile at the O-acyl bond, liberating the intermediate pilocarpic acid ester, which spontaneously undergoes lactonization to regenerate pilocarpine quantitatively (Scheme 9).[14] Besides solving the stability problem of pilocarpic acid monoesters, pilocarpic acid diesters penetrate the cornea more readily and are in action longer than the monoesters.[12,15]

The double prodrug concept has also been applied to N-α-hydroxyalkylated derivatives of peptides[50] and to oxazolidines. Oxazolidines are cyclic condensation products of aldehydes (or ketones) and β-aminoalcohols present in various sympathomimetic amines and β-blockers.[153-155] Such oxazolidines undergo facile and complete hydrolysis in aqueous solution (Scheme 10). For ephedrine, the half-lives were 5 s to 30 min. By contrast, N-acylated or N-benzoylated oxazolidines derived from primary aminoalcohols are highly stable in aqueous solution; unfortunately, they are also quite resistant to enzymatic hydrolysis.

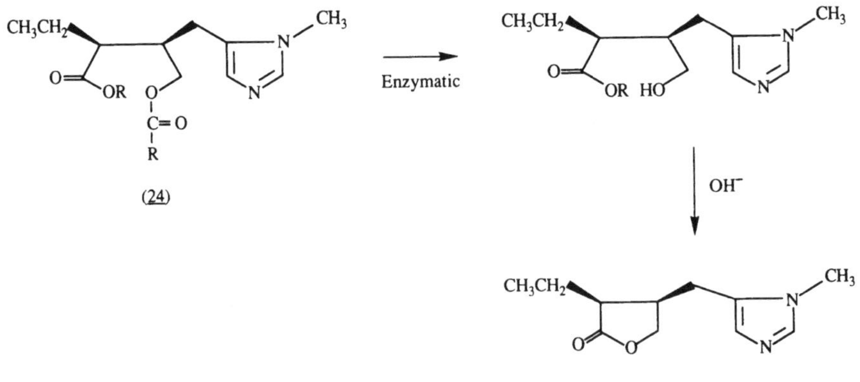

Scheme 9.

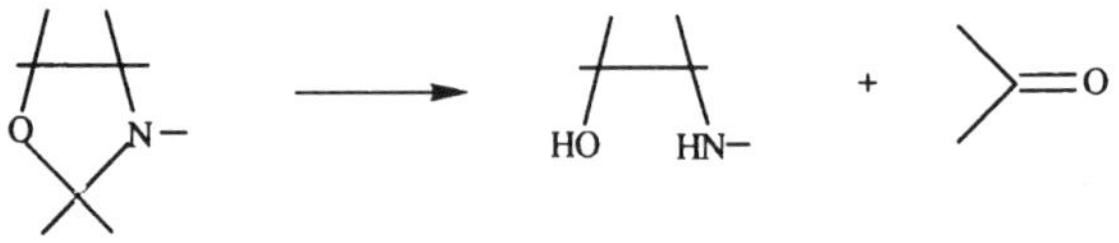

Scheme 10.

VI. FORMULATION CONSIDERATIONS

Because of the important role played by the corneal epithelium in modulating the penetration and conversion of the prodrug, its integrity is anticipated to affect prodrug efficacy. Preservatives, which are included in all multidose ophthalmic formulations to maintain sterility, are notorious for the damaging effects on the corneal epithelium.[156] Alexander et al.[112] and Chien et al.[10] have demonstrated that de-epithelializing the cornea adversely affected the corneal penetration of an (acyloxy)alkyl carbamate prodrug and aliphatic prodrugs of timolol. It is, therefore, not surprising that benzalkonium chloride reduced the corneal permeability of the isopropyl ester prodrug of $PGF_{2\alpha}$ by a factor of two, even though it enhanced the corneal permeability to its parent compound tenfold.[157] The factor of reduction was, however, less than the ninefold reduction observed with de-epithelializing the cornea.[20] The reason underlying the negative effect of benzalkonium chloride on the permeation of this prostaglandin prodrug has not been revealed, but may be related to the inhibitory effect of the preservative on esterase activity or to saturation of the esterases by the higher concentration of prodrug exposed to the enzyme, as has been reported for levobunolol,[158] which undergoes reduction during corneal penetration.[125,158] The fact that preservatives affect the corneal permeation of certain prodrugs raises the question of whether other formulation ingredients would exert a similar effect.

VII. TOXICITY CONSIDERATIONS

An important aspect in the development of ophthalmic drugs is possible contact sensitization potential of the compounds. As a case in point, although several benzofuran- and indole-2-sulfonamides were found to be potent carbonic anhydrase inhibitors following topical administration, they showed such strong allergenic activities that further development of the compounds for clinical use was precluded.[159]

The possibility of corneal toxicity associated with higher than usual drug concentration achieved in the cornea due to improved corneal penetration must be considered. This was the case for several pilocarpic acid diesters of pilocarpine (H. Bundgaard, personal communication, 1992). Further work with over 20 pilocarpic acid diesters has led to the selection of the O-benzoyl pilocarpic acid methyl ester which has the optimal balance of ocular safety and efficacy. When administered repeatedly to albino rabbits, this compound showed no acute ocular toxicity and was nonirritating to the conjunctiva.[160] At the same time, it reduced intraocular pressure significantly in both normotensive Owl monkey and glaucomatous Cynomolgus monkey, while producing a much smaller miosis than a 0.5% equivalent dose of pilocarpine.[160] The latter finding suggests that a greater pilocarpine concentration is required at the pupillary muscle to cause constriction than is required at the ciliary muscle, the suggested site of action for intraocular pressure reduction.

VIII. CONCLUSIONS

Drug development for ocular diseases has traditionally relied on drugs originally developed for systemic use. Unfortunately, few of them are optimal for ocular absorption. This is because they possess few of the physicochemcial properties that are required to overcome the constraints imposed by the eye on drug absorption, which are far more severe than those imposed by the skin or by the gastrointestinal tract. In spite of their proven utility in overcoming the constraint due to poor corneal penetration, prodrugs have received surprisingly little attention, when compared with vehicle optimization, for improvement of ocular drug delivery. Nevertheless, prodrug derivatization deserves more attention in the future. This is because of their potential in achieving the aims of modifying the duration of drug action, reducing the extent of systemic drug absorption, reducing the incidence of ocular side effects, and maximizing the ratio of drug concentrations in the target to nontarget tissues.

ACKNOWLEDGMENTS

This work was supported in part by grants EY-3816 and EY-7389 from the National Institutes of Health, and in part by the Gavin S. Herbert Professorship.

REFERENCES

1. **Sinkula, A. A. and Yalkowsky, S. H.**, Rationale for design of biologically reversible drug derivatives: prodrugs, *J. Pharm. Sci.*, 64, 181, 1975.
2. **Apt, L., Henrick, A., and Silverman, L. M.**, Patient compliance with use of topical ophthalmic corticosteroid suspensions, *Am. J. Ophthalmol.*, 87, 210, 1979.
3. **Mandell, A. I., Stentz, F., and Kitabchi, A. E.**, Dipivalyl epinephrine: a new prodrug in the treatment of glaucoma, *Ophthalmology*, 85, 268, 1978.
4. **Bundgaard, H., Buur, A., Chang, S. C., and Lee, V. H. L.**, Prodrugs of timolol for improved ocular delivery: synthesis, hydrolysis kinetics and liphophilicity of various timolol esters, *Int. J. Pharm.*, 33, 15, 1986.
5. **Bundgaard, H., Buur, A., Chang, S. C., and Lee, V. H. L.**, Timolol prodrugs: synthesis, stability and lipophilicity of various alkyl, cycloalkyl and aromatic esters of timolol, *Int. J. Pharm.* 46, 77, 1988.
6. **Chang, S. C., Bundgaard, H., Buur, A., and Lee, V. H. L.**, Improved corneal penetration of timolol by produgs as a means to reduce systemic drug load, *Invest. Ophthalmol. Vis. Sci.*, 28, 487, 1987.
7. **Sasaki, H., Chien, D. S., Lew, K., Bundgaard, H., and Lee, V. H. L.**, Timolol prodrugs: enhanced potency and duration of ocular beta adrenergic blockage following topical solution instillation in the pigmented rabbit, *Invest. Ophthalmol. Vis. Sci.*, 29, 83, 1988.

8. **Chang, S. C., Chien, D. S., Bundgaard, H., and Lee, V. H. L.**, Relative effectiveness of prodrug and viscous solution approaches in maximizing the ratio of ocular to systemic absorption of topically applied timolol, *Exp. Eye Res.*, 46, 59, 1988.

9. **Chang, S. C., Bundgaard, H., Buur, A., and Lee, V. H. L.**, Low dose O-butyryl timolol improves the therapeutic index of timolol in the pigmented rabbit, *Invest. Opthalmol. Vis. Sci.*, 29, 626, 1988.

10. **Chien, D. S., Bundgaard, H., and Lee, V. H. L.**, The influence of corneal integrity in the ocular absorption of timolol prodrugs, *J. Ocular Pharmacol.*, 4, 137, 1988.

11. **Duzman, E., Chen, C. C., Anderson, J., Blumenthal, M., and Twizer, H.**, Diacetyl derivative of nadolol. I. Ocular pharmacology and short-term ocular hypotensive effect in glaucomatous eyes, *Arch. Ophthalmol.*, 100, 1916, 1982.

12. **Bundgaard, H., Falch, E., Larsen, C., Mosher, G. L., and Mikkelson, T. J.**, Pilocarpic acid esters as novel sequentially labile pilocarpine prodrugs for improved ocular delivery, *J. Med. Chem.*, 28, 979, 1985.

13. **Bundgaard, H., Falch, E., Larsen, C., and Mikkelson, T. J.**, Pilocarpine prodrugs. I. Synthesis, physicochemical properties and kinetics of lactonization of pilocarpic acid esters, *J. Pharm. Sci.*, 75, 36, 1986.

14. **Bundgaard, H., Falch, E., Larsen, C., Mosher, G., and Mikkelson, T. J.**, Pilocarpine prodrugs of sequentially labile pilocarpic acid diesters, *J. Pharm. Sci.*, 75, 775, 1986.

15. **Mosher, G. L., Bundgaard, H., Falch, E., Larsen, C., and Mikkelson, T. J.**, Ocular bioavailability in pilocarpic acid mono- and diester prodrugs as assessed by miotic activity in the rabbit, *Int. J. Pharm.*, 39, 113, 1987.

16. **Bito, L. Z., Draga, A., Blanchs, J., and Camras, C. B.**, Long term maintenance of reduced ocular pressure by daily or twice daily topical application of prostaglandins to cat and monkey eyes, *Invest. Ophthalmol. Vis. Sci.*, 24, 312, 1983.

17. **Bito, L.**, Comparison of the ocular hypotensive efficacy of eicosanoids and related compounds, *Exp. Eye Res.*, 38, 181, 1984.

18. **Bito, L. Z. and Baroody, R. A.**, The ocular pharmacokinetics of eicosanoids and their derivatives. 1. Comparison of ocular eicosanoid penetration and distribution following the topical application of $PGF_{2\alpha}$, $PGF_{2\alpha}$-1-methyl ester, and $PGF_{2\alpha}$-1 isopropyl ester, *Exp. Eye Res.*, 44, 217, 1987.

19. **Camber, O., Edman, P., and Olsson, L. I.**, Permeability of prostaglandin $F_{2\alpha}$ and prostaglandin $F_{2\alpha}$ esters across cornea in vitro, *Int. J. Pharm.*, 29, 259, 1986.

20. **Camber, O. and Edman, P.**, Factors influencing the corneal permeability of prostaglandin $F_{2\alpha}$ and its isopropyl ester *in vitro*, *Int. J. Pharm.*, 37, 27, 1987.

21. **Bergamini, M. V. W., Murray, D. L., and Krause, P. D.**, Pivalyl phenylephrine (PPE), a mydriatic prodrug of phenylephrine with reduced cardiovascular effects, *Invest. Ophthalmol. Vis. Sci.*, 20 (Suppl.), 187, 1979.

22. **Mindel, J. S., Shaikewitz, S. T., and Podos, S. M.**, Is phenylephrine pivalate a prodrug? *Arch. Ophthalmol.*, 98, 2220, 1980.

23. **Yuan, S. S. and Bodor, N.**, Synthesis and activity of (R)-(−)-m-trimethylacetoxy-alpha-[(methylamino)methyl]benzyl alcohol hydrochloride: a prodrug form of (R)-(−)-phenylephrine, *J. Pharm. Sci.*, 65, 929, 1976.

24. **Chien, D. S. and Schoenwald, R. D.**, Improving the ocular absorption of phenylephrine, *Biopharm. Drug Disp.*, 7, 453, 1986.

25. **Phipps, T. L., Potter, D. E., and Rowland, J. M.**, Effects of ibuterol, a beta-2-adrenergic prodrug, on intraocular pressure, *J. Ocular Pharmacol.*, 2, 225, 1986.

26. **Bonomi, L., Perfetti, S., Bellucci, R., De Franco, I., and Massa, F.**, Effect of ibuterol on the intraocular pressure in glaucoma, *Glaucoma*, 10, 45, 1988.

27. **Bar-Ilan, A., Pessah, N. I., and Maren, T. H.**, Ocular penetration and hypotensive activity of the topically applied carbonic anhydrase inhibitor L-645,151, *J. Ocular Pharmacol.*, 2, 109, 1986.

28. **Sugrue, M. F., Gautheron, P., Schmitt, C., Viader, M. P., Conquet, P., Smith, R. L., Share, N. N., and Stone, C. A.**, On the pharmacology of L-645,151: a topically effective ocular hypotensive carbonic anhydrase inhibitor, *J. Pharmacol. Exp. Ther.*, 232, 534, 1985.

29. **Maudgal, P. C., Clercq, K. D., Descamps, J., and Missotten, L.**, Topical treatment of experimental herpes simplex keratouveitis with 2′-O′-glycylacyclovir, *Arch. Ophthalmol.*, 102, 140, 1984.

30. **Pavan-Langston, D., North, R. D., Geary, P. A., and Kinkel, A.**, Intraocular penetration of the soluble antiviral, ara AMP, *Arch. Ophthalmol.*, 94, 1585, 1976.

31. **Narurkar, M. M. and Mitra, A. K.**, Synthesis, physicochemical properties, and cytotoxicity of a series of 5′-ester prodrugs of 5-iodo-2′-deoxyuridine, *Pharm. Res.*, 5, 734, 1988.

32. **Narurkar, M. M. and Mitra, A. K.**, Prodrugs of 5-iodo-2′-deoxyuridine for enhanced ocular transport, *Pharm. Res.*, 6, 887, 1989.

33. **Shih, R. L. and Lee, V. H. L.,** Rate limiting barrier to the penetration of ocular hypotensive beta blockers across the corneal epithelium in the pigmented rabbit, *J. Ocular Pharmacol.,* 6, 329, 1990.

34. **Hull, D. S., Hine, J. E., Edelhauser, H. F., and Hyndiuk, B. A.,** Permeability of the isolated rabbit cornea to corticosteroids, *Invest. Ophthalmol.,* 13, 457, 1974.

35. **Wang, W., Bundgaard, H., Buur, A., and Lee, V. H. L.,** Corneal penetration of 5-fluorouracil and its improvement by prodrug derivatization in the albino rabbit: implication in glaucoma filtration surgery, *Curr. Eye Res.,* 10, 87, 1991.

36. **Lee, V. H. L., Carson, L. W., Dodda Kashi, S., and Stratford, R. E.,** Metabolic and permeation barriers to the ocular absorption of topically applied enkephalins in albino rabbits, *J. Ocular Pharmacol.,* 2, 345, 1986.

37. **Dodda Kashi, S. and Lee, V. H. L.** Hydrolysis of enkephalins in anterior segment tissue homogenates of the albino rabbit eye, *Invest. Ophthalmol. Vis. Sci.,* 27, 1300, 1986.

38. **Lee, V. H. L., Carson, L. W., and Takemoto, K. A.,** Macromolecular drug absorption in the albino rabbit eye, *Int. J. Pharm.,* 72, 1272, 1983.

39. **Schaeffer, H. J., Beauchamp, L., De Miranda, P. Elion, G. B., Bauer, D. J., and Collins, P.,** 9-(2-hydroxyethoxymethyl) guanine activity against viruses of the herpes group, *Nature,* 272, 583, 1978.

40. **Chien, D. S. and Schoenwald, R. D.,** Ocular pharmacokinetics and pharmacodynamics of phenylephrine and phenylephrine oxazolidine in rabbits eyes, *Pharm. Res.,* 7, 476, 1990.

41. **Miller-Meeks, M. J., Farrell, T. A., Munden, P. M., Folk, J. C., Rao, C., and Schoenwald, R. D.,** Phenylephrine prodrug. Report of clinical trials, *Ophthalmology,* 98, 222, 1991.

42. **Schoenwald, R. D., Folk, J. C., Kumar, V., and Piper, J. G.,** In vivo comparison of phenylephrine and phenylephrine oxazolidine instilled in the monkey eye, *J. Ocular Pharmacol.,* 3, 333, 1987.

43. **Ashton, P., Clark, D. S., and Lee, V. H. L.,** A mechanistic study on the enhancement of corneal penetration of phenylephrine by flurbiprofen in the rabbit, *Curr. Eye Res.,* 11, 85, 1992.

44. **Bundgaard, H.,** Prodrugs as a means to improve the delivery of peptide drugs, *Adv. Drug Deliv. Rev.,* 8, 1, 1992.

45. **Bundgaard, H. and Moss, J.,** Prodrugs of peptides. 4. Bioreversible derivatization of the pyroglutamyl group by N-acylation and N-aminomethylation to effect protection against pyroglutamyl aminopeptidase, *J. Pharm. Sci.,* 78, 122, 1989.

46. **Moss, J. and Bundgaard, H.,** Prodrugs of peptides. 5. Protection of the pyroglutamyl residue against pyroglutamyl aminopeptidase by bioreversible derivatization with glyoxylic acid derivatives, *Int. J. Pharm.,* 52, 255, 1989.

47. **Muranishi, S., Sakai, A., Yamada, K., Murakami, M., Takada, K., and Kiso, Y.,** Lipophilic peptides: synthesis of lauroyl thyrotropin-releasing hormone and its biological activity, *Pharm. Res.,* 8, 649, 1991.

48. **Klixbüll, U. and Bundgaard, H.,** Prodrugs as drug delivery systems. 30. 4-imidazolidinones as potential bioreversible derivatives for the α-aminoamide moiety in peptides, *Int. J. Pharm.,* 20, 273, 1984.

49. **Bundgaard, H. and Rasmussen, G. J.,** Prodrugs of peptides. 9. Bioreversible N-α-hydroxyalkylation of the peptide bond to effect protection against carboxypeptidase or other proteolytic enzymes, *Pharm. Res.,* 8, 313, 1991.

50. **Bundgaard, H. and Rasmussen, G. J.,** Prodrugs of peptides. 11. Chemical and enzymatic hydrolysis kinetics of A-acyloxymethyl derivatives of a peptide-like bond, *Pharm. Res.,* 8, 1238, 1991.

51. **Sasaki, H., Chien, D. S., Lew, K., Bundgard, H., and Lee, V. H. L.,** Timolol prodrugs: enhanced potency and duration of ocular beta adrenergic blockade following topical solution instillation in the pigmented rabbit, *Invest. Ophthalmol. Vis. Sci.,* 29 (Suppl.), 83, 1988.

52. **Chrai, S. S. and Robinson, J. R.,** Ocular evaluation of methylcellulose vehicle in albino rabbits, *J. Pharm. Sci.,* 63, 1218, 1974.

53. **Patton, T. F. and Robinson, J. R.,** Ocular evaluation of polyvinyl alcohol vehicle in rabbits, *J. Pharm. Sci.,* 64, 1312, 1975.

54. **Camber, O., Edman, P., and Gurny, R.,** Influence of sodium hyaluronate on the meiotic effect of pilocarpine in rabbits, *Curr. Eye Res.,* 6, 779, 1987.

55. **Davies, N. M., Farr, S. J., Hadgraft, J., and Kellaway, I. W.,** Evaluation of mucoadhesive polymers in ocular drug delivery. I. Viscous solutions, *Pharm. Res.,* 8, 1039, 1991.

56. **Gurny, R., Ibrahim, H., Aebi, A., Buri, P., Wilson, C. G., Washington, N., Edman, P., and Camber, O.,** Design and evaluation of controlled release systems for the eye, *J. Controlled Release,* 6, 367, 1987.

57. **Mitra, A. K. and Mikkelson, T. J.,** Ophthalmic solution buffer systems. I. The effect of buffer concentration on the ocular absorption of pilocarpine, *Int. J. Pharm.,* 10, 219, 1982.

58. **Ticho, U., Blumenthal, M., Zonis, S., Gal, A., Blank, I., and Mazor, Z. W.,** Piloplex, a new long-acting pilocarpine polymer salt. A: long-term study, *Br. J. Ophthalmol.,* 63, 45, 1979.

59. **Ellis, P. P. and Riegel, M. A.,** Comparative intraocular levels of pilocarpine achieved with drops and repository preparations, *J. Ocular Pharmacol.,* 3, 121, 1987.

60. **Robinson, J. R. and Eriksen, S. P.,** Drug delivery from soft lens materials, in *Soft Contact Lenses: Clinical and Applied Technology,* Ruben, M., Ed., John Wiley & Sons, New York, 1978, 265.
61. **Van Buskirk, E. M.,** Adverse reactions from timolol administration, *Ophthalmology,* 87, 447, 1980.
62. **Nelson, W. L., Fraunfelder, F. T., Sills, J. M., Arrowsmith, J. B., and Kruitsky, J. N.,** Adverse respiratory and cardiovascular events attributed to timolol ophthalmic solution, *Am. J. Ophthalmol.,* 102, 606, 1986.
63. **Phan, T.-M. M., Nguyen, K. P. V., Giacomini, J. C., and Lee, D. A.,** Ophthalmic beta-blockers: determination of plasma and aqueous humor levels by a radioreceptor assay following multiple doses, *J. Ocular Pharmacol.,* 7, 243, 1991.
64. **Anderson, J. A.,** Systemic absorption of topical ocularly applied epinephrine and dipivefrin, *Arch. Ophthalmol.,* 98, 350, 1980.
65. **Kumar, V., Schoenwald, R. D., Barcellos, W. A., Chien, D.-S., Folk, J. C., and Weingeist, T. A.,** Aqueous vs. viscous phenylephrine. I. Systemic absorption and cardiovascular effects, *Arch. Ophthalmol.,* 104, 1189, 1988.
66. **Duzman, E., Anderson, J., Vita, J. B., Lue, J. C., Chen, C.-C., and Leopold, I. H.,** Topically applied oxymetazoline. Ocular vasoconstrictive activity, pharmacokinetics, and metabolism, *Arch. Ophthalmol.,* 101, 1122, 1983.
67. **Bundgaard, H. and Lasen, J. D.,** N-sulfonyl imidates as a novel prodrug form for an ester function of a sulfonamide group, *J. Pharmacokinet. Biopharm.,* 14, 175, 1986.
68. **Urtti, A., Salminen, L., and Miinalainen, O.,** Systemic absorption of ocular pilocarpine is modified by polymer matrices, *Int. J. Pharm.,* 23, 147, 1985.
69. **Janes, R. B. and Stiles, J. F.,** The penetration of cortisol into normal and pathologic rabbit eyes, *Am. J. Ophthalmol.,* 56, 84, 1963.
70. **Tang-Liu, D. D.-S., Liu, S. S., and Weinkam, R. J.,** Ocular and systemic bioavailability of ophthalmic flurbiprofen, *J. Pharmacokinet. Biopharm.,* 12, 611, 1984.
71. **Chiang, C. W. N., Barnett, G., and Brine, D.,** Systemic absorption of Δ9-tetrahydrocannabinol after ophthalmic administration to the rabbit, *J. Pharm. Sci.,* 72, 136, 1983.
72. **Mosteller, M. W., Gebhardt, B. M., Hamilton, A. M., and Kaufman, H. E.,** Penetration of topical cyclosporine into the rabbit cornea, aqueous humor, and serum, *Arch. Ophthalmol.,* 103, 101, 1985.
73. **Zimmerman, T. J., Kooner, K. S., Kandarakis, A. S., and Ziegler, L. P.,** Improving the therapeutic index of topically applied ocular drugs, *Arch. Ophthalmol.,* 102, 551, 1984.
74. **Kaila, T., Huupponen, R., and Salminen, L.,** Effects of eyelid closure and nasolacrimal duct occlusion on the systemic absorption of ocular timolol in human subjects, *J. Ocular Pharmacol.,* 2, 365, 1986.
75. **Podder, K., Moy, K. C., and Lee, V. H. L.,** Improving the safety of topically applied timolol in the pigmented rabbit through manipulation of formulation composition, *Exp. Eye Res.,* 54, 747, 1992.
76. **Kyyrönen, K. and Arto, U.,** Improved ocular:systemic absorption ratio of timolol by viscous vehicle and phenylephrine, *Invest. Ophthalmol. Vis. Sci.,* 31, 1827, 1990.
77. **Lee, V. H. L., Luo, A. M., Li, S., Podder, S. K., Chang, S. C., Ohdo, S., and Grass, G. M.,** Pharmacokinetic basis for nonadditivity of IOP lowering in timolol combinations, *Invest. Ophthalmol. Vis. Sci.,* 32, 2948, 1991.
78. **Urtti, A., Pipkin, J. D., Rork, G., Sendo, T., Finne, U., and Repta, A. J.,** Controlled drug delivery devices for experimental ocular studies with timolol. 2. Ocular and systemic absorption in rabbits, *Int. J. Pharm.,* 61, 241, 1990.
79. **Luo, A. M., Sasaki, H., and Lee, V. H. L.,** Ocular drug interactions involving topically applied timolol in the pigmented rabbit, *Curr. Eye Res.,* 10, 231, 1991.
80. **Ohdo, S., Grass, G. M., and Lee, V. H. L.,** Improving the ocular:systemic ratio of topical timolol by varying the dosing time, *Invest. Ophthalmol. Vis. Sci.,* 32, 2790, 1991.
81. **Kompella, U., Ohdo, S., Gurny, R., Martenet, M., Bundgaard, H., and Lee, V. H. L.,** Varying the dosing time to further improve the ocular:systemic ratio of 0-1'-methylcyclopropanoyl timolol in the pigmented rabbit, *Invest. Ophthalmol. Vis. Sci.,* 32 (Suppl.), 733, 1991.
82. **Ohdo, S., Podder, S. P., and Lee, V. H. L.,** Ocular chronopharmacology in the pigmented rabbit: ocular timolol concentrations are dependent on the time of drop instillation, *Invest. Ophthalmol. Vis. Sci.,* 31, (suppl.), 232, 1990.
83. **Lee, V. H. L., Zhu, J., Kompella, U., and Huang, C.-L.,** Diurnal changes in ocular and systemic absorption of topically applied betaxolol in the pigmented rabbit, *Invest. Ophthalmol. Vis. Sci.,* 32 (Suppl.), 1296, 1991.
84. **Lee, V. H. L.,** Minimizing the systemic absorption of topically applied ophthalmic drugs, *STP Pharma.,* 2, 5, 1992.
85. **Sasaki, H., Bundgaard, H., and Lee, V. H. L.,** Design of prodrugs to selectively reduce systemic timolol absorption on the basis of the differential lipophilic characteristics of the cornea and the conjunctiva, *Invest. Ophthalmol. Vis. Sci.,* 30 (Suppl.), 25, 1989.

86. **Hussain, A. and Truelove, J. E.**, Prodrug approaches to enhancement of physicochemical properties of drugs IV: novel epinephrine prodrug, *J. Pharm. Sci.*, 65, 1510, 1976.
87. **Sasaki, H., Chien, D.-S., Bundgaard, H., and Lee, V. H. L.**, Reduction of systemic absorption of ocularly applied timolol by prodrugs, *Pharm. Res. Suppl.*, 5, S164, 1988.
88. **Sasaki, H., Chien, D. S., and Lee, V. H. L.**, Differential conjunctival and corneal permeability of β blockers and its influence on the ratio of systemic to ocular drug absorption, *Pharm. Res.*, 5, S98, 1988.
89. **Sugrue, M. F., Gautheron, P., Grove, J., Mallorga, P., Viader, M. P., Baldwin, J. P., Ponticello, G. S., and Varga, S. L.**, L-653,328: an ocular hypotensive agent with modest beta receptor blocking activity, *Invest. Ophthalmol. Vis. Sci.*, 29, 776, 1988.
90. **Bodor, N.**, Soft drugs: principles and methods for the design of safe drugs, *Med. Res. Rev.*, 4, 449, 1984.
91. **Bodor, N., ElKoussi, A., Kano, M., and Nakamura, T.**, Improved delivery through biological membranes. 26. Design, synthesis, and pharmacological activity of a novel chemical delivery system for β-adrenergic blocking agents, *J. Med. Chem.*, 31, 100, 1988.
92. **Bodor, N., Oshiro, Y., Loftsson, T., Katovich, M., and Cladwell, W.**, Soft drugs. VI. The application of the inactive metabolite approach for design of soft β-blockers, *Pharm. Res.*, 1, 120, 1984.
93. **Bodor, N. and Prokai, L.**, Site- and stereospecific ocular drug delivery by sequential enzymatic bioactivation, *Pharm. Res.*, 7, 723, 1990.
94. **Himber, J., Sallee, V. L., Andermann, G., Bouzoubaa, M., Leclerc, G., and De Santis, L.**, Effects of topically applied falintolol: a new beta-adrenergic antagonist for treatment of glaucoma, *J. Ocular Pharmacol.*, 3, 111, 1987.
95. **Bodor, N., Kaminski, J. J., and Selk, S.**, Soft drugs. I. Labile quaternary ammonium salts as soft antimicrobials, *J. Med. Chem.*, 23, 469, 1980.
96. **Bodor, N., Woods, R., Raper, C., Kearney, P., and Kaminski, J. J.**, Soft drugs. 3. A new class of anticholinergic agents, *J. Med. Chem.*, 23, 474, 1980.
97. **Bodor, N. and Varga, M.**, Effect of a novel soft steroid on the wound healing of rabbit cornea, *Exp. Eye Res.*, 50, 183, 1990.
98. **Bodor, N. and ElKoussi, A.**, Novel 'soft' beta-blockers as potential safe antiglaucoma agents, *Curr. Eye Res.*, 7, 369, 1988.
99. **Kaback, M. B., Podos, S. M., Harbin, T. S., Mandell, A. I., and Becker, B.**, The effects of dipivalyl epinephrine on the eye, *Am. J. Ophthalmol.*, 81, 768, 1976.
100. **Yablonski, M. E., Shin, D. H., Kolker, A. E., Kass, M., and Becker, B.**, Dipivefrin use in patients with intolerance to topically applied epinephrine, *Arch. Ophthalmol.*, 95, 2157, 1977.
101. **Kohn, A. N., Moss, A. P., Hargett, N. A., Ritch, R., Smith, H., and Podos, S. M.**, Clinical comparison of dipivalyl epinephrine and epinephrine in the treatment of glaucoma, *Am. J. Ophthalmol.*, 87, 196, 1979.
102. **Theodore, J. and Leibowitz, H. M.**, External ocular toxicity of dipivalyl epinephrine, *Am. J. Ophthalmol.*, 88, 1013, 1979.
103. **Petersen, P. E., Evans, R. B., Johnstone, M. A., and Henderson, W. R.**, Evaluation of ocular hypersensitivity to dipivalyl epinephrine by component eye-drop testing, *J. Allergy Clin. Immunol.*, 85, 954, 1990.
104. **Lee, P.-Y., Shao, H., Xu, L., and Qu, C.-K.**, The effect of prostaglandin $F_{2\alpha}$ on intraocular pressure in normotensive human subjects, *Invest. Ophthalmol. Vis. Sci.*, 29, 1474, 1988.
105. **Bito, L. Z. and Baroody, R. A.**, The penetration of exogenous prostaglandin and arachidonic acid into, and their distribution within, the mammalian eye, *Curr. Eye Res.*, 1, 659, 1982.
106. **Wang, R.-F., Camras, C. B., Lee, P.-Y., Podos, S. M., and Bito, L. Z.**, Effects of prostaglandins $F_{2\alpha}$, A_2, and their esters in glaucomatous monkey eyes, *Invest. Ophthalmol. Vis. Sci.*, 31, 2466, 1990.
107. **Camras, C. B., Siebold, E. C., Lustgarten, J. S., Serle, J. B., Frisch, S. C., Podos, S. M., and Bito, L. Z.**, Maintained reduction of intraocular pressure by prostaglandin $F_{2\alpha}$-1-isopropyl ester applied in multiple doses in ocular hypertensive and glaucoma patients, *Ophthalmology*, 96, 1329, 1989.
108. **Gum, G. G., Kingsbury, S., Whitley, R. D., Garcia, A., and Gelatt, K. N.**, Effect of topical prostaglandin PGA_2, PGA_2, PGA_2 isopropyl ester, and $PGF_{2\alpha}$ isopropyl ester on intraocular pressure in normotensive and glaucomatous canine eyes, *J. Ocular Pharmacol.*, 7, 107, 1991.
109. **Bito, L. Z., Miranda, O. C., Tendler, M. R., and Resul, B.**, Eicosanoids as a new class of ocular hypotensive agents. 3. Prostaglandin A_2-1-isopropyl ester is the most potent reported hypotensive agent on feline eyes, *Exp. Eye Res.*, 50, 419, 1990.
110. **Bundgaard, H.**, Design of prodrugs: bioreversible derivatives for various functional groups and chemical entities, in *Design of Prodrugs*, Bundgaard, H., Ed., Elsevier, Amsterdam, 1985, 1.
111. **Gogate, U. S., Repta, A. J., and Alexander, J.**, N-(Acyloxyalkoxycarbonyl) derivatives as potential prodrugs of amines. I. Kinetics and mechanism of degradation in aqueous solutions, *Int. J. Pharm.*, 40, 235, 1987.

112. **Alexander, J., Cargill, R., Michelson, S. R., and Schwam, H.,** (Acyloxy)alkyl carbamates as novel bioreversible prodrugs for amines: increased permeation through biological membranes, *J. Med. Chem.*, 31, 318, 1988.
113. **Amsberry, K. L., Gerstenberger, A. E., and Borchardt, R. T.,** Amine prodrugs which utilize hydroxy amide lactonization. II. A potential esterase-sensitive amide prodrug, *Pharm. Res.*, 8, 455, 1990.
114. **Amsberry, K. L. and Borchardt, R. T.,** Amine prodrugs which utilize hydroxy amide lactonization. I. A potential redox-sensitive amide prodrug, *Pharm. Res.*, 8, 323, 1991.
115. **Larsen, J. D. and Bundgaard, H.,** Prodrug forms for the sulfonamide group. Part III. Chemical and enzymatic hydrolysis of various N-sulfonyl imidates — novel prodrug form for a sulfonamide group or an ester function, *Int. J. Pharm.*, 51, 27, 1989.
116. **Larsen, J.D., Bundgaard, H., and Lee, V. H. L.,** Prodrug forms for the sulfonamide group. Part 2. Water-soluble amino acid derivatives of N-methylsulfonamides as possible prodrugs, *Int. J. Pharm.*, 47, 103, 1988.
117. **Bundgaard, H. and Larsen, J. D.,** N-sulfonyl imidates as a novel prodrug form for an ester function or a sulfonamide group, *J. Med. Chem.*, 31, 2066, 1988.
118. **Larsen, J. D. and Bundgaard, H.,** Prodrug forms for the sulfonamide group, IV. Kinetics of hydrolysis of N-sulfonyl pseudoures derivatives, *Acta Pharm. Nord.*, 1, 31, 1989.
119. **Larsen, J. D. and Bundgaard, H.,** Prodrug forms for the sulfonamide group. I. Evaluation of N-acyl derivatives, N-sulfonylamidines, N-sulfonylsulfilimines and sulfonylureas as possible prodrug derivatives, *Int. J. Pharm.*, 37, 87, 1987.
120. **Lee, V. H. L.,** Esterase activities in adult rabbit eyes, *J. Pharm. Sci.*, 72, 239, 1983.
121. **Redell, M. A., Yang, D. C., and Lee, V. H. L.,** The role of esterase activity in the ocular disposition of dipivalyl epinephrine in rabbits, *Int. J. Pharm.*, 17, 299, 1983.
122. **Lee, V. H. L., Morimito, K. W., and Stratford, R. E.,** Esterase distribution in the rabbit cornea and its implications in ocular drug bioavailability, *Biopharm. Drug Disp.*, 3, 291, 1982.
123. **Lee, V. H. L., Chang, S.-C., Oshiro, C. M., and Smith, R. E.,** Ocular esterase composition in albino and pigmented rabbits: possible implications in ocular prodrug design and evaluation, *Curr. Eye Res.*, 4, 1117, 1985.
124. **Lee, V. H. L. and Bundgaard, H.,** Improved ocular drug delivery with prodrugs, in *Prodrugs: Topical and Ocular Drug Delivery*, Sloan, K. B., Ed., Marcel Dekker, New York, 1992, 221.
125. **Lee, V. H. L., Chien, D. S., and Sasaki, H.,** Ocular ketone reductase distribution and its role in the metabolism of ocularly applied levobunolol in the pigmented rabbit, *J. Pharmacol. Exp. Ther.*, 246, 871, 1988.
126. **Duffel, M. W., Ing, I. S., Segarra, T. M., Dixson, T. M., Barfknecht, C. F., and Schoenwald, R. D.,** N-Substituted sulfonamide carbonic anhydrase inhibitors with topical effects on intraocular pressure, *J. Med. Chem.*, 29, 1488, 1986.
126a. **Lee, V. H. L. and Bundgaard, H.,** unpublished observations.
127. **Schoenwald, R. D., Eller, M. G., Dixson, J. A., and Barfknecht, C. F.,** Topical carbonic anhydrase inhibitors, *J. Med. Chem.*, 27, 810, 1984.
128. **Bodor, N. and Visor, G.,** Formation of adrenaline in the iris-ciliary body from adrenalone diesters, *Exp. Eye Res.*, 38, 621, 1984.
129. **Lee, V. H. L., Stratford, R. E., and Morimoto, K. W.,** Age-related changes in esterase activity in rabbit eyes, *Int. J. Pharm.*, 13, 183, 1983.
130. **Lee, V. H. L. and Li, V. H. K.,** Prodrugs for improved ocular drug delivery, *Adv. Drug Deliv. Rev.*, 3, 1, 1989.
131. **Schoenwald, R. D. and Ward, R. L.,** Relationship between steroid permeability across excised rabbit cornea and octanol/water partition coefficients, *J. Pharm. Sci.*, 67, 786, 1981.
132. **Mosher, G. L. and Mikkelson, T. J.,** Permeability of the n-alkyl p-aminobenzoate esters across the isolated corneal membrane of the rabbit, *Int. J. Pharm.*, 2, 239, 1979.
133. **Kishida, K. and Otori, T.,** A quantitative study on the relationship between transcorneal permeability of drugs and their hydrophobicity, *Jpn. J. Opthalmol.*, 24, 251, 1980.
134. **Schoenwald, R. D. and Huang, H. S.,** Corneal penetration behavior of β_2-blocking agents. I. Physicochemical factors, *J. Pharm. Sci.*, 72, 1266, 1983.
135. **Chien, D. S., Sasaki, H., Bundgaard, H., Buur, A., and Lee, V. H. L.,** Role of enzymatic lability in the corneal and conjunctival penetration of timolol ester prodrugs in the pigmented rabbit, *Pharm. Res.*, 8, 728, 1991.
136. **Wang, W., Sasaki, H., Chien, D. S., and Lee, V. H. L.,** Lipophilicity influence on conjunctival drug penetration in the pigmented rabbit: a comparison with corneal penetration, *Curr. Eye Res.*, 10, 571, 1991.
137. **Grass, G. M. and Robinson, J. R.,** Relationship of chemical structure to corneal penetration and influence of low-viscosity solution on ocular bioavailability, *J. Pharm. Sci.*, 73, 1021, 1984.

138. **Hobden, J. A., Reidy, J. J., O'Callaghan, R. J., Insler, M. S., and Hill, J. M.,** Quinolones in collagen shields to treat aminoglycoside-resistant pseudomonal keratitis, *Invest. Ophthalmol. Vis. Sci.*, 31, 2241, 1990.

139. **Mitra, A. K. and Mikkelson, T. J.** Mechanism of transcorneal permeation of pilocarpine, *J. Pharm. Sci.*, 77, 771, 1988.

140. **Jankowska, L. M., Bar-Ilan, A., and Maren, T. H.,** The relations between ionic and non-ionic diffusion of sulfonamides across the rabbit cornea, *Invest. Ophthalmol. Vis. Sci.*, 27, 29, 1986.

141. **Grass, G. M., Wood, R. W., and Robinson, J. R.,** Effects of calcium chelating agents on corneal permeability, *Invest. Ophthalmol. Vis. Sci.*, 26, 110, 1985.

142. **Suhonen, P., Järvinen, T., Rytkönen, P., Peura, P., and Urtti, A.,** Improved corneal pilocarpine permeability with O,O'-(1,4-xylylene) bispilocarpic acid ester double prodrugs, *Pharm. Res.*, 8, 1539, 1991.

143. **Usayapant, A., Karara, A. H., and Narurkar, M. M.,** Effect of 2-hydroxy-propyl-β-cyclodextrin on the ocular absorption of dexamethasone and dexamethasone acetate, *Pharm. Res.*, 8, 1494, 1991.

144. **Colla, L., DeClercq, E., Busson, R., and Vanderhaeghe, H.,** Synthesis and antiviral activity of water-soluble esters of acyclovir [9((2-hydroxyethoxy)methyl)guanine], *J. Med. Chem.*, 26, 602, 1983.

145. **Kaufman, H. E., Varnell, E. D., Centifanto, Y. M., and Rheinstrom, S. D.,** Effect of 9-(2-hydroxyl-ethoxymethyl)guanine on herpes virus-induced keratitis and iritis in rabbit, *Antimicrob. Agents Chemother.*, 14, 842, 1978.

146. **Varnell, E. D. and Kaufman, H. E.,** Antiviral agents in experimental herpetic stromal disease, in *Herpetic Eye Diseases,* Bergmann, J. F., Ed., Verlag, Munich, 1981, 303.

147. **Bundgaard, H., Falch, E., and Jensen, E.,** A novel solution-stable, water-soluble prodrug type for drugs containing a hydroxyl or an NH-acidic group, *J. Med. Chem.*, 32, 2503, 1989.

148. **Powell, M. F., Magill, A., Chu, N., Hama, K., Mau, C. I., Foster, L., and Bergstrom, R.,** Chemical and enzymatic degradation of ganciclovir prodrugs: enhanced stability of the diadamantoate prodrug under acid conditions, *Pharm. Res.*, 8, 1418, 1991.

149. **Kirby, A. J. and Lloyd, G. J.,** Intramolecular general base catalysis in the hydrolysis of 3-dimethyl-aminopropionates, *J. Chem. Soc. Perkin Trans.*, 2, 1748, 1976.

150. **Bundgaard, H., Jensen, E., and Falch, E.,** Water-soluble, solution-stable, and biolabile N'substituted(aminomethyl)benzoate ester prodrugs of acyclovir, *Pharm. Res.*, 8, 1087, 1991.

151. **Bundgaard, H.,** Design of bioreversible drug derivatives and the utility of the double prodrug concept, in *Bioreversible Carriers in Drug Design,* Roche, E. B., Ed., Pergamon Press, New York, 1987, 13.

152. **Bundgaard, H.,** The double prodrug concept and its applications, *Adv. Drug Deliv. Rev.*, 3, 39, 1989.

153. **Bundgaard, H. and Johansen, M.,** Prodrugs as drug delivery systems. Part 20. Oxazolidines as potential prodrugs types for beta-amino alcohols, aldehydes or ketones, *Int. J. Pharm.*, 10, 165, 1982.

154. **Johansen, M. and Bundgaard, H.,** Prodrugs as drug delivery systems XXV: hydrolysis of oxazolidines — a potential new prodrug type, *J. Pharm. Sci.*, 72, 1294, 1983.

155. **Buur, A. and Bundgaard, H.,** Prodrugs as drug delivery systems. XXVIII. Structural factors influencing the rate of hydrolysis of oxazolidines — a potential prodrug type, *Int. J. Pharm.* 18, 325, 1984.

156. **Green, K., Chapman, J. M., Cheeks, L., Clayton, M. R., Wilson, M., and Zehir, A.,** Detergent penetration into young and adult rabbit eyes: comparative pharmacokinetics, *J. Toxicol. Cutan. Ocular Toxicol.*, 6, 89, 1987.

157. **Kane, A., Barza, M., and Baum, J.,** Intravitreal injection of gentamicin in rabbits: effects of inflammation and pigmentation on half-life and ocular distribution, *Invest. Ophthalmol. Vis. Sci.*, 20, 593, 1981.

158. **Ashton, P., Wang, W., and Lee, V. H. L.,** Location of penetration and metabolic barriers to levobunolol in the pigmented rabbit, *J. Pharmacol. Exp. Ther.*, 259, 719, 1991.

159. **Graham, S. K., Hoffman, J. M., Gautheron, P., Michelson, S. R., Scholz, T. H., Schwan, H., Shepard, K. L., Smith, A. M., Smith, R. L., and Sondey, J. M.,** Topically active carbonic anhydrase inhibitors. 3. Benzofuran- and idole-2-sulfonamides, *J. Med. Chem.*, 33, 749, 1990.

160. **Weinkam, R. J., Bundgaard, H., WaldeMussie, E., Ruiz, G., Feldman, B., Dino, J., Ismail, I., and Bundgaard, H.,** Pilocarpine prodrugs: O-benzoyl pilocarpic acid methyl ester ocular metabolism and effects on miosis and intraocular pressure, *Pharm. Res.*, 7, S-64, 1990.

Chapter 9

BIOADHESIVES IN OCULAR DRUG DELIVERY

Eliot M. Slovin and Joseph R. Robinson

TABLE OF CONTENTS

I.   Introduction 146

II. Anatomical Aspects of Ocular Drug Delivery 146

III. Ocular Drug Disposition 148

IV. Bioadhesion 150

V.   Ocular Bioadhesives 152

VI. Factors Affecting Ocular Mucoadhesive Drug Delivery 154

References 155

0-8493-7296-8/93/$0.00 + $.50
© 1993 by CRC Press, Inc.

I. INTRODUCTION

Bioadhesive polymers have generated considerable interest in recent years as a way to substantially improve the performance of controlled delivery systems. The reasons for this interest are that these polymers can improve drug delivery through: (1) their ability to localize a dosage form within a particular region, to enhance drug bioavailability, and for local treatment; (2) optimum contact with the absorbing surface to permit modification of tissue permeability in a restricted region, as might be required for absorption of certain drugs; and (3) prolonged residence time/reduced dosing frequency, which promotes patient compliance.[1]

Given the considerable challenge of ocular drug delivery, i.e., short contact time and low drug bioavailability, it is not surprising that alternatives to simple ocular solutions have been sought. A number of systems, intended to improve contact time and drug bioavailability, e.g., soluble and insoluble ocular inserts, are not user-friendly in that patient compliance is low and/or the system is often very uncomfortable. This chapter will focus on a relatively new way to deliver drugs to the eye, namely employing a polymer that attaches, in non-covalent form, to tissues in the front of the eye, i.e., a bioadhesive dosage form. Such systems can be used in suspension form and thus offer the advantage of simplicity of instillation (user-friendly), yet provide for longer contact time.

II. ANATOMICAL ASPECTS OF OCULAR DRUG DELIVERY

Table 1 gives a description of the general mechanisms of drug movement through the cornea.

Specifically, the cornea is a transparent, approximately circular tissue that makes up the forward 1/6 of the eyeball, and is the membrane through which drugs must pass if they are to reach the inner areas of the eye.

The cornea is an avascular, three-layer tissue, approximately 0.5 to 0.7 mm thick and about 11.5 mm in diameter.[2] The first layer, the epithelium, is a tight junction tissue that is approximately six cell layers thick and has a cell turnover rate of approximately one layer per day. This layer has been found to be relatively hydrophobic.[2-4]

The anterior corneal stroma is condensed into a thin membrane separating the top epithelium from the stroma. This interfacial layer is known as Bowman's membrane and is continuous with the stroma. The stroma constitutes 85 to 90% of the cornea and consists of migrant cells and fine collagen fibrils able to hold a substantial quantity of water while remaining optically transparent.[2,3]

Loosely attached to the back surface of the stroma is another interfacial layer known as Descemet's membrane. Descemet's membrane is a glossy membrane which is secreted by the endothelial cells and may, following an injury, form a double layer.[2,3]

The bottom layer of the cornea, the endothelium, consists of a single cell layer which houses an active water pump that regulates corneal thickness through hydration. It is a very porous tissue with an open intercellular network. Endothelial cells do not undergo mitosis. In addition, the flat cells of the corneal endothelium are seen to be continuous with the endothelial covering of the iris.[2-4]

The cornea and conjunctiva are coated with a thin layer of mucin, approximately 0.02 to 0.05 μm[5] and 1.4 μm[6] thick, respectively. Mucin, secreted by the goblet cells in the conjunctiva, consists of a polypeptide backbone lined with sugar groups that terminate in a sialic acid or a sulfate residue. These are acidic functional groups and, as a result, mucin, at physiological pH, acts as an anionic polyelectrolyte capable of picking up 40 to 80 times its weight in water. On the surface of the mucosal tissue mucin molecules are found to be tightly packed, but as one moves outward from the epithelial surface of the cornea, the

TABLE 1
Mechanisms of Drug Permeability Through the Cornea

A. Organ level

- Rate-limiting membrane for most drugs is the corneal epithelium.
- Stroma is rate limiting for very lipid-soluble drugs.
- Molecular weight cutoff for relatively rapid permeation of most drugs is around 5000.

B. Cellular level

- Small molecules, e.g., water, methanol, ethanol, propanol, and butanol, readily traverse the cornea through assumed aqueous pores. Permeability constants are very large.
- Water soluble compounds traverse the cornea by the paracellular route. The smaller the o/w partition coefficient, the smaller the permeability constant. Very lipid-soluble compounds, e.g., progesterone, permeate the cornea via the paracellular route.
- The rate-limiting barrier for most drugs appears to reside in the top two cell layers of the epithelium.
- Peptides and other charged compounds appear to penetrate the cornea by the paracellular route.

From Robinson, J. R., *Bioadhesion — Possibilities and Future Trends,* Gurny, R. and Junginger, H. E., Eds., Wissenschaftliche Verlagsgesellschaft mbH, Stuttgart, 1990, chap. 8. With permission.

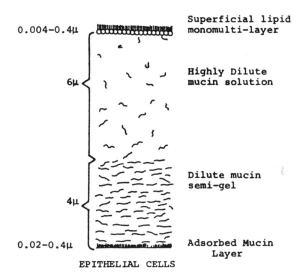

FIGURE 1. Proposed structure of tear film. (From Holly, F. J. and Lemp, M. A., *Contact Lens Soc. Am. J.,* 5, 1, 1971. With permission.)

mucin becomes less densely packed. This is accompanied by a corresponding decrease in viscosity and ion content. It is important to note, though, that while the mucous layers covering the cornea are thin, they are still thick enough for significant interpenetration of the bioadhesive polymer to occur.[4,7]

As previously described, the cornea is a complex membrane through which drugs must pass in order to reach the interior regions of the eye. This would suggest that the bioavailability and duration of the action of drugs which must penetrate the cornea to gain access to its site of action, or whose site of action is the cornea itself, would be improved by prolonging contact between the cornea and the drug. Unfortunately, to complicate matters, the cornea is the window of the vision system and many adhering systems interfere with vision. Thus,

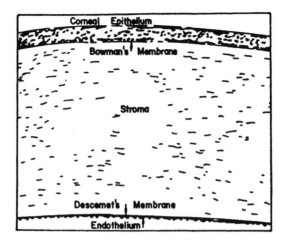

FIGURE 2. Depiction of the cornea in cross-section. (From Robinson, J. R., in *Bioadhesion — Possibilities and Future Trends*, Gurny, R. and Junginger, H. E., Eds., 1990, chap. 8. With permission.)

while direct attachment of the drug delivery system to the cornea is preferred, an alternative approach exists in which the delivery system is placed on, or adhered to, the conjunctiva. The released drug is then able to bathe the cornea.

III. OCULAR DRUG DISPOSITION

A variety of protective physiological events in the front of the eye are responsible for the removal of instilled solution products. The more important of these are listed in Table 2. Collectively these processes lead to a typical corneal contact time of about 1 to 2 min in humans, for an instilled solution, and an ocular bioavailability that is commonly less than 10%.[3,4]

To appreciate the overall importance of these protective mechanisms to drug loss it is helpful to examine the kinetics of the corneal absorptions and precorneal loss processes. Such an examination can permit an estimation of the magnitude of change needed to substantially influence the time course of drug in the eye.

The simplest kinetic model of drug disposition in the eye following dosing is shown in Figure 3.[4]

The k_{loss} term is an overall k_{loss} term, assuming all of the loss systems are first order.[4]

$$k_{loss} = k_m + k_{N.P.A.} + k_{T.T.} + \ldots$$

Independent *in vitro* measurements of corneal absorption for many drugs provide a range of corneal absorption rate constants in the neighborhood of $k_{absorption} = 0.001$ to 0.01 min^{-1}.[3,4] In contrast, $k_{elimination}$ for many drugs is in the range of $k_{elimination} = 0.02$ to 0.008 min^{-1}.[8,9] Without the k_{loss} portion of the model we would have what is shown in Figure 5. Based on the above description and given the relative magnitudes of k_{abs} and k_{elim}, this is a classic "flip-flop" pharmacokinetic model, i.e., the $k_{absorption}$ term is smaller in magnitude than the $k_{elimination}$ term. However, the addition of the k_{loss} term converts the flip-flop model to a conventional model because $k_{absorption}^{observed} = k_{absorption} + k_{loss}$. Given that the typical magnitude of k_{loss} is in the neighborhood of 0.2 to 0.5 min^{-1},[8,9] the overall observed absorption term is thus

$$k_{abs}^{obs} = (0.01—0.001) + (0.5—0.2) = (0.501—0.2001) \text{ min}^{-1}$$

TABLE 2
Precorneal Factors Causing Loss of Drug from the Front of the Eye

Precorneal factor	Explanation
Tear turnover	• Tears replace themselves at a rate of 16%/min, except during periods of sleep or during anesthesia. Normal tear volume is only 7 μl so drug loss can be substantial.
Instilled solution drainage	• The precorneal area can hold approximately 20 μl, including resident tears. Excess instilled volumes will spill onto the cheek or rapidly drain.
	• From the moment of solution instillation, solution drains from the front of the eye into the nasolacrimal duct with subsequent absorption into the systemic circulation.
	• Rate of solution drainage is proportional to the instilled volume and for low viscosity solutions is generally complete in 1 to 2 min in the human.
Protein binding	• Tears normally contain only about 0.2% protein, as compared to approximately 7.0% in blood, but can rise dramatically if an infection or inflammation is present. Unlike the blood, where the drug-protein complex continues to circulate, tears replace themselves quickly thus removing both free and bound forms of the drug from the front of the eye.
	• Protein content in the aqueous humor is normally low, about 0.02%, but the level can rise dramatically during certain anterior segment pathologies. Aqueous humor replaces itself at a rate of 1%/min and drug levels in the anterior segment are typically quite low.
Non-productive drug absorption	• From the moment of drug instillation into the eye, drug is absorbed into the cornea and conjunctiva and, in the case of rabbits, into the nictitating membrane.
	• The surface area of the conjunctiva is about five times that of the cornea with a slightly greater permeability to many drugs. If the target tissue is the interior of the eye, all tissue absorption other than the cornea is perceived as nonproductive loss.

From Robinson, J. R., *Bioadhesion — Possibilities and Future Trends*, Gurny, R. and Junginger, H. E., Eds., Wissenschaftliche Verlagsgesellschaft mbH, Stuttgart, 1990, chap. 8. With permission.

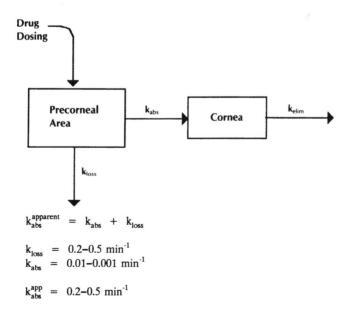

FIGURE 3. Precorneal parallel elimination loss pathway. (From Robinson, J. R., *STP Pharma*, 5(12), 839, 1989. With permission.)

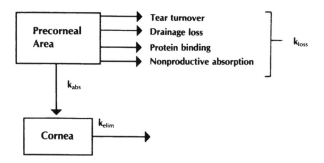

FIGURE 4. Pathways of potential drug loss from the front of the eye. (From Robinson, J. R., *STP Pharma*, 5(12), 839, 1989. With permission.)

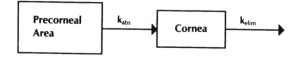

FIGURE 5. Ocular drug delivery.

This is the reason why the peak time of most drugs in aqueous humor, irrespective of their physicochemical properties, is usually short, signifying a large absorption rate constant when, indeed, the true absorption rate constant is very small.[8] In addition, there is a general compression of C_{max} values for many drugs. This is also the reason why ocular drug bioavailability is relatively insensitive to dosage form modification. Thus, to have a substantial influence on ocular drug bioavailability it will be necessary to

1. Increase corneal drug absorption by one to two orders of magnitude through prodrugs or corneal penetration enhancers to make the k_{abs} term larger and thus competitive with k_{loss} and k_{elim}.
2. Decrease precorneal pocket loss by one to two orders of magnitude by minimizing solution drainage/tear turnover effect on drug loss, etc. This then makes k_{abs} competitive with k_{loss} by making k_{loss} smaller.

IV. BIOADHESION

Bioadhesion is an interfacial phenomenon in which a synthetic or natural polymer is attached to a biological substrate by means of interfacial forces. When the adhesive bond is established, the total surface energy of the system is diminished, and upon destruction of the two free surfaces, a new interface is created.

The adhesive interaction between two materials or surfaces, at least one of which is biological, is called bioadhesion.[10] If one of these surfaces is a mucous-covered membrane, or if one of the substances involved is mucin, the interaction is classified more narrowly and the term mucoadhesion is employed.

It is interesting to note that the concept of bioadhesion is not new, given that cells can strongly attach to one another and bacteria are known to attach to mucosal tissues. In addition, the attachment of natural and synthetic polymers to biological substrates is also old, as demonstrated with the use of the bioadhesive, polymerized maleic anhydride for denture retention. However, what is novel is the renewed interest in the employment of bioadhesive polymers for drug delivery purposes since 1984 when Nagai[11] demonstrated the successful commercial use of a buccal bioadhesive.

An important limitation in ocular drug delivery is the short residence time of a topically applied drug. It has recently been shown,[12] through calculations of the passive permeation of drug through a biological membrane, that permeability is not necessarily the major barrier to peptide delivery. To achieve therapeutic levels of the drug via ocular delivery, one needs to extend the residence time of the dose. Bioadhesives have been shown to have the potential of giving enhanced drug availability[13,14] through their ability to increase the residence time of a drug.

Many researchers[15-19] active in the field of drug delivery have reported on attempts to identify potential bioadhesives. From these numerous studies, a number of polymers possessing mucoadhesive properties have been discovered. In addition, a variety of tests have been reported in the literature[20] to assess the bioadhesive strength of a number of natural and synthetic polymers. Most of these tests provide the same rank order of adhesiveness for the polymers tested. A short list of the best of the adhesives currently used in pharmaceutical products includes

- carboxymethylcellulose
- carbopol
- polycarbophil
- hydroxypropylcellulose

Note that in the above list some of the polymers are neutral, while others are charged. Moreover, some are water soluble and others are crosslinked and water insoluble. All of these are macromolecular hydrocolloids with numerous hydrophilic functional groups, e.g., carboxyl, hydroxyl, amide, and sulfate. It has been reported[15,21] that (1) the mucoadherence of neutral polymers is usually much weaker than that seen with either anionic or cationic polymers, and (2) cationic polymers are usually more toxic than their anionic counterparts. Therefore, on the basis of the most effective balance between adhesiveness and toxicity, anionic polymers, in general, are preferred over neutral and cationic. In addition, crosslinked polymers give longer residence times than their linear, water soluble counterparts.

Water soluble and water insoluble mucoadhesives have been observed to attach through noncovalent bonds to the mucin covering of the eye. Once attached, it would be expected that the water soluble mucoadhesive would slowly be dissolved and cleared by the bathing tears, while the insoluble mucoadhesive would remain attached until either the shear force of blinking causes the mucoadhesive to be dislodged or until the mucous layer goes through its natural turnover cycle (estimated to be approximately 15 to 20 h in the human), dislodging the polymer.[3] Indeed, residence time for crosslinked polymers, e.g., polycarbophil, appears to be limited by the turnover time of the underlying epithelial cell layer or mucin.

The mechanism(s) of attachment of these polymers to the membrane surface has been explored by a number of investigators.[16,22,23] The possible forces of interactions include

- covalent bonds such as in cyanoacrylates
- hydrogen bonds
- electrostatic interactions
- hydrophobic interactions

Cyanoacrylates are not approved for use in the U.S. because of the formation of formaldehyde. However, assuming that toxicity is not an issue, there is nothing fundamentally wrong with covalent bioadhesives. Of the remaining three forces, hydrogen bonding appears to be the most important followed by electrostatic and hydrophobic.

It would appear that the adhesion process begins as a surface phenomenon where the closeness in surface tension between the adhesive polymer and the biological substrate determines initial contact and interaction. Additional forces then stabilize the interactions. There is also some contribution from entanglement of the swollen polymer network and the hydrated mucin, i.e., interpenetration.

The molecular weight of the polymer has also been found to be important in the design of a drug delivery system. Adhesive strength increases with molecular weight until a critical limit is reached beyond which little improvement in bioadhesive strength is seen. This adhesive strength/molecular weight relationship is related to the chain length and configuration of the polymer, as borne out by studies[16,24] in which optimal interpenetration and molecular entanglement between the polymer and the substrate were examined. For example, for polyethylene oxide, a highly linear polymer, improvement in adhesive strength is observed[24] upon increases in molecular weight to 4 million, whereas the characterization of the adhesive properties of dextrans shows that polymers with molecular weights of 19.5 million had bioadhesive strengths similar to polymers of 200,000. This has been explained[25] as mainly being due to the many adhesively active groups shielded within the coiled configuration of the dextrans. This coiled configuration prevents these groups from participating in the formation of secondary chemical bonds. Thus, molecular weight, chain length, and configuration of the polymer are all factors critical in the optimization of the interpenetration and entanglement of the polymer and substrate.

V. OCULAR BIOADHESIVES

A viscous gel containing pilocarpine base and 0.77% w/v polyacrylic acid produced a significant increase in bioavailability over an aqueous solution of pilocarpine nitrate.[26] The area under the curve (pupillary diameter vs. time) was seen to be 2.4 times greater. When a lightly crosslinked (0.3%) polyacrylic acid was used as a delivery system, bioavailability studies showed that the area under the curve was 4.2 times greater than a conventional suspension.[27]

Similarly, the administration of pilocarpine incorporated into solid inserts of polyvinyl alcohol placed into the conjunctival sac produced bioavailability increases of 1.7 to 2.3 over an aqueous solution.[26] When similar inserts containing polyacrylic acid in addition to the polyvinyl alcohol were used, the bioavailability was seen to be 2.7 to 4.3 times greater than an aqueous solution.[26] Therefore, it appears that polyacrylic acid, as well as its lightly cross-linked analog, possesses good bioadhesive character, indicating prolonged residence time in the precorneal region with a greater chance for ocular absorption.

Investigations of ocular therapy with nanoparticulate systems have resulted in the observation that some nanoparticles are able to adhere to corneal and conjunctival surfaces. This adhesiveness enables them to resist the complex precorneal fluid dynamics, thereby increasing drug absorption and bioavailability.[28-31] Nanoparticles are solid, colloidal particles ranging in size from 0.01 to 1.0 μm that are made up of macromolecular materials in which drug may be dissolved, entrapped, or adsorbed.[28,31] Unfortunately, the loading capacity of nanoparticles is usually low; thus, the thin layer of particles on the corneal surface is able to deliver only small quantities of drug.

To date, two general nanoparticle systems have been developed for ophthalmic delivery.[28] The first uses a charged polymethacrylate[30] and the second, a polyalkylcyanoacrylate system.[28] In the charged polymethacrylate system pilocarpine containing nanoparticles, normally at a pH around 4.4, coagulates within seconds of being placed in the cul-de-sac of the eye. It was suggested that this was due to the pH change of some 2.8 units upon instillation into the tear fluids normally at pH 7.2. The resulting gel cannot easily be washed out of the cul-de-sac by the lacrimal fluid and a retardation in the release of pilocarpine is observed. Therefore, it was shown that by temperature, pH, and electrolyte changes there is an alteration in vicosity of the instilled polymer resulting in prolongation of the residence time of a drug in the tear film.

In the polyalkylcyanoacrylate system the nanoparticles have a tendency to accumulate on the mucous membranes by binding to the cornea and the conjunctival tissues resulting in a prolonged residence time and an increased biological response. In addition, a mucolytic agent, used to demonstrate that the polyhexylcyanoacrylate nanoparticles adhered directly to the epithelial surface of the corneal and conjunctival tissues, led the authors[29] to conclude that the mucin layer was not a barrier to drug permeation.

The potential of using adhesive liposomes as a means of facilitating the transport of drugs through the cornea and enhancing the bioavailability of the entrapped drug has also been studied.[32-36] Liposomes are highly ordered collections of water-insoluble polar lipids that are formed when these lipids are combined with water under suitable conditions. If the liposomes are formed in the presence of a drug, the drug, depending on its solubility characteristics, will be incorporated in either the aqueous or lipid layer.[37] In general, polar or hydrophilic drugs are largely found to incorporate within the internal, aqueous portion of the liposome, while neutral or lipophilic drugs are more often found in the lipid layer of the liposome.

The behavior of liposomes as an ocular drug delivery system has been observed to be in part due to surface charge. The binding affinity of liposomes to the cornea has been shown to be greatest for positively charged liposomes, less for negatively charged liposomes, and least for neutral liposomes[32] suggesting that the interaction between the cornea and the liposomes is probably electrostatic in nature. Hence, while positively charged liposomes work best to enhance bioavailability and prolong the uptake of incorporated drug into the cornea, significant increases were also seen for the negatively charged and neutral liposomal systems.[36] From this evidence it appears that liposomes can interact with the corneal epithelium resulting in an increase in their precorneal residence time and, in turn, the pharmacological effect of the incorporated drug.

Lectins are plant and animal extracts found to have a strong tendency to bind to specific carbohydrate groups.[38,39] Some researchers[40-42] have reported isolating purified lectins that selectively bind to sialic acids. This seems very promising from a mucoadhesive point of view since sialic acid is seen prominently in the structural backbone of mucin.

In addition, pretreatment of the cornea with wheat germ agglutinin (a plant lectin) produced a 2.5-fold increase in the binding of liposomes to the cornea,[43] suggesting that lectin might mediate the specific binding of the liposomes to the corneal surface. This observation further suggests that lectin, when applied in concert with liposomes, may be found to be an effective ocular delivery system.

Fibrin film, a biodegradable polymer prepared from human plasma, has also been evaluated as a possible carrier that will prolong drug activity in the eye.[44] Prepared as a biodegradable insert loaded with pilocarpine, the fibrin film showed good biocompatibility with ocular tissues in an *in vivo* rabbit study. The pharmacological contribution of the pilocarpine-loaded system was seen to last longer than 8 h as compared with the 4 to 5 h seen with an ophthalmic solution.

A similar erodible insert made of reconstituted, solubilizable collagen polymer has been reported[45] for the long-term ocular delivery of therapeutic levels of gentamicin. The data suggests that the inserts offer a convenient, atraumatic method of treating infected, ulcerated corneal tissues with antimicrobial medications. The collagen wafer showed the highest and most sustained concentration of the drug when compared to gentamicin administered by drops, ointment, or periocular injection.

The bioadhesive properties of fibrin have also been proven to be useful in preventing bleeding and reestablishing attachment and adhesion of the conjunctiva in retinal detachment, strabismus, and cataract surgery.[46] Strands of fibrin are produced through the interaction of thrombin and fibrinogen containing human cryoprecipitate. Calcium and factor XII, both present in the cryoprecipitate, catalyze the chemical conversion of fibrinogen to fibrin and activate fibrin for reattachment of conjunctiva cells.

Fibronectin, a glycoprotein found in plasma and the extracellular matrix is responsible for cellular adhesion and the attachment of fibroblasts to the extracellular matrix. Fibronectin has been observed to bind lectin,[47] collagen,[48-51] glycosaminoglycans,[52] other cell surfaces, granulocytes, monocytes, and bacteria.[53,54] Re-epitheliation of corneal ulcers has been clinically facilitated upon treatment with autologous, purified fibronectin eye drops.[55] Fibronectin and hyaluronic acid have been shown[56] to decrease the healing time of dermal wounds when used in conjunction with a collagen-based dressing.

VI. FACTORS AFFECTING OCULAR MUCOADHESIVE DRUG DELIVERY

As previously stated, it is generally accepted that to improve ocular drug bioavailability it is necessary to extend the period of contact between the drug and the cornea. In order to be able to design a dosage form which will be able to increase this contact time, one needs to understand the physicochemical nature of the cornea and the corneal surface.

At the corneal surface it has been found that there is a preferential uptake of cationic over anionic and neutral liposomes.[32] It is therefore likely that electrostatic interactions occur at the negatively charged corneal surface with the possible involvement of the negatively charged groups on the mucous covering of the surface of the cornea.

In the precorneal region, the physiological pH has been found to be between 7.3 and 7.7.[7] pH effect has been shown[57] to affect ocular drug penetration through the epithelial layers by altering the ionic form of the drug. In addition, the hydration of anionic bioadhesives, e.g., polycarbophil, a lightly crosslinked polyacrylic acid, is often maximum at physiological pH, and while the formation of hydrogen bonds and mucoadhesive strength is seen to be less than at a more acidic pH where carboxyl groups are protonated, attachment is still strong enough for an excellent retention of the drug delivery system in the eye.[57-60] This implies that while hydrogen bonding is the primary force, interpenetration and physical entanglement of the polymer chains and mucin also play an important role in the establishment of bioadhesive bonds.[61,62]

Viscosity in aqueous media is one of the most important properties of a mucoadhesive polymer. Polymer-solvent and polymer-solvent-tear film interactions depend upon molecular flexibility, type of solvent, degree of ionization, polymer concentration, and pH.[60,63] In addition, the degree of entanglement between the polymer chains also affects viscosity as demonstrated by a correlation between molecular weight and viscosity[64] in which it was seen that the more extended the polymer form, the higher its viscosity.

In general, it is seen that upon an increase in viscosity of the delivery system, the rate of precorneal loss of drug is decreased. This is most probably due to the ability of the vehicle to retain the drug in the precorneal region for an extended period of time. This extended contact time has been observed to result in increased drug absorption and therapeutic effect.[65-68] Since increases in precorneal contact time may be due to both the mucoadhesive and viscosity effects of the polymer, it may be advisable that when a delivery system is designed, a polymer should be chosen that, in addition to possessing good mucoadhesive strength, is also seen to increase the viscosity at a reasonably low concentration.

In the precorneal area, the increase in the lacrimation produced in response to an external insult to the eye can result in a dilution of the instilled drug and a decrease in bioavailability due to the continual tear turnover. Tear secretions have been seen to be affected by the pH, tonicity, anesthesia, and the instillation of drug and/or its dosage form. This effect of increased lacrimation is important to consider, especially when the bioadhesive system is designed in a liquid form in which an increased production of tears increases the rate of clearance of the delivery system.[4,7,69-71]

REFERENCES

1. **Gu, J. M., Robinson, J. R., and Leung, S.-H., S.,** Binding of acrylic polymers to mucin/epithelial surfaces: structure-property relationships, *CRC Critical Reviews in Therapeutic Drug Carrier Systems,* Vol. 5 (1), 1988, 21.
2. **Cumming, J. S.,** Relevant anatomy and physiology of the eye, in *Ophthalmic Drug Delivery Systems,* Robinson, J. R., Ed., American Pharmaceutical Association, Washingtons, D.C., 1980., 1980, chap. 1.
3. **Robinson, J. R.,** Mucoadhesive ocular drug delivery systems, in *Biadhesion — Possibilities and Future Trends,* Gurny, R. and Junginger, H. E., Eds., Wissenschaftliche Verlagsgesellschaft mbH, Stuttgart, 1990, chap. 8.
4. **Robinson, J. R.,** Ocular drug delivery. Mechanism(s) of corneal drug transport and mucoadhesive delivery systems, *STP Pharma* , 5 (12), 839, 1989.
5. **Sade, J., Eliezer, N., Silberberg, A., and Nevo, J.,** The role of mucin transport by cilia, *Am. Rev. Resp. Dis.,* 102, 48, 1970.
6. **Nichols, B. A., Chiappino, M. L., and Dawson, C. R.,** Determination of the mucous layer of the tear film by electron microscope, *Invest. Ophthalmol. Vis. Sci.,* 26, 464, 1985.
7. **Leung, S.-H. S. and Robinson, J. R.,** Bioadhesives in drug delivery, *Polym. News,* 15, 333, 1990.
8. **Makoid, M. C., Sieg, J. W., and Robinson, J. R.,** Corneal drug absorption: an illustration of parallel first-order absorption and rapid loss of drug from absorption depot, *J. Pharm. Sci.,* 65, 150, 1976.
9. **Middleton, D. L. and Robinson, J. R.,** Design and evaluation of an ocular bioadhesive delivery system, *STP Pharma,* 1, 200, 1991.
10. **Good, R. J.,** Definition of bioadhesion, *J. Adhes.,* 8, 1, 1976.
11. **Nagai, T. and Machida, Y.,** Advances in drug delivery. Mucosal adhesive dosage forms, *Pharm. Int.,* 6, 652, 1985.
12. **Harris, D. and Robinson, J. R.,** Bioadhesive polymers in peptide drug delivery, *Biomaterials,* 11, 652, 1990.
13. **Rozier, A., Mazuel, C., Grove, J., and Plazonnet, B.,** Gelrite®: a novel, ion-activated, *in situ* gelling polymer for ophthalmic vehicles. Effect on bioavailability of timolol, *Int. J. Pharm.,* 57, 163, 1989.
14. **Gurny, R., Ibrahim, H., Aebi, A., Buri, P., and Wilson, C.,** Design and evaluation of controlled release systems for the eye, *J. Controlled Release,* 6, 367, 1987.
15. **Park, K. and Robinson, J. R.,** Bioadhesive polymers as platforms for oral controlled drug delivery: method to study bioadhesion, *Int. J. Pharm.,* 19, 107, 1984.
16. **Smart, J. D., Kellaway, I. W., and Worthington, H. E. C.,** An in-vitro investigation of mucosa-adhesive materials for use in controlled drug delivery, *J. Pharm. Pharmacol.,* 36, 295, 1984.
17. **Ching H. S., Park, H., Kelly, P., and Robinson, J. R.,** Bioadhesive polymers as platforms for oral controlled drug delivery. II. Synthesis and evaluation of some swelling, water insoluble bioadhesive polymers, *J. Pharm. Sci.,* 74, 399, 1985.
18. **Bindschaedler, C., Gurny, R., and Doelker, E.,** Mechanically strong films produced from cellulose acetate latexes, *J. Pharm. Pharmacol.,* 39, 335, 1987.
19. **Mikos, A. G. and Peppas, N. A.,** Comparison of experimental techniques for the measurement of the bioadhesive forces of polymeric material with soft tissues, in *Proc. Int. Symp. Controlled Release Bioact. Mater.,* 13, 97, 1986.
20. **Park, K. and Park, H.,** Test methods of bioadhesion, in *Bioadhesive Drug Delivery Systems,* Lenaerts, V. and Gurny, R., Eds., CRC Press, Boca Raton, FL, 1990, chap. 3.
21. **Park, K., Ch'ng, H. S., and Robinson, J. R.,** Alternate approaches to oral controlled drug delivery. Bioadhesives and in-situ systems, in *Recent Advances in Drug Delivery Systems,* Anderson, J. M. and Kim, S. W., Eds., Plenum Press, 1984, 163.

22. **Peppas, N. A. and Buri, P. A.,** Surface, interfacial, and molecular aspects of polymer bioadhesion on soft tissues, *J. Controlled Release,* 2, 257, 1985.

23. **Leung, S.-H. S. and Robinson, J. R.,** The contribution of anionic polymer structural features to mucoadhesion, *J. Controlled Release,* 5, 223, 1988.

24. **Chen, J. L. and Cyr, G. N.,** Compositions producing adhesion through hydration, in *Adhesive Biological System,* Manly, R. S., Ed., Academic Press, New York, chap. 10.

25. **Gurny, R., Meyer, J. M., and Peppas, N. A.,** Bioadhesive intraoral release systems: design, testing, and analysis, *Biomaterials,* 5, 336, 1984.

26. **Saettone, M. F., Giannaccini, B., Chetoni, P., Galli, G., and Chiellini, E.,** Vehicle effects in ophthalmic bioavailability: an evaluation of polymeric inserts containing pilocarpine, *J. Pharm. Pharmacol.,* 36, 229, 1983.

27. **Hui, H.-W. and Robinson, J. R.,** Ocular delivery of progesterone using a bioadhesive polymer, *Int. J. Pharm.,* 26, 203, 1985.

28. **Kreuter, J.,** Nanoparticles as bioadhesive ocular drug delivery systems, in *Bioadhesive Drug Delivery Systems,* Lenaerts, V. and Gurny, R., Eds., CRC Press, Boca Raton, FL, 1990, chap. 11.

29. **Wood, R. W., Li, V. H. K., Kreuter, J., and Robinson, J. R.,** Ocular disposition of poly-hexyl-2-cyano-[3–14C]-acrylate nanoparticles in the albino rabbit, *Int. J. Pharm.,* 23, 175, 1985.

30. **Gurny, R., Boye, T., and Ibrahim, H.,** Ocular therapy with nanoparticulate systems for controlled drug delivery, *J. Controlled Release,* 2, 353, 1985.

31. **Kreuter, J.,** Evaluation of nanoparticles as drug delivery systems. I. Preparation methods, *Pharm. Acta Helv.,* 58, 196, 1983.

32. **Schaeffer, H. E. and Krohn, D. L.,** Liposomes in topical drug delivery, *Invest. Ophthalmol. Vis. Sci.,* 22, 220, 1982.

33. **Stratford, R. E., Yang, D. C., Redell, M. A., and Lee, V. H. L.,** Effects of topically applied liposomes on disposition of epinephrine and inulin in the rabbit eye, *Int. J. Pharm.,* 13, 263, 1983.

34. **Singh, K. and Mezei, M.,** Liposomal ophthalmic drug delivery system. I. Triamcinolone acetonide, *Int. J. Pharm.,* 16, 339, 1983.

35. **Fitzgerald, P., Hadgraft, J., and Wilson, C. G.,** A gamma scintigraphic evaluation of the precorneal residence of liposomal formations in the rabbit, *J. Pharm. Pharmacol.,* 39, 487, 1987.

36. **Lee, V. H. L., Takemoto, K. A., and Iimoto, D. S.,** Precorneal factors influencing the ocular disposition of topically applied inulin, *Curr. Eye Res.,* 3, 585, 1984.

37. **Shell, J. W.,** Ophthalmic drug delivery systems, *Drug. Dev. Res.,* 6, 245, 1985.

38. **McCoy, J. P.,** Contemporary laboratory applications of lectins, *Biotechniques,* 4, 252, 1986.

39. **Barondes, S. H.,** Soluble lectins: a new class of extracellular proteins, *Science,* 223, 1259, 1984.

40. **Marchalonis, J. J. and Edelman, G. M.,** Isolation and characterization of hemaglutinin from Limulus polyphemus, *J. Mol. Biol.,* 32, 453, 1968.

41. **Bishayee, S. and Dorai, D. T.,** Isolation and characterization of a sialic-binding lectin (Carcinoscoporin) from Indian horseshoe crab, Carcinoscoporus rotunda cauda, *Biochim. Biophys. Acta,* 623, 89, 1980.

42. **Miller, R. L., Colawn, J. F., Jr., and Fish, W. W.,** Purification and macromolecular properties of a sialic acid specific lectin from the slug Limax flavus, *J. Biol. Chem.,* 257, 7574, 1982.

43. **Schaeffer, H. E., Breitfeller, J. M., and Krohn, D. L.,** Lectin-mediated attachment of liposomes to cornea: influence on transcorneal flux, *Invest. Ophthalmol. Vis. Sci.,* 23, 530, 1982.

44. **Miyazaki, S., Ishii, K., and Takada, M.,** Use of fibrin film as a carrier for drug delivery: a long-acting delivery system for pilocarpine into the eye, *Chem. Pharm. Bull,* 30, 3405, 1982.

45. **Bloomfield, S. E., Miyata, T., Dunn, M. W., Bueser, N., Stenzel, K. H., and Rubin, A. L.,** Soluble gentamicin ophthalmic inserts as a drug delivery system, *Arch. Ophthalmol.,* 96, 885, 1978.

46. **Zauberman, H. and Hemo, I.,** Use of fibrin glue in ocular surgery, *Ophthalmic Surg.,* 19, 132, 1988.

47. **Peters, B. P. and Goldstein, I. J.,** The use of fluorescein conjugated Bandeireaea simplicifolia B4-isolectin as a histochemical reagent for the detection of α-D-galactopyranosyl groups. Their occurrence in basement membranes, *Expl. Cell. Res.,* 120, 321, 1979.

48. **Dessau, W., Jilek, F., Adelman, B. C., and Hormann, H.,** Similarity of antigelatin factor and cold insoluble globulin, *Biochim. Biophys. Acta,* 533, 227, 1978.

49. **Fyrand, O.,** Studies on fibronectin in the skin. I. Indirect immunofluorescence studies in normal human skin, *Br. J. Dermatol.,* 101, 263, 1979.

50. **Yamada, K. M.,** Immunological characterization of a major transformation sensitive fibroblast cell surface glycoprotein, *J. Cell Biol.,* 78, 520, 1978.

51. **Ruoslahti, E., Engvall, E., and Hayman, E. G.,** Fibronectin: current concepts of its structure and function, *Collagen Res.,* 1, 95, 1981.

52. **Strathakis, N. E. and Mosesson, M. W.,** Interaction among heparin, cold insoluble globulin, and fibrinogen in the formation of the heparin-precipitate fraction of plasma, *J. Clin. Invest.,* 60, 855, 1988.

53. **Snyder, E. L. and Luban, N. L. C.**, Fibronectin: applications to clinical medicine, *CRC Crit. Rev. Clin. Lab. Sci.*, 23, 15, 1986.
54. **Hasty, D. L. and Simpson, W. A.**, Effects of fibronectin and other salivary macromolecules on the adherence of Escherichia coli to buccal epithelial cell, *Infect. Immun.*, 55, 2103, 1987.
55. **Nishida, T., Ohashi, Y., Awata, T., and Manabe, R.**, Fibronectin: a new therapy for corneal trophic ulcer, *Arch. Ophthalmol.*, 101, 1046, 1983.
56. **Doillon, C. J. and Silver, F. H.**, Collagen-based wound dressing: effects of hyaluronic acid and fibronectin on wound healing, *Biomaterials*, 7, 3, 1986.
57. **Leibowitz, H. and Kupferman, A.**, Pharmacology of topically administered corticosteroids, presented at 79th Annu. Meet, Am. Acad. Ophthalmol. and Otolaryngol., October 1974.
58. **Park, H. and Robinson, J. R.**, Physico-chemical properties of water insoluble polymers important to mucin/epithelial adhesion, *J. Controlled Release*, 2, 47, 1985.
59. **Park, H.**, Synthesis and Evaluation of Some Bioadhesive Hydrogels, M.S. thesis, University of Wisconsin, Madison, 1984.
60. **Middleton, D. L., Leung, S.-H. S., and Robinson, J. R.**, Ocular mucoadhesive delivery systems, in *Bioadhesive Drug Delivery Systems*, Lenaerts, V. and Gurny, R., Eds., CRC Press, Boca Raton, FL, 1990, chap. 10.
61. **Peppas, N. A. and Buri, P. A.**, Surface, interfacial and molecular aspects of polymer adhesion on soft tissues, *J. Controlled Release*, 2, 257, 1985.
62. **Mikos, A. G. and Pappas, N. A.**, Scaling concepts and molecular theories of adhesion of synthetic polymers to glycoproteinic networks, in *Bioadhesive Drug Delivery Systems*, Lenaerts, V. and Gurny, R., Eds., CRC Press, Boca Raton, FL, 1990, chap. 2.
63. **Florence, A. T. and Attwood, D.**, Polymeric system, in *Physicochemical Principles of Pharmacy*, 3rd ed., Chapman and Hall, New York, 1982, chap. 8.
64. **Hiemenz, P. C.**, The viscous state, in *Polymer Chemistry*, Hiemenz, P. C., Ed., Marcel Dekker, New York, 1984, chap. 2.
65. **Madger, H. and Boyaner, D.**, The use of a longer acting pilocarpine in the management of chronic simple glaucoma, *Can. J. Ophthalmol.*, 9, 285, 1984.
66. **Haas, J. and Merrill, D. L.**, The effects of methyl cellulose on responses to solutions of pilocarpine, *Am. J. Ophthalmol.*, 54, 21, 1962.
67. **Hardberger, R. E., Hanna, C., and Goodart, R.**, Effects of drug vehicles on ocular uptake of tetracycline, *Am. J. Ophthalmol.*, 80, 133, 1974.
68. **Gurny, R., Boye, T., and Ibrahim, H.**, Ocular therapy with nanoparticles for controlled drug delivery, *J. Controlled Release*, 2, 353, 1985.
69. **Patton, T. F.**, Ocular drug disposition, in *Ophthalmic Drug Delivery Systems*, Robinson, J. R., Ed., American Pharmaceutical Association, Washington, D.C., 1980, chap. 2.
70. **Sieg, J. and Robinson, J. R.**, Vehicle effects on ocular drug availability II: evaluation of pilocarpine, *J. Pharm. Sci.*, 66, 1222, 1977.
71. **Sieg, J. and Robinson, J. R.**, Corneal absorption of fluorometholone in rabbits. A comparative evaluation of corneal drug transport characteristics in anesthetized and unanesthetized rabbits, *Arch. Ophthalmol.*, 92, 240, 1974.

Chapter 10

PHARMACOKINETICS IN OCULAR DRUG DELIVERY

Ronald D. Schoenwald

TABLE OF CONTENTS

I.   Introduction 160

II.   Classical Pharmacokinetic Modeling 160
       A.   Application to the Eye 160
             1.   Compartmental Modeling 160
                   a.   Fluorescein 161
                   b.   Pilocarpine 161
                   c.   Cefotaxime 164
                   d.   Clonidine 165
             2.   Noncompartmental Modeling 165
             3.   Physiologic Modeling 169
       B.   Limitations to the Ocular Use of Classical Modeling
             Approaches 172

III.   Precorneal Loss 173

IV.   Absorption into the Anterior Chamber 176
       A.   Cornea 176
       B.   Sclera 183

V.   Anterior Chamber Disposition (Distribution and Elimination) 185
       A.   Distribution 185
             1.   Iris 185
             2.   Ciliary Body 186
             3.   Lens 186
       B.   Elimination 187

References 188

0-8493-7296-8/93/$0.00 + $.50
© 1993 by CRC Press, Inc.

I. INTRODUCTION

The pharmacokinetics of drugs intended for systemic use has been extremely useful in the design of an improved therapeutic agent. Specifically, pharmacokinetics has aided in the design of new chemical structures with optimal transport characteristics. It has also been an indispensable tool in establishing bioequivalent drug products and in determining therapeutic dosing regimens. The individual processes of pharmacokinetics are absorption, distribution, metabolism, and excretion (i.e., ADME). These individual processes, which occur in a sequential manner, can be quantitated from measurement of tissue concentrations of drug and are almost always expressed mathematically as a summation of exponentials. The classical approach to quantifying ADME is to divide the body into a series of reversibly connected compartments. This approach often permits an accurate mathematical description of the data, but suffers from the disadvantage that the compartments do not strictly represent physiological or anatomical regions of the body. An alternate approach, e.g., noncompartmental analysis, only requires that the data fit into sums of exponentials. Another method, referred to as physiologic modeling, is based upon clearance concepts. These approaches allow for the development of equations to calculate parameter values representing the rate and extent of each of the processes.

Although the eye can be easily divided into compartments representing anatomical or physiological regions, classical pharmacokinetic modeling has not been very useful in improving therapeutic agents intended for ocular use. Nevertheless, numerous studies have been published in the ophthalmic literature in which various tissue concentrations of drug have been measured over time. Despite the lack of modeling, these studies have been indispensable to both the design and delivery of ocular drugs. The lack of success in applying classical pharmacokinetic modeling to the eye is a result of a number of limitations, all unique to the eye. However, prior to discussing these limitations, the following section summarizes the ocular applications of classical pharmacokinetic modeling.

II. CLASSICAL PHARMACOKINETIC MODELING

A. APPLICATION TO THE EYE

For drugs administered systemically, three modeling systems have been extensively studied; they are the multicompartmental approach, noncompartmental analysis based on statistical moment theory, and physiologic models.[1] The first two approaches have been successful in new drug design, helping to establish bioavailability parameters and to predict multiple dosing regimens in the clinic. The latter approach, physiologic modeling, has led to a better understanding of clearance concepts when applied to various organ systems, but has not been very useful for predictive purposes.

1. Compartmental Modeling

There are a number of assumptions that must be met for the successful application of the classical compartmental model. First, the approach requires that the data be described by a sum of exponentials (i.e., linear kinetics). Second, in order to correctly assign parameter values to each process, the relative magnitude of the exponentials has to correspond to a known rank order for the rate processes. Once these assumptions have been verified, a continuous curve must ensue from the experimental observations or a poor fit (or no fit) will result. Once a statistically valid fit is obtained, the model must be validated, usually by determining parameter values in an independent experiment. In this manner, one can gain confidence in extrapolating the model beyond the experimentally obtained data. Nevertheless, when disagreement with predictions from the model occurs, the results can provide a lead in designing another compartmental scheme or in identifying nonlinear behavior. Hence, one may gain additional knowledge of the pharmacokinetic behavior of a drug. Although somewhat simplified, the requirements outlined above for the compartmental modeling approach are, more often than not, successfully realized for systemically administered drugs, but not when applied to the eye.

In the eye the classical modeling approach has been applied to fluorescein,[2] pilocarpine,[3-5] cefotaxime,[6] and clonidine[7] with reasonably good results with the exception of clonidine. Figure 1 shows the various compartmental schemes that have been proposed for these compounds.

a. Fluorescein

The compartmental scheme used to explain the ocular pharmacokinetics of fluorescein following the instillation of a 10% solution by iontophoresis shows aqueous humor reversibly connected with the cornea and a single exit pathway to plasma. Drug enters the plasma indirectly as a result of bulk aqueous humor turnover via the trabecular meshwork, but also from distribution into the anterior uvea and subsequent uptake by blood vessels residing in these tissues.

In the model, k_e is the first order rate constant representing loss of fluorescein from the anterior chamber, most of which is by bulk aqueous flow. However, for fluorescein an additional 10% of k_e is lost via uptake by fenestrated anterior uvea blood vessels.[8] No tear drainage or scleral absorption is presumed to occur because of the method of administration. This scheme accounts for no significant distribution to peripheral tissues, which is reasonable based upon the very high hydrophilicity of fluorescein. Also, its high hydrophilicity would predict little or no penetration across the epithelial and endothelial barriers by the transcellular pathway, but alternatively would enter the anterior chamber by "pore" transport (i.e., intercellular or between the cells).

The uniqueness of the physicochemical properties of fluorescein as well as the method of administration clearly justify the model shown in Figure 1. As a result, the following equations were proposed by Jones and Maurice:[2]

$$Ca = \frac{M_o k_{c.ca}}{V_a(B-A)} [e^{-At} - e^{-Bt}] \tag{1}$$

$$A + B = k_{c.ca} + k_{a.ca} + k_e \tag{2}$$

$$AB = k_o k_{c.ca} \tag{3}$$

where Ca is the fluorescein concentration in aqueous humor; $k_{c.ca}$ and $k_{ca.a}$ are the first order rate constants for the transfer of drug to and from the cornea and aqueous humor, respectively. V_a is the volume of distribution, which for fluorescein is equal or nearly equal to the aqueous humor volume. A and B are equation parameters representing slopes of ln(Ca) vs. t, where A is assigned to the larger of the two slopes. These equations provided the basis for the determination of the rate of fluorescein turnover in the aqueous humor. A value of 0.0153 (± 0.0011) min^{-1} was determined for 11 subjects,[2] which is remarkably close to the loss of aqueous humor by bulk flow in the human eye, 1.5%/min.

b. Pilocarpine

The most extensive ocular modeling has been applied to pilocarpine by Robinson and co-workers.[3-5] Makoid and Robinson[3] reported on tissue drug concentrations of ^{3}H-pilocarpine nitrate measured up to 12 h following topical instillation of drug to the rabbit eye. A

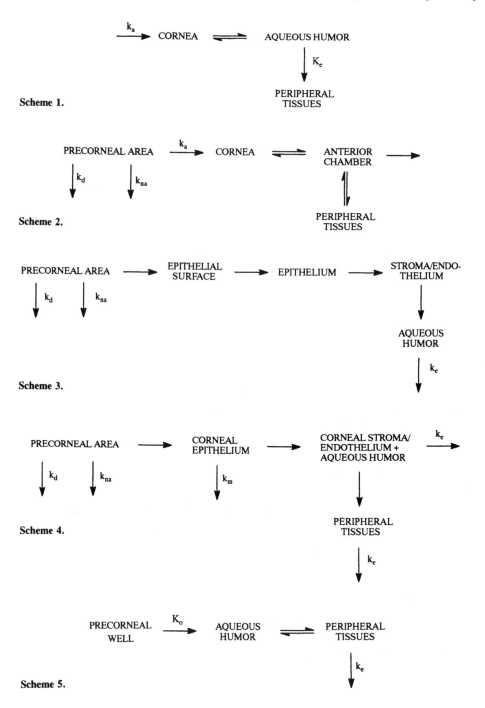

FIGURE 1.   Pharmacokinetic models used to define the ocular pharmacokinetics of fluorescein (Scheme 1), pilocarpine (Schemes 1 through 4 and 7), cefotaxime (Scheme 1), clonidine (Scheme 5), and phenylephrine (Scheme 6). k_{ij} = first rate constant between compartments i and j; Q_{AH} and K_O are the aqueous humor turnover rate and the constant rate infusion across the cornea. In particular, k_d, k_{na}, k_m, and k_e represent first order rate constants for lacrimal drainage, nonabsorptive pathways, metabolism, and elimination, respectively.

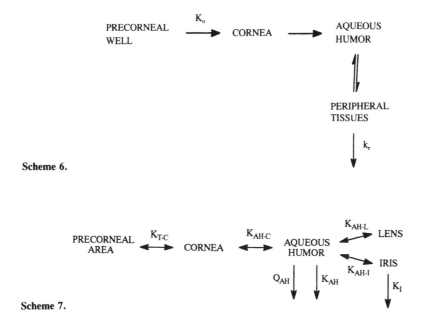

Scheme 6.

Scheme 7.

FIGURE 1 (continued).

four-compartment model (see Figure 1, Scheme 2) described the disposition of drug to cornea, aqueous humor, iris, ciliary body, lens, and vitreous humor. Simultaneous computer fitting of tissue concentrations identified the precorneal area, cornea, anterior chamber, and reservoir as separate compartments. As a result of their work, it was found that the drainage rate at the precorneal area was one to two orders of magnitude larger than the corneal absorption rate constant. Because of the magnitude of the drainage rate, the sum of the two processes is large and therefore justifies the assumption that the loss of drug from the absorption site (but not the absorption rate) > the rate of elimination.

This information is critical in assigning slopes to either the absorption or elimination phases. For systemic drugs, absorption is generally considered the faster process. Whenever the reverse is true, the model has been referred to as a "flip-flop" model.[8] Makoid and Robinson[3] also concluded that aqueous humor turnover accounted for the elimination of drug from the anterior chamber.

The influence of drainage rate and aqueous humor turnover on the pharmacokinetics of ^{3}H-pilocarpine nitrate are independent of drug and suggest that many drugs may have relatively similar disposition kinetics in the eye, despite differences in their physicochemical properties. For example, a consequence of the relatively fixed residence time for applied solutions is that the time to peak (t_p) for nearly all ophthalmic drugs is 20 to 60 min. Makoid and Robinson[3] developed Equation 4 below which showed the relationship between the nonabsorptive (k_{na}) and absorptive (k_a) rate constants:

$$t_p = \frac{\ln\frac{k_{na}}{k_a}}{k_{na} - k_a} \qquad (4)$$

For pilocarpine, and likely for most other ophthalmic drugs, k_{na} is many-fold larger than k_a and therefore predominates in determining t_p.

In another study which focused on the transcorneal penetration of ^{3}H-pilocarpine nitrate, Seig and Robinson[4] measured drug concentrations in the rabbit epithelium, stroma/endothelium, and aqueous humor. Their model, shown in Figure 1, Scheme 3, separated the cornea into a series of three compartments: the epithelium within which the outer and inner layers were separated, and the stroma/endothelium. The epithelium was identified as a barrier to penetration as well as a reservoir for drug. More significantly, the stroma/endothleium was found to be kinetically very similar to the aqueous humor. Consequently, the endothelium, in contrast to the outer layers of the epithelium, was not considered a controlling factor in the corneal penetration of pilocarpine.

Lee and Robinson[5] extended the knowledge of the ocular pharmacokinetics of pilocarpine from the two previous studies to include a detailed analysis of the precorneal disposition of pilocarpine based upon clearance concepts. A pharmacokinetic model was developed which described pilocarpine pharmacokinetics as a four-compartmental model in series. The compartments were identified as the precorneal area with accompanying parallel loss routes, the epithelium, a single compartment comprising stroma, endothelium and aqueous humor, and a fourth compartment referred to as a reservoir. The latter three compartments had single exit rate constants (see Figure 1, Scheme 4).

Results from these studies clearly explain why only 1 to 2% of an administered dose of pilocarpine reaches the anterior chamber.[9,10] The results also show the difficulty one encounters in optimizing ocular bioavailability, either by formulation control or by changes in chemical structure. Nevertheless, the proper assignment of tissues to compartments and the development of a mathematical model to predict the effect of various physiological constraints on bioavailability allow for the development of effective drug delivery approaches. If up to 10% of an administered dose of pilocarpine can be absorbed, this results in a fivefold improvement or more.

c. Cefotaxime

Cefotaxime is very water soluble and therefore expected to possess pharmacokinetic behavior similar to fluorescein. Significant distribution to lipophilic tissue depots does not occur for this drug and justifies a relatively simple, open, two-compartment model for which the cornea and aqueous humor represent each compartment (see Figure 1, Scheme 1). In a study by Vigo et al.,[6] cefotaxime concentrations in the cornea and aqueous humor were measured over 2 h following topical (2.5 mg) and subconjunctival (50 mg) administration. Keratitis was induced by injecting *Pseudomonas aeruginosa* intrastromally 24 h prior to drug administration; considerable loss of the corneal epithelium was observed. The absorption and elimination of the drug was adequately predicted by Equations 1 through 3 for aqueous humor concentrations following subconjunctival administration, but the equations were of questionable validity following topical administration because the drainage rate and other noncontributing parallel routes were not accounted for by the model. However, the lack of a significant barrier (i.e., epithelium) observed in the infected eyes may have resulted in rapid corneal uptake of the topical dose and minimal nonabsorptive loss. This was evident from the fact that no absorptive phase was apparent (see Figure 2); corneal concentrations showed a monoexponential decline from 5 through 120 min.

Even though the subconjunctival dose was 20-fold higher, cornea and aqueous humor levels were only 50 to 100% higher for the conjunctival dose compared to the topical dose. The authors concluded that scleral as well as corneal absorption may have occurred following the topical route since the profiles following either topical or subconjunctival routes of administration for both cornea and aqueous humor were dissimilar. If leakage of drug through

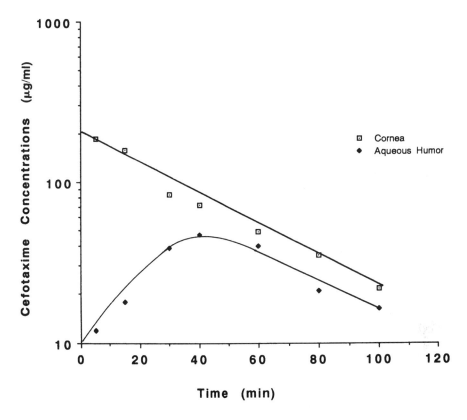

FIGURE 2. Ocular disposition of cefotaxime (5%) administered as a single drop to the infected eye of 25 rabbits. (Compiled from Vigo, J. F., Rafart, J., Concheiro, A., Martinez, R., and Cordido, M., *Curr. Eye Res.*, 7, 1149, 1988. With permission.)

the injection site into the tear film had occurred, the curves would have been somewhat similar.

d. Clonidine

A topical instillation of 3H-clonidine (30 μl, 0.2%) was administered to the rabbit eye after which eight different tissues and plasma were excised and measured for drug concentration.[7] A simple pharmacokinetic model could not be devised for the resulting data. Tissue concentrations over time were sufficiently different from one another in either the latter log linear slope or in the absorptive phase (i.e., time to peak and initial slopes). This result prevented the grouping of tissues into kinetically homogenous compartments (see Figure 3).

Tissue concentrations as separate compartments (n = 8) could not be fit to integrated exponential equations because initial estimates could not be obtained for the multitude of transfer coefficients. However, a stepwise procedure for building the model generated estimates of parameter values when differential equations for the complex model were fit simultaneously to tissue levels. Nevertheless, the estimates for parameter values representing ADME were unreasonable. Even though tissue concentrations over time provided useful information concerning the ocular pharmacokinetics of clonidine, the model was considered too complex and not useful.

2. Noncompartmental Modeling

The noncompartmental approach was adapted for systemic pharmacokinetic use in the 1970s[1] and obviated the necessity for compartments to determine ADME. The noncom-

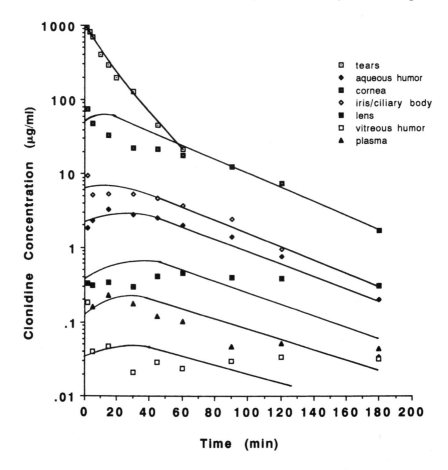

FIGURE 3.   Computer-generated fit of clonidine to various eye tissues following topical administration of 30 μl of a 0.2% solution. (Compiled from Vigo, J. F., Rafart, J., Concheiro, A., Martinez, R., and Cordido, M., *Curr. Eye Res.*, 7, 1149, 1988. With permission.)

partmental approach in estimating ADME required the calculation of areas under the tissue concentration vs. time curves as well as the tissue concentration × time vs. time curves. By this method of calculating areas, parameters are not severely compensated by a lack of a smooth curve as can occur with the compartmental modeling approach.

For a bolus intravenous dose, the resulting plasma profile was assumed to be a log normal distribution of the drug molecules over time and could be expressed as a mean residence time (MRT). MRT was defined as the time for 63.2% of the drug to be eliminated. Clearance, volumes of distribution, mean absorption time (MAT), fraction absorbed, and other useful parameters were developed from area calculations. As long as linear pharmacokinetics are correctly assumed, the noncompartmental approach can be applied.

In the eye, Eller et al.[11] developed Equations 5 through 8 below using the noncompartmental approach to estimate the corneal absorption rate constant, k_a(min^{-1}); the ocular volume of distribution at steady state, v_{ss} (ml); and the ocular clearance, Cl.

$$k_a = \frac{V_A(dC_A/dt)_t}{C_W V_W} \tag{5}$$

$$Cl_e = \frac{K_o T}{AUC} \tag{6}$$

$$V_{ss} = \frac{K_oT\,(AUMC)}{(AUC)^2} - \frac{K_oT^2}{(2AUC)} \qquad (7)$$

$$K_o = (dC_A/dt)_I V_A \qquad (8)$$

In the above equations, V_w is the volume of drug solution maintained on the cornea (ml); AUC and AUMC are the areas to infinity under the aqueous humor concentration-time curve and concentration × time-time curve, respectively ($\mu g \cdot min \cdot ml^{-1}$ and $\mu g \cdot min^2 \cdot ml^{-1}$); C_w is the constant concentration maintained on the cornea over time, T; K_o is the constant rate input into the cornea; and $(dC_A/dt)_I$ is the initial rate of appearance of drug in aqueous humor independent of lag time [$\mu g \cdot (ml \cdot min)^{-1}$].

In order to apply Equations 5 through 8, Eller et al.[11] devised a procedure for maintaining a constant concentration on the corneal surface of anesthetized rabbits. A plastic cylinder, the base of which was shaped like a contact lens, was placed over the cornea so that only the cornea was exposed to drug solution. The well, which held 0.7 ml, remained on the cornea until steady state concentrations could be reached in the aqueous humor. Figure 4 shows a plot of ibufenac (300 $\mu g/ml$) obtained from the topical infusion method in which drug was maintained on the cornea for 120 min. Equations 4 through 7 are independent of compartmental modeling and the use of the well eliminates the effect of drainage and parallel loss from the absorption site.

Table 1 lists the k_a values of drugs[5,7,11-15] for which this procedure has been used. These values are small and represent a range of absorption half-lives of 7.7 h for ethoxzolamide up to 46 d for phenylephrine. These half-lives are exceptionally long, but because of the short residence time for drugs applied to the eye, which is approximately 2 to 5 min for solutions, only a small fraction of the administered dose is absorbed. It is clear that if a greater percent of an ophthalmic dose is to be absorbed, one of two general approaches must be followed. Either one must develop a formulation that is retained at the absorption site for a relatively long period of time or design a very rapidly penetrating drug. In order to design optimal dosing regimens, calculations must depend on an accurate estimate of the volume of distribution (V_d). The V_d has been an elusive parameter to determine because it requires a knowledge of the absorbed dose. Reasonable estimates have been obtained from either an instantaneous input (i.e., intracameral injection)[9,16-18] or from a known constant rate of input (i.e., topical infusion method).[7,11-15] Both procedures permit an estimate of the dose reaching the anterior chamber. Table 2 lists values obtained from either an intracameral injection (V_E) or from topical infusion (V_{ss}). Compared to the aqueous humor volume of 0.311 ml,[10,19] none of the tabulated values are significantly larger which suggests that distribution to peripheral tissues is not extensive.

For systemic drugs, V_d is often 5- to 100-fold larger than blood or extracellular volume, whereas the largest ocular values were obtained from ketorolac tromethamine and levobunolol which are 1.65 and 1.94 ml, respectively, or about 5- to 6-fold larger than aqueous humor volume. It is surprising that ocular V_d values are not larger since tissues in the anterior and posterior chambers are directly adjacent to aqueous humor allowing for extensive distribution, should it be possible. Also, protein concentration in aqueous humor is about 10% of plasma concentrations and therefore would not be expected to hinder distribution because of extensive binding as compared to systemically administered drugs. However, the expectation of a relatively large V_d, which is based upon a knowledge of systemic pharmacokinetic behavior, may be unrealistic for ophthalmic drugs because the ratio of circulating fluid to tissues is much smaller in the eye than in the whole body.

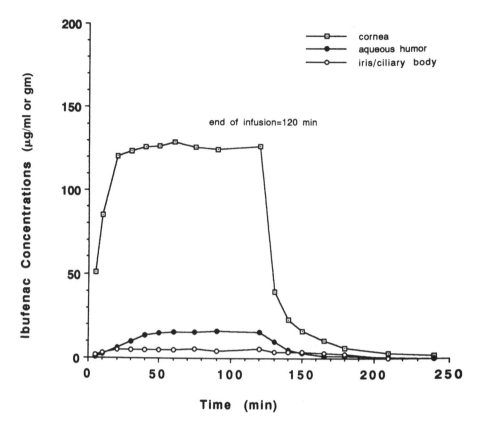

FIGURE 4.   Cornea, aqueous humor, and iris/ciliary body concentrations of ibufenac following topical infusion of 300 μg/ml maintained on the cornea of an anesthetized rabbit for 120 min. (From Chiang, C. H. and Schoenwald, R. D., *J. Pharmacokinet. Biopharm.*, 14, 175, 1986. With permission.)

Elimination from the eye can be expressed as ocular clearance (Cl_e), and in addition to Equation 6, two other equations can be used:

$$Cl_e = k_e V_d \tag{9}$$

$$Cl_e = \frac{D}{AUC} \tag{10}$$

In Equation 9, k_e is the elimination rate constant obtained from the latter log linear slope of the concentration-time curve. It does not depend on compartmental modeling, but is most reliably determined from concentrations of drug in aqueous humor determined over sufficient time to clearly represent the elimination phase. The V_d is either V_{ss} or V_E; and in Equation 10, D is the absorbed dose which represents the intracameral dose. AUC has been defined previously.

Table 3 contains Cl_e values calculated from Equations 6, 9, or 10.[11-17] Assuming an aqueous chamber volume of 0.311 ml, clearance of aqueous humor due exclusively to aqueous humor turnover is 4.67 μl/min or expressed another way, 1.5% of aqueous humor/ min. Values for Cl_e vary from 13 to 28.7 μl/min which are approximately 3 to 6 times higher than aqueous humor turnover. The significantly higher values suggest that other pathways contribute to ocular drug elimination (see Section V).

TABLE 1
Transcorneal Absorption Rate Constant and Half-Life

Compound of interest	k_a (min^{-1})	$t_{1/2}$ (h)	Ref.
Pilocarpine	0.004	2.88	5
Clonidine	0.0014	8.25	7
Phenylephrine	0.00001	1155	12
Ibuprofen	0.0013	8.88	13
Ibufenac	0.00061	18.9	13
2-[4'-(2"-Hydroxyethoxy) phenyl]acetic acid	0.000095	122	13
2-[4'-(2"-Hydroxyethoxy) phenyl]proprionic acid	0.00039	29.6	13
Ethoxzolamide	0.0015	7.7	11
Aminozolamide	0.0014	8.25	14
2-Benzothiazolesulfonamide	0.0013	8.88	11
6-Hydroxyethoxy-2-benzothiazolesulfonamide	0.0042	5.37	11
N-methylacetazolamide	0.00126	9.17	15
Acetazolamide	0.000153	75.5	15

TABLE 2
Volumes of Distribution (V_d) for Drugs of Ophthalmic Interest

Compound of interest	V_d (ml)	Procedure	Ref.
Pilocarpine	0.58	EX[a]	9
Clonidine	0.53	SS[b]	7
Phenylephrine	0.42	SS	12
Flurbiprofen	0.62	EX	16
Levobunolol	1.65	EX	17
Dihydrolevobunolol	1.68	EX	17
Ibuprofen	0.527	SS	13
Ibufenac	0.206	SS	13
2-[4'-(2"-Hydroxyethoxy)phenyl]acetic acid	0.929	SS	13
2-[4'-(2"-Hydroxyethoxy)phenyl]proprionic acid	1.71	SS	13
Ketorolac tromethamine	1.93	EX	18
Ethoxzolamide	0.28	SS	11
Aminozolamide	0.53	SS	14
2-Benzothiazolesulfonamide	0.24	SS	11
6-Hydroxyethoxy-2-benzothiazolesulfonamide	0.33	SS	11
N-methylacetazolamide	0.42	SS	15
Acetazolamide	0.47	SS	15

[a] EX = extrapolated method; determined by extrapolating log-linear elimination phase to C to t_0 and dividing into the intracameral dose.

[b] SS = steady state method; determined by maintaining a constant concentration of drug on the cornea of an anesthetized rabbit and measuring aqueous humor concentrations of drug over time during infusion and post-infusion. See Equation 7 for the determination of F_{ss}.

3. Physiologic Modeling

A number of physiological phenomena, particularly the blinking rate and turnover of tears and aqueous humor, significantly impact on the ocular pharmacokinetic behavior of drugs. Table 4 lists a comparison between the human and rabbit eye for anatomical as well as physiological factors. Because of rapid and extensive drainage and tearing in both human and rabbit eyes, most therapeutic agents have relatively similar behavior with regard to absorption and disposition as evidenced by the narrow range of parameter values reported for these events in Tables 1 through 3. Consequently, the application of a modeling technique

TABLE 3
Ocular Clearances (Cl$_e$) for Drugs of Ophthalmic Interest

Compound of Interest	Cl$_e$ (μl/min)	Ref.
Pilocarpine	13.0	21
Clonidine	14.9	7
Phenylephrine	14.6	12
Flurbiprofen	14.4	16
Levobunolol	28.7	17
Dihydrolevobunolol	19.7	17
Ketorolac tromethamine	11.0	18
Ibuprofen	18.7	13
Ibufenac	8.4	13
2-[4'-(2"-Hydroxyethoxy)phenyl]acetic acid	1.2	13
2-[4'-(2"-Hydroxyethoxy)phenyl]proprionic acid	1.5	13
Ethoxzolamide	9.0	11
2-Benzothiazolesulfonamide	1.15	11
6-Hydroxyethoxy-2-benzothiazolesulfonamide	3.0	11
N-methylacetazolamide	1.56	15
Acetazolamide	5.27	15

TABLE 4
Physiological Differences Between the New Zealand Rabbit and the Human Eye Pertinent to Ophthalmic Pharmacokinetics

Physiological factor	Rabbit eye	Human eye
Tear volume with blinking	7-10 μl	12-15 μl
Tear volume without blinking	25-30 μl	25 + [a] μl
Tear turnover rate	0.6-0.8 μl/min	0.5–2.2 μl/min
Spontaneous blinking rate[b]	4-5 times/min	15 times/min
Nictitating membrane[c]	Present	Absent
pH of tears	[d]	7.14-7.82
Milliosmolarity of tears	[d]	305 mOsm/l
Corneal thickness	0.40 mm	0.52 mm
Corneal diameter	15 mm	12 mm
Aqueous humor volume	[d]	310 μl
Aqueous humor turnover rate	[d]	1.53 μl/min

[a]   Varies depending on conjunctival sac volume.
[b]   Occurs during normal waking hours without apparent external stimuli.
[c]   Significance of nictitating membrane is small relative to overall loss rate from precornea area.
[d]   Approximately same measurement as human.

that emphasizes the use of clearance concepts clearly provides a rational basis for filling the void between mathematical description and physiological reality.

In studies by Himmelstein and co-workers,[20,21] a physiologic model was developed to describe the ocular disposition of pilocarpine in tears, cornea, aqueous humor iris/ciliary body, and lens. The model for pilocarpine[21] (Figure 1, Scheme 7) shows a series of compartments representing eye tissues. The compartments are arranged in a flow diagram with arrows representing flow rates or clearances of drug between compartments. The information needed to verify a physiologic model are the concentration of drug in tissue over time, flow

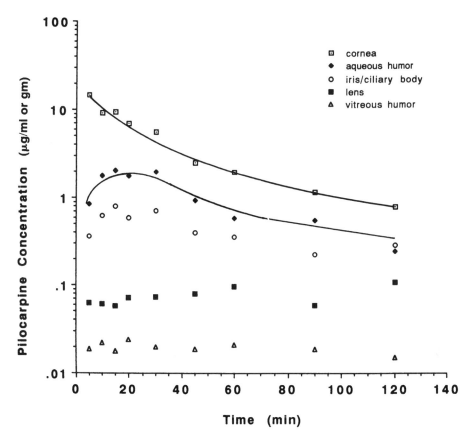

FIGURE 5. Comparisons of ocular tissues following the topical administration of 25 μl of pilocarpine nitrate (0.01 *M*) to the rabbit eye. Computerized fits of both cornea and aqueous humor are shown. (Modified from Miller, S. C., Himmelstein, K. J., and Patton, T. F., *J. Pharmacokinet. Biopharm.*, 9, 671, 1981. With permission.)

rates and/or clearances of drug between compartments, and partition coefficients (at equilibrium) between adjacent tissues (ie., compartments). Generally, the rate equations for physiologic models are numerous, complex, and cannot be integrated directly. However, numerical solutions using computer algorithms are available and concentrations of drug in the various tissues can be predicted over time and compared to experimentally obtained values.[1,7,21]

Figure 5 shows various tissue concentrations of pilocarpine[21] over time. With the exception of corneal and aqueous humor concentrations, computer-generated fits to pilocarpine concentrations in the other tissues were poor and not shown in Figure 5. Likewise, computer-generated fits of clonidine to various tissue concentrations,[7] shown in Figure 3, are also poor. Although physiologic models are experimentally difficult to confirm, the original expectation for these models was to substitute human flow rates and/or clearances for animal values. Moreover, partitioning of drug between animal tissues was to be used in human calculations and along with plasma (or aqueous humor in the eye) concentrations of drug measured over time, be able to predict therapeutic tissue concentrations in patients. However, the approach suffers from inadequate predictability, particularly for drug concentrations in tissues other than plasma (or aqueous humor). In the eye, computer fits for pilocarpine and clonidine are good for some tissues, but poorly fit for others, namely, iris/ciliary body and lens for pilocarpine, and cornea and aqueous humor for clonidine.

Nevertheless, clearance concepts have been successfully applied to the precorneal area[5] and represent a rather precise description of the pharmacokinetics of the precorneal region of the eye. Although drainage quickly removes a significant portion of an administered dose from the precorneal area, Lee and Robinson[5] established that drainage accounted for only about one third of the loss and many other factors were also contributing. These factors and their relative importance in removing drug from the absorption site were drainage $\cong$ vasodilation due to pilocarpine $>$ uptake of drug by the nictitating membrane $>$ induced lacrimation diluting drug concentration at the absorption site $\cong$ conjunctival absorption $>$ normal tear flow.

B. LIMITATIONS TO THE OCULAR USE OF CLASSICAL MODELING APPROACHES

Eye tissues cannot be continuously sampled over time without severely compromising the results. Once the eye is invaded blood-aqueous or blood-vitreous barriers are disrupted and a prostaglandin-induced increase in protein occurs.[22] The increase in protein can alter the disposition of drug in the eye because of an increase in binding to the circulating proteins. Since these proteins are changing in concentration over time, a nonlinear behavior can also potentially result. However, for nonsteroidal anti-inflammatory drugs (NSAID) which inhibit prostaglandin formation, particularly diclofenac, flurbiprofen, and indomethacin, no differences in protein concentration are likely to occur when intracameral injections of these drugs are made.[23]

It is common practice for one animal to be used in determining drug concentration at a single time interval. As a result, in order to construct a complete kinetic profile of drug concentration over time, as many as 150 to 250 rabbits may be required. By using a large number of animals to construct the curve, it is assumed that a representative profile will prevail and that conventional fitting techniques can be applied. The consequence of this approach is that averaged results do not always produce a kinetic profile which is typical of an individual determination.

The inability to continuously measure drug concentrations in eye tissues impacts all pharmacometric approaches. However, the classical compartmental modeling approach in particular has rather limited use when applied to the eye. When a topical dose is instilled in the eye, the precorneal loss routes overwhelmingly dictate the t_p and fraction absorbed, as discussed previously. In addition, the largest rate constant associated with the computer-fitted sum of exponentials is not the absorption rate (k_a) constant, but instead is a a sum of all the parallel loss rate constants including k_a. Therefore, in order to determine k_a by this approach, it is necessary to subtract values for all other loss phenomena.

Also, without accurate knowledge of the fraction absorbed, it is not possible to determine V_d if only a topical dose is administered. Consequently, the only pharmacokinetic constant that can be reliably determined is the half-life for ocular elimination of drug ($t_{1/2}$). It can be determined from the latter log-linear portion of the drug concentration vs. time curve (i.e., postdistributive phase). However, even the half-life may be incorrectly estimated if drug is slowly redistributing back into aqueous humor from a depot compartment. This phenomenon, sometimes referred to as "back-diffusion", has been observed for pilocarpine[3,21] and has led to half-life determinations that were overestimated. Measurements of pilocarpine in aqueous humor through 8 h have produced reliable estimates of the half-life of pilocarpine (2.9 h).[21]

Although two input methods allow for the calculation of V_d (i.e., V_{ss} determined from topical infusion of V_E determined from intracameral injection), the volume of distribution is a general measurement and does not differentiate between a reservoir site and the site of action. Nevertheless, when V_d is multiplied by the ocular elimination constant (Equation

9), an estimate of ocular clearance (Q_e) is provided which, if greater than 4.67 μl/min, suggests an alternate elimination pathway other than bulk aqueous flow. This information may be useful in the design of a derivative with a greater or lesser ocular clearance.

A lack of assay sensitivity often complicates the process of measuring reasonable pharmacokinetic parameters values. Generally, eye tissues contain micrograms or smaller concentrations of drug per gram of tissue weight. This expression of concentration is somewhat misleading because eye tissues (e.g., conjunctiva, sclera, cornea, iris/ciliary body, lens, aqueous or vitreous humor) weigh below 50 mg, so that the absolute amount of drug that is measured is often below 100 ng. Over a decade ago it was most common to prepare a radioactive tracer in order to achieve the necessary assay sensitivity. In recent years, significant advances have been made in instrumentation. High pressure liquid chromatography (HPLC) equipped with ultraviolet (including diode ray), radioactive, or fluorescence detectors, or gas-liquid chromatography using nitrogen or electron capture detectors have allowed for adequate sensitivity.[24-27]

Once pharmacometric measurements are made, it is desirable to accurately predict human ocular kinetics, and in particular, predict the therapeutic effect in patients. At this time, pharmacokinetic determinations in the human eye can only be made in subjects undergoing eye surgery. This is accomplished by administering the drug just prior to surgery and at an appropriate time removing a sample of aqueous humor for storage and subsequent assay analysis. Unfortunately, a complete profile cannot be easily obtained except from samples removed at various time intervals from a number of patients.

Lee and Robinson,[10] in an extensive review, discussed the suitability of using the albino rabbit as a model in predicting human ocular pharmacokinetics. Because of the difficulty in measuring human ocular pharmacokinetics, a large body of data for interspecies comparison is not available. From Table 4 it is apparent that major differences exist in tear turnover rate and the blinking rate which is more frequent in the human eye. The "third eyelid" of the rabbit, which is not present in man, is a nictitating membrane capable of removing foreign objects from the precorneal area of the rabbit eye. Also, the rabbit has an active retractor bulbi muscle, not present in man. This muscle allows the rabbit to increase or decrease the conjunctival sac volume by slightly moving its eye in or out of its orbit. Relatively similar between the rabbit and human eye are the pH and milliosmolarity of the tears, tear volume, corneal thickness and diameter, as well as the aqueous humor and aqueous humor turnover rate.

Ocular studies of prednisolone acetate[28] in both species indicate similar disposition properties. On the other hand, Saettone and co-workers[29,30] cited precorneal dynamics as a likely reason for interspecies differences in pharmacological response intensities due to vehicular effects for tropicamide and pilocarpine. Although the albino rabbit is a relatively good model for predicting toxicological effects in the human eye,[31] it is not entirely clear whether or not it is an acceptable model for predicting ADME.[10,32,33]

III. PRECORNEAL LOSS

The loss of drug from the precorneal area is a net effect of drainage, tear secretion, noncorneal absorption, and corneal absorption rate processes. As discussed previously, the drainage rate is about 100 times faster than the corneal absorption rate.[3,5] In a series of studies, Robinson and co-workers[3,5,34-36] determined that in the rabbit eye the instilled volume is directly proportional to the volume of fluid above the normal lacrimal fluid volume. This phenomenon is predicted by Equation 11 below:[5]

$$V_t = V_O + V_i e^{-k_d t} \qquad (11)$$

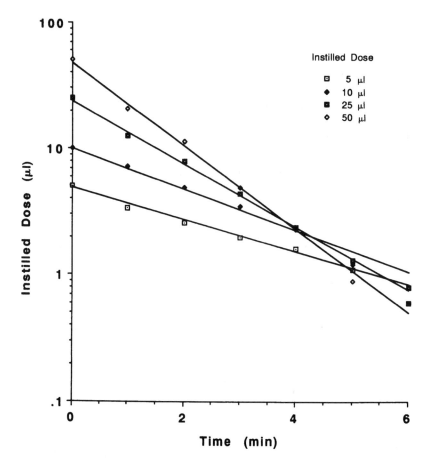

FIGURE 6. Precorneal loss from the rabbit eye of instilled volumes from 5 to 50 μl of radioactive technetium colloidal suspensions. (Modified from Miller, S. C., Himmelstein, K. J., and Patton, T. F., *J. Pharmacokinet. Biopharm.*, 9, 653, 1981. With permission.)

where V_t is the volume remaining in the conjunctival sac at time t, V_o is the normal lacrimal tear volume, V_i is the instilled drop volume, and k_d is the drainage rate constant. Figure 6 shows the influence of drainage rates on various volumes ranging from 50 to 5 μl. From this plot it was possible for the authors[5,34] to determine the value for k_d as it decreases with V_i:

$$k_d = 0.25 \ (\text{min}^{-1}) + [0.0113 \ \mu\text{l/min})] \ V_i \qquad (12)$$

Figure 6 is significant to drug delivery applications for a number of reasons. First, it is apparent that the residence time at the absorption site is exceptionally short compared to other routes of administration in the body. Therefore, it is imperative that either the drug be designed for very rapid absorption or a dosage form be formulated to significantly prolong the retention time. This is not a particularly revealing fact to those who routinely develop drugs for ophthalmic use.[10,37-40] In fact, two commercially successful dosage forms which prolong the retention of pilocarpine in the conjunctival sac are the Ocusert®, a solid insert, and Pilopine H.S.®, a rigid gel. Molecular modification has also been found to be a commercially viable option. For example, dipivefrin is a dipivalyl ester of epinephrine which represents a rapidly absorbed prodrug of epinephrine. Its major clinical advantage is a tenfold reduction in dose with a significant lowering of systemic side effects.[41,42]

Second, Figure 6 clearly indicates that the smaller the drop instilled, the lower the drainage rate, and the greater the extent of ophthalmic absorption. This principle was demonstrated by Patton and Francoeur[43] who found equal bioavailability of pilocarpine nitrate solutions in the rabbit eye following instillation of 25 μl of a 0.01 M solution (67.8 μg) or 5μl of a 0.092 M solution (26 μg). This results in a 2.6-fold improvement in bioavailability from a 5-fold reduction in drop size. Brown and co-workers[44,45] extended the obvious benefits of this phenomenon to the clinical use of phenylephrine, a highly effective mydriatic, but with significant cardiovascular risk in certain patients. Eleven neonates, considered a high risk group, were administered an 8 μl dose of 2.5% phenylephrine hydrochloride in one eye and a 30 μl dose in the other eye. The mean pupillary diameters (4.86 vs. 4.57 mm) were the same, however, the plasma concentration of phenylephrine was 0.9 ng/ml for the 8 μl dose and 1.9 ng/ml for the 30 μl dose.[45]

Clinical application of the benefits of small-volume dosing has also been reported by Hanna and co-workers[46-48] for dosing mydriatic solutions to children and adults. Nevertheless, no commercial application of small-volume dosing is presently available, likely because of the cost of routinely supplying a small volume drop on a large scale production basis. The drop size of a commercial product is approximately 30 μl which is the largest volume that the conjunctival sac can hold. However, upon blinking the eye retains only about 10 μl. Obviously, much of an instilled drop is either squeezed out of the eye from reflex blinking or never reaches the lower conjunctival sac, since most patients are not efficient in instilling a drop themselves.

If a smaller drop size was technologically feasible, bioavailability would be improved, however, the product would have to be reformulated as a more concentrated solution in order to maintain the same absolute dose. There is a danger in marketing a more concentrated product. In practice, patients might perceive that the small drop did not adequately enter their eye and then proceed to instill another drop. With a more concentrated drug solution a greater chance of overdose and/or toxicity might result.

From the results of Figure 6 (studied more extensively in other publications[35,43,45]) is the implication that two drops instilled immediately after one another will show a reduced bioavailability compared to separating the doses by 3 to 5 min. This implies that combination products may be more efficient unless sufficient time is allowed to elapse between instillations.

Robinson and co-workers[3-5,33-36] have systematically studied the factors responsible for precorneal loss of pilocarpine. Rate constants have been individually determined for drainage, induced lacrimation, conjunctival uptake, vasodilation due to pilocarpine, and nonconjunctival loss. Table 5 gives the influence of each factor on the absorption of pilocarpine in the anterior chamber. From Table 5 it is observed that if the drainage rate is suppressed, the area under the aqueous humor concentration-time curve is increased fourfold compared to the normal physiological conditions with all factors operating (0.007 in Table 5).

In a study by DeSantis and Schoenwald,[48a] it was shown that removal of the rabbit nictitating membrane had no significant effect on miosis following instillation of 50 μl of a 2% pilocarpine hydrochloride solution. Although the membrane is a competitive depot for channeling topically applied pilocarpine away from the cornea, the removal of the membrane possibly altered nictitans glandular secretions which are important to tear stability, tear volume, and turnover and were not measured in the study.

TABLE 5
Parallel Loss Factors and Their Effect on the Ocular
Bioavailability of Pilocarpine

Parallel loss factor	Fraction of dose absorbed when only indicated factor is operative[a]
Drainage rate	0.24
Basal tear flow	0.18
Induced lacrimation	0.13
Conjunctival absorption	0.16
Vasodilation (due to pilocarpine)	0.03
Nonconjunctival loss	0.05
All factors present	0.007

[a] Data reproduced from Reference 5.

IV. ABSORPTION INTO THE ANTERIOR CHAMBER

A. CORNEA

Traditionally the cornea has been regarded as the major route of entry for drugs into the anterior chamber. Whereas physiological factors largely determine ocular bioavailability, once the drug enters the cornea, drug-related factors, e.g., partitioning behavior, solubility, concentration, and pKa have a predominating influence on the rate of absorption across the cornea. Table 6 differentiates between membrane and drug and formulation-related factors influencing corneal penetration.

The cornea consists of five layers, however, only three of the layers are significant with respect to barrier resistance, namely the epithelium, stroma, and endothelium. Specifically, the outer epithelium provides the greatest resistance to penetration. Because the epithelium is lipophilic, low in porosity, and relatively high in tortuosity, a rapidly penetrating drug must possess a log octanol/buffer (pH 7.2 to 7.7) partition coefficient (log PC) greater than 1 in order to achieve a sufficient penetration rate.[49-57] On the other hand, the stroma is basically acellular, hydrophilic in nature (76 to 80% water), high in porosity, and low in tortuosity, but because it represents 90% of the thickness of the cornea, the stroma is significant in overall contribution to resistance.[58] Although the endothelium is cellular, it is only one cell thick and is less significant in overall barrier resistance when compared to the other layers.

Kinetic models (as discussed in Section II) have not been particularly useful in helping formulators design optimally penetrating drugs. Models that have been most useful in understanding corneal penetration are multiple linear regression models, particularly models relating either partitioning or structural parameters to penetration.

Multiple linear regression models have been applied to a series of β-blocking agents,[49,51] naphthyl esters,[60] steroids,[54,61] and n-alkyl p-aminobenzoate ester homologs.[56,61] Partition coefficient, molecular weight, and degree of ionization were the major determinants to passive diffusion across the cornea. In these examples, partition coefficient was the most important determinant of penetration with degree of ionization and molecular weight only minimally contributing. Degree of ionization is a factor only because of its indirect relationship to partition coefficient, whereas, molecular weight is a less critical factor because it is related to the cube root of diffusional forces and because most drugs used in the eye have a relatively small and narrow range of molecular weight.

TABLE 6
Membrane, Drug, and Formulation Factors
that Influence Corneal Permeability

Membrane Factors

Area available for absorption (cornea and/or sclera)
Thickness
Porosity
Tortuosity
Lipophilicity/hydrophilicity balance

Drug Factors

Concentration instilled into eye
Solubility
Partition coefficient
Molecular weight
pKa

Formulation Factors

Retention time at absorption site
pH
Tonicity
Viscosity
Adjuvant effect (e.g., surfactant)
Release rate (if semisolid or insert)

In these studies as well as most other *in vitro* studies measuring drug penetration across an isolated cornea, a relative measure is obtained from the permeability coefficient (PC) which is independent of concentration and area of the absorbing surface:

$$PC = \frac{(flux)}{C_o A} \tag{13}$$

In equation 13, PC is expressed in units of cm/s from flux studies of drug penetration across excised rabbit corneas,[51] whee C_o is the initial concentration of drug placed on the epithelial side and A is the surface area of the cornea exposed to drug.

Table 7 lists PC values for drugs of ophthalmic interest determined for an intact but excised rabbit cornea. From the table it is observed that drugs with PC values of about 10×10^{-6} cm/s or less, must be formulated in relatively high concentrations to achieve therapeutic activity (e.g., phenylephrine, sulfacetamide, epinephrine, or cromolyn). For drugs which are highly potent, a low concentration will suffice in spite of poor penetrability (e.g., tobramycin, chloramphenicol, and cyclosporin). In practice, the penetration rate (PR) is a more critical determinant to drug activity:

$$PR = (PC)\, t_{conc} \tag{14}$$

In Equation 14, t_{conc} is the concentration of drug in the tears; the maximum PR (MPR) is represented by Equation 15 in which tear solubility (t_{sol}) is substituted for t_{conc}:

$$MPR = (PC)\, t_{sol} \tag{15}$$

TABLE 7
Corneal Permeability Coefficients (PC) Across Excised Rabbit Corneas

Compound of interest	PC (cm/s × 10^{-6})	Ref.
[1,2,3]Thiadiazolo[5,4-h]-6,7,8,9-tetrahydroisoquinoline	78.8	85
6-Chloro-3-methyl-2,3,4,5-tetrahydro-1H-3-benzazepine	70.8	85
Bufurolol	72.4	15
4-Chloro-N-methylbenzenesulfonamide	65.1	15
Bevantolol	57.0	51
4-Chlorobenzenesulfonamide	54.6	15
O-Butyryl timolol	53.0	86
O-Propionyl timolol	48.9	86
5,8-Dimethoxy-1,2,3,4-tetrahydroisoquinoline	48.5	85
Propranolol	47.6	51
	30.9	86
6-Benzyloxy-2-benzothiazolesulfonamide	47.0	55
Penbutolol	44.9	51
Clonidine	44.0	7
	36.3	66
Ethoxzolamide	43.9	55
6-Chloro-2-benzothiazolesulfonamide	42.8	55
Testosterone	41.7	54
Desoxycorticosterone	39.8	54
4,6-Dichloro-2-benzothiazolesulfonamide	38.8	15
O-Acetyl timolol	38.3	86
Dexamethasone acetate	36.7	54
Prednisolone acetate	33.3	54
2-Benzothiazolesulfonamide	36.2	55
Cortexolone	30.2	54
Oxprenolol	25.1	51
O-Pivalyl timolol	24.4	86
α-Yohimbine	23.4	85
Ibuprofen	22.4	13
Metoprolol	22.0	51
Ibufenac	21.2	13
Yohimbine	18.4	85
Progesterone	17.8	88
	19.5	54
Pilocarpine	17.4	87
Fluorometholone	16.5	54
Levbunolol	16.4	51
Triamcinolone acetonide	15.9	88
4,7-Dimethyl-6-ethoxy-2-benzothiazolesulfonamide	13.7	55
Timolol	11.7	51
	18.2	86
Corynanthine	11.4	85
Cyclophosphamide	11.3	89
6-Quinoxalyinyl derivative of clonidine (AGN 190342)	9.8	66
Rauwolfine	9.2	85
2-Deoxy-glucose	7.4	90
Chloramphenicol	6.8	87
6-Amino-2-benzothiazolesulfonamide	6.7	55
6-Nitro-2-benzothiazolesulfonamide	6.6	55
2-[4'-(2"-Hydroxyethoxy)phenyl]acetic acid	6.2	13
Cocaine	6.1	53
2-[4'-(2"-Hydroxyethoxy)phenyl]proprionic acid	6.0	13
6-Hydroxy-2-benzothiazolesulfonamide	5.6	55

TABLE 7 (continued)
Corneal Permeability Coefficients (PC) Across Excised Rabbit Corneas

Compound of interest	PC (cm/s × 10^{-6})	Ref.
Dexamethasone	5.0	54
Nadolol diacetate	4.8	51
6-Acetamido-2-benzothiazolesulfonamide	4.7	55
1-α-Methyl-2-deoxy-glucose	4.6	90
Glycerin	4.5	88
Procaine	4.2	53
Methazolamide	4.2	15
Acetazolamide	4.1	15
Prednisolone	3.7	54
Hydrocortisone	3.5	88
	8.5	54
2-Benzimidazolesulfonamide	3.0	90
1-α-Ethyl-2-deoxy-glucose	2.9	90
Mannitol	2.4	88
N-Methylacetazolamide	2.3	15
7-Amino-6-ethoxy-2-benzothiazolesulfonamide	2.2	55
1-α-Cyclopropyl-2-deoxy-glucose	2.2	90
Tetrasodium edetate	2.1	88
Sulfacetamide	1.9	87
1-α-Isopropyl-2-deoxy-glucose	1.8	90
Sotalol	1.6	51
Tetracaine	1.5	53
6-Hydroxyethoxy-2-benzothiazolesulfonamide	1.5	55
Water	1.5	88
Cyclosporin	1.1	91
Cromolyn	1.1	88
Nadolol	1.0	52
Phenylephrine	0.94	55
Acebutolol	0.85	52
Atenolol	0.67	52
Tobramycin	0.52	87
p-Aminoclonidine	0.44	66

Note: Averages of 4 to 10 determinations at pH 7.4 to 7.65 using the experimental procedure of Reference 51; standard deviations range from 5 to 25% of mean.

Data modified from Reference 37.

Although micronized drug particles are retained in the eye two- to threefold longer than solutions,[62-64] if a drug is poorly soluble, its penetration rate may be limited and therefore not high enough to achieve adequate concentration for therapeutic activity.

From studies using excised rabbit corneas, the percentage contribution of each barrier layer has been determined for β-blocking agents and a few other drugs.[37] Table 8 summarizes the results and shows that for hydrophilic drugs (log DC < 0) the epithelium provides a large percentage of the resistance to corneal penetration. For lipophilic drugs with log distribution coefficient (DC) between 1.6 and 2.5, the stroma contributes a significant percentage of the resistance. For the remaining lipophilic drugs (log DC > 0 and < 1.6), the sum of the stromal and endothelial resistances equaled the epithelial resistance. Figure 7 shows that for any corneal layer (PC$_i$) a plot of log PC$_i$ vs. log DC is linear, but when PC of an intact cornea is determined, a curvilinear plot will result. A mathematical

TABLE 8
Percent Resistance of Corneal Layers to Drug Penetration

	Log DC[a]	Epithelium	Stroma	Endothelium
Bevantolol	2.2	7	44	49
Bufurolol	2.3	18	50	32
Penbutolol	2.5	1	48	53
Corynanthine	1.9	71	15	14
6-Chloro-3-methyl-2,3,4,5-tetrahydro-1H-3-benzazepine	1.9	16	35	49
Yohimbine	1.8	12	20	68
Propranolol	1.6	7	45	48
Rauwolfine	1.2	71	8	21
Clonidine	1.0	60	20	20
Oxprenolol	0.7	45	21	34
Levobunolol	0.7	58	15	27
[1,2,3]Thiadiazolo[5,4-h]-6,7,8,9-tetrahydroisoquinoline	0.32	42	35	22
Cyclophosphamide	0.4	72	10	13
Metoprolol	0.3	48	18	34
Timolol	0.34	68	9	23
5,8-Dimethoxy-1,2,3,4-tetrahydroisoquinoline	0.32	38	38	24
Acebutolol	0.2	91	1	8
Nadolol	−0.82	95	1	4
Phenylephrine	−1.0	95	1	4
Sotolol	−1.25	95	1	4
Atenolol	−1.5	97	1	2
Tobramycin	< −2.0	95	1	4

[a] Log DC is the octanol/buffer (pH 7.65) distribution coefficient. Data compiled from References 52, 37, and 85.

representation of the permeability observed in Figure 7 was derived by Huange et al.[52] and is given in Equations 16 through 18:

$$P_{app} = \frac{1}{R} = \cfrac{1}{\cfrac{h_1}{D_1(PC_1)} + \cfrac{h_2}{D_2(PC_2)} + \cfrac{h_3}{D_3(PC_3)}} \tag{16}$$

$$\log (PC)_i = \log (DC)_i + b_i \tag{17}$$

Equation 17 represents a linear relationship between PC, the biological partition coefficient between the membrane and adjacent biological fluid, and DC, the distribution coefficient for octanol/buffer. In Equations 16 and 18, P_{app} is the apparent permeability coefficient for the intact cornea, shown in Figure 7; R is the sum of the resistances for permeability across epithelium, stroma, and endothelium; the numerical subscripts 1 through 3 represent each layer, respectively; h is the effective barrier thickness; D is the diffusion coefficient; the subscript "i" represents any layer, and "a" and "b" are equation parameters for the semilogarithmic linear transformation of PC and DC.

$$P_{app} = \frac{1}{R} = \cfrac{1}{\cfrac{h_1}{D_1 b_1 (DC_1)^{a1}} + \cfrac{h_2}{D_2 b_2 (DC_2)^{a2}} + \cfrac{h_3}{D_3 b_3 (DC_3)^{a3}}} \tag{18}$$

Equation 18 is derived by substituting PC in equation 16 for the antilogarithmic relationship of Equation 17.

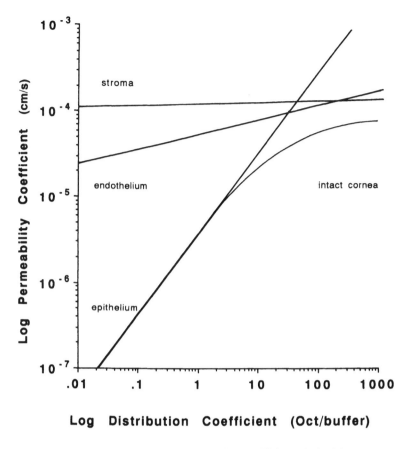

FIGURE 7. Computer-generated log-log plots of permeability coefficients obtained from separate and intact layers of excised rabbit cornea vs. the distribution coefficient of a homolog series of β-blocking agents. (From Huang, H. S., Schoenwald, R. D., and Lach, J. L., *J. Pharm. Sci.*, 72, 1272, 1983. With permission.)

The curvilinear plot for intact cornea shown in Figure 7 was determined from parameter values obtained from individual permeability experiments for β-blocking agents for each corneal layer and predicted from Equation 18.[52] The plateau for the intact cornea occurs over a range of DC from about 1.5 to 2.5 because of the small slope for the endothelium and particularly the stroma. As analog behavior approaches the plateau region (i.e., increases in lipophilicity), primary barrier resistance begins to shift from epithelium to endothelium and finally to the stroma for the most lipophilic analogs.

The stroma, as a barrier to drug penetration, is depicted in Figure 8. The collagen fibrils, 300 Å in diameter, are arranged nearly parallel to one another with an open spacing of 300 Å between each fibril.[58] Based upon the dimensions given in Figure 8, tortuosity (τ) and porosity (ε) can be estimated as 1.21 and 0.773, respectively, giving a ratio of 1.56. Huang et al.[52] estimated the ratio to be 1.58 by experimentally determining R from the penetration of β-blocking agents across isolated stromal tissue, estimating D_2 from the Sutherland-Einstein Equation, and calculating τ/ε from equation 19[52]:

$$R_2 = \frac{h_2 \tau}{D_2 \epsilon} \tag{19}$$

Knowledge of the partitioning behavior of drugs penetrating the individual layers of the cornea can be useful in developing a prodrug. For example, a lipophilic prodrug will rapidly

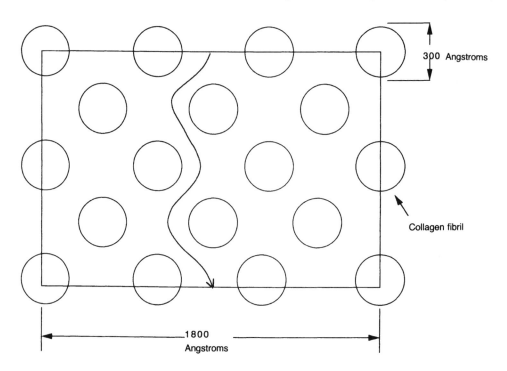

FIGURE 8. Geometric arrangement of collagen fibrils in the stroma as proposed for the calculation of the ratio of tortuosity/porosity ($=1.56$). The curved arrow between the collagen fibrils represents the proposed path of least resistance for a drug molecule penetrating the stroma. (Modified from Huang, H. S., Schoenwald, R. D., and Lach, J. L., *J. Pharm. Sci.*, 72, 1272, 1983. With permission.)

penetrate the corneal epithelium, and if enzymatic hydrolysis is rapid, the hydrophilic drug can accumulate in the stroma. As a result, the hydrophilic drug will slowly cross the endothelium and anterior chamber over a prolonged period of time. This phenomenon likely explains the long duration of miosis of diester prodrugs of pilocarpine.[39] On the other hand, if a prodrug cannot be developed for a particular hydrophilic drug, then an improvement in therapy must come from a formulation that can be retained well in the conjunctival sac.

Although penetrability can be characterized on the basis of correlating partitioning behavior to drug behavior in various layers, this approach does not identify an exact optimal structure. Partitioning can be identified with a specific functionality, but in addition to partitioning behavior, electronic effects of a particular substituent influence penetrability through pKa or polarity. In order to more accurately define an optimally penetrating structure, Eller et al.[55] related the partitioning behavior (Π) and electronic effects (σ) of substituents to changes in MPR for an analog series of 2-benzothiazolesulfonamide. These analogs were related in structure to ethoxzolamide which was effective in treating glaucoma when taken orally, but inactive when instilled in the eye. Ethoxzolamide was presumed to be topically inactive in lowering intraocular pressure (IOP) because of poor corneal penetrability.

Equation 15 identified the maximum penetration rate (MPR) as a function of corneal permeability (CP) and solubility (S). From an individual analysis of S and CP at pH 7.65, it was possible to identify which parameter was contributing to a low penetration rate, as judged by a calculation of MPR. Table 9 lists CP, S, Π, σ, and MPR values for the series studied by Eller et al.[55] From the use of the mathematical definitions of Π and σ (Equations 20 and 21 below) and through a series of algebraic substitutions interrelating the physico-chemical parameters, the authors were able to express MPR as a function of Π and σ.

TABLE 9
In Vitro Parameter Values for Determining and Optimizing Maximum Penetration
Rate (MPR) Across the Excised Rabbit Cornea

Compound of interest[a]	CP^b (cm/s × 10⁶)	S^c (µg/ml)	MPR^d (Ng/cm²/s)	Π	σ
6-Hydrogen	36.2	792.2	26.7	0	0
6-Hydroxy	5.64	1349.	7.61	−0.67	−0.37
6-Chloro	42.8	156.4	6.69	0.71	0.23
4,6-Dichloro	38.8	56.0	2.17	1.42	0.48
6-Amino[e]	6.7	269.4	1.8	−1.23	−0.66
6-Ethoxy[f]	43.9	40.9	1.79	0.38	−0.24
6-Nitro	6.57	176.0	1.16	−0.28	0.78
6-Hydroxyethoxy	1.48	310.4	0.46	−0.97	—
6-Benzyloxy	47.0	2.2	0.103	1.66	−0.23
6-Acetamido	4.74	209.1	0.99	−0.97	0

[a] Derivatives of 6-substituted benzothiazole-2-sulfonamides; data compiled from Reference 55.
[b] Corneal permeability.
[c] Total solubility measured at pH 7.65 (phosphate buffer).
[d] Maximum penetration rate predicted for excised rabbit corneas and calculated from MPR = (CP × S)/1000.
[e] Also referred to as aminozolamide.
[f] Ethoxzolamide.

$$pKa = r\ (\sigma_p) + (pKa)_H \tag{20}$$

$$\log\ (PC)_X = c\ (\Pi)_X + \log\ (PC)_H \tag{21}$$

In Equations 20 and 21, r and c are equation parameters determined from regression analysis of the experimental data for pKa and PC. The subscript H represents the 6-hydrogen substituent and X refers to any substituent at the same position of 2-benzothiazolesulfon-amide. Values of Π and σ can be obtained for many different substituent groups.[65] Therefore, once an optimal range is established for a particular series, substituents can be chosen to optimize MPR. Figure 9 is a three-dimensional plot showing the relationship between MPR, Π, and σ for the 2-benzothiazolesulfonamide series. An optimal range of Π (−0.8 to 0.1) and σ (−0.2 to 0.95) was identified. The approach reduces the syntheses to relatively few derivatives that are likely to show optimal corneal penetration.

B. SCLERA

For many years researchers have attempted to develop ocular drugs based on the premise that drugs enter the anterior chamber by penetration through the cornea. In recent years more definitive studies[66-71] have been conducted to suggest that high concentrations of drug found in iris/ciliary body tissue were a result of scleral absorption. Logically, it is not unreasonable to expect significant absorption via the scleral pathway.

Although drug entering conjunctival tissue could be removed by systemic uptake from vessels embedded in that tissue, evidence suggests that scleral resistance to penetration is less than the resistance from the multilayered corneal tissue. The exact pathway is not clear at this time. If ciliary process is the target site, direct access requires that drug must penetrate the conjunctiva, sclera, and finally the ciliary muscle to reach the ciliary process. On the other hand, the sclera contains vessels which lead to the uvea and retina and, in opposition to direct diffusion across tissue layers, are a more reasonable representation of a means by which drugs could reach the uvea, and particularly, the retina.

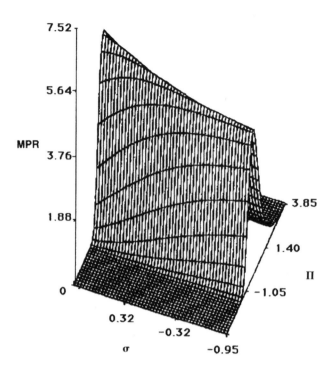

FIGURE 9. A three-dimensional relationship between the maximum penetration rate (MPR) obtained from measurements of 2-benzothiazolesulfonamide analogs across excised rabbit corneas vs. σ and II values of 6-substituted functionalities. (Modified from Eller, M. G., Schoenwald, R. D., Dixson, J. A., Segarra, T., and Barfknecht, C. F., *J. Pharm. Sci.*, 74, 155, 1985. With permission.)

Conversely, drugs entering the anterior chamber by corneal penetration must diffuse against the flow of aqueous humor. Also, when drug is instilled in the eye, it resides in the conjunctival sac in direct contact with conjunctival/scleral tissue and only reaches the cornea via spreading of the tear film across the cornea during blinking. Moreover, once absorbed across the cornea, drug is diluted by aqueous humor prior to reaching ciliary body tissue. Additional arguments against drug diffusing toward the ciliary body in high concentrations are that adjacent tissues compete for drug, and the force of aqueous humor flow is in the opposite direction.

Edelhauser and Maren[70] compared corneal and scleral permeability for ethoxzolamide and methazolamide, the latter a much more hydrophilic compound. They found that scleral permeability was about sixfold faster than corneal permeability for methazolamide, but about equal for the two tissues for ethoxzolamide. Although neither drug is active in lowering IOP when given topically to the eye, their differences in physicochemical properties suggest that topical application of a derivative optimized for scleral penetration could lead to a thera-peutically active drug.

In a study by Ahmed et al.[67] both corneal and scleral penetration were evaluated for propranolol, timolol, nadolol, penbutolol, sucrose, and inulin. Their results showed that for the hydrophilic drugs, i.e., nadolol, sucrose, and inulin, the outer layer of the sclera was much less resistant to penetration than the epithelium of the cornea. For the lipophilic drugs, i.e., propranolol, timolol, and penbutolol, there were no significant differences in penetration for the two tissues.

Chien et al.[66] compared scleral and corneal absorption for an analog series. Clonidine, *p*-aminoclonidine, and a 6-quinoxalinyl derivative of clonidine (AGN 190342) were each administered to the eye of anesthetized rabbits with a plastic cylinder (0.7 ml) affixed to the corneoscleral junction by cyanoacrylate adhesive. Drug solution was placed for 90 min either within the well in contact with the cornea or outside the well, excluding the cornea but exposed to conjunctiva. When drug solution was in contact with conjunctiva, the order of highest to lowest concentration was conjunctiva > cornea > ciliary body > aqueous humor. Following contact with the cornea, the order was cornea > aqueous humor > ciliary body > conjunctiva. Their results further showed that drug absorption in the conjunctiva and sclera was more significant for the most polar compound, p-aminoclonidine, than for clonidine and the 6-quinoxalinyl derivative of clonidine. The corneal route was the major pathway for absorption into ciliary body for the latter two compounds.

One other study by Lee and Schoenwald[72] used the well described above and compared the corneal and scleral routes of entry for ethoxzolamide and 6-hydroxy-2-benzothiazole-sulfonamide. The two drugs have similar physicochemical properties and *in vitro* inhibition of carbonic anhydrase, yet only the 6-hydroxy derivative was capable of lowering IOP when administered topically to either the rabbit or monkey eye.[73,74] Iris/ciliary body tissues were found to be 80 times higher for the scleral route than the corneal route for the 6-hydroxy derivative, suggesting why the latter was active when given topically.

Additional studies are necessary to determine which drugs may preferentially enter the anterior chamber via the scleral pathway and also to precisely define the physicochemical properties which are optimal.

V. ANTERIOR CHAMBER DISPOSITION (DISTRIBUTION AND ELIMINATION)

In the following sections the kinetics of distribution and elimination will be discussed from the perspective of tissues within the anterior chamber. Many anterior and, to a lesser extent, posterior tissues have been measured for drug concentration following topical, periocular, oral, or parenteral routes of administration. The iris/ciliary body represents the biophase for many drugs administered topically to the eye. Also of interest is the lens, since drug accumulation has been known to induce cataract formation.[75] These tissues are easily removed but are often treated as kinetically homogenous tissues, even though they are anatomically quite different and therefore can potentially accumulate drug in different concentrations. Although tissues within the anterior chamber are often measured for drug concentration over time following various methods of administration, specific information is lacking regarding the ability of these tissues to accumulate drug by partitioning and/or binding.

A. DISTRIBUTION
1. Iris

Iris tissue is highly vascular, porous, and possesses a large surface so that distribution equilibrium with drug dissolved in aqueous humor is expected to occur rapidly. Whenever the iris has been studied separately from the ciliary body, drug concentrations from topical application have been nearly equal to aqueous humor levels.[76] The sphincter and dilator muscles of the iris are the target sites for miotics and mydriatics, whereas, the ciliary body is the target site for the carbonic anhydrase inhibitors. Yet when studied, the iris and ciliary body are often removed without further separation since the iris is continuous with the anterior part of the ciliary body and difficult to isolate in the rabbit eye. Consequently, tissue concentrations, which are reported on a mass/unit weight basis, are sometimes of questionable interpretation because the tissue that is reported is not homogeneous.

It has been shown that dark-eyed individuals have a delayed onset and a reduced, but prolonged response to catecholamines and atropine.[78] This is likely a result of increased binding to the pigmented iris that occurs for these drugs, presumably to melanin. In addition, drugs may bind to autonomic receptors located in the iris. Binding to an inactive site can act as a reservoir (e.g., cornea, iris, or lens), releasing drug over time and acting to sustain the effect much like a sustained-release preparation for the intramuscular or oral routes of administration.

Because of the binding characteristics of melanin, the use of the pigmented rabbit may be a more suitable model for studying ocular diposition than the albino rabbit. Also, it has been shown that drugs with linkages capable of hydrolysis, namely dipivalyl epinephrine and pilocarpine, are degraded more rapidly in the pigmented rabbit eye.[10]

2. Ciliary Body

For many drugs given topically, drug concentration in the ciliary body is relatively high, often higher than that found in aqueous humor. As discussed previously, these high tissue levels are suspected to have reached ciliary body directly from the sclera and not via a diffusional gradient from corneal penetration and transfer from aqueous humor. The anatomy of the ciliary body supports the notion that drug enters this tissue by the former and not the latter route. The portion of the ciliary body exposed to the posterior chamber contains two epithelial layers. The outer layer is pigmented, whereas the inner layer is nonpigmented and responsible for secretion of aqueous humor. It is the nonpigmented layer that contains carbonic anhydrase (CA), consequently, CA inhibitors must reach this interior layer of cells in order to lower IOP. Between the epithelial layers the junctions are tight and therefore not easily traversed by drug. However, beneath the epithelial layers is the stroma that contains a rich supply of capillaries that are fenestrated and allow penetration of large molecules.[76] Blood flow through these capillaries is high and therefore encourages a rapid exchange of drug between the blood and the stroma. Clearly, drugs given systemically have access to the ciliary body. For example, the commercially available CA inhibitors are effective in lowering IOP when given orally, but not when administered topically. Manipulation of the physicochemical properties and the potency of CA inhibitors has yielded topically active derivatives, but as discussed previously, their route of access to the ciliary body is not clear.

3. Lens

Although the lens is continuously bathed by aqueous humor, it does not accumulate drug as one might expect. In part, lack of accumulation is a result of its structure. The lens is an epithelial tissue consisting of tightly packed layers indicating high tortuosity and low porosity for drugs that cannot directly penetrate cells. The nucleus is composed of hard, condensed cellular material which would be expected to resist drug penetration. Less than expected accumulation in the lens may also be a consequence of the rapid turnover of aqueous humor.[21,78] Nevertheless, when accumulation does occur, cataract formation is of obvious concern. Chlorpromazine, eosin, and sulfonamides have been thought to induce cataract formation.[75]

A detailed study of the diffusional properties of various lens tissues has not been reported. Because the lens is easy to remove, it is often treated, albeit incorrectly, as a kinetically homogeneous tissue. Maurice and Mishima[79] have observed that fluorescein, a watersoluble dye, diffuses laterally within the outermost layers of the lens more rapidly than it diffuses to the inner layers. On the other hand, rhodamine B, a lipophilic dye, diffuses the lens more readily than fluorescein.[80] In various studies,[21,78,81] and in particular for pilocarpine,[21] distribution into and out of the lens is slow and has resulted in incorrectly identifying the

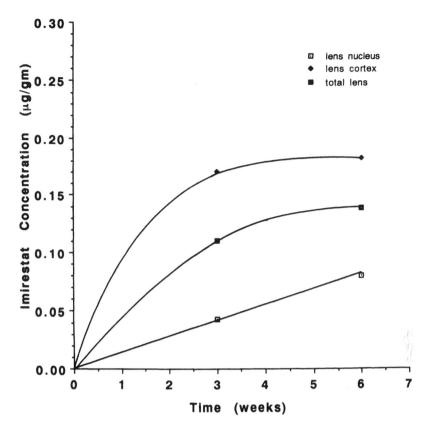

FIGURE 10. Accumulation of imirestat in lens tissues following once-daily dosing of 30 μl of 0.05% to the rabbit eye for 6 weeks. (Modified from Brazzell, R. K., Wooldridge, C. B., Hackett, R. B., and McCue, B. A., *Pharm. Res.*, 7, 197, 1990. With permission.)

elimination phase for the log-linear latter portion of the aqueous humor concentration of drug vs. time curve.

The ocular pharmacokinetics of imirestat, a new drug being studied for its ability to prevent cataract formation, has been evaluated for lens accumulation following topical administration of a 0.05% suspension to the rabbit eye.[78] In this study, the concentration of drug was followed in the lens cortex and nucleus as well as cornea, aqueous humor, vitreous humor, and plasma. Elimination half-lives of drug in the cornea and lens were exceptionally long: 130 and 140 h, respectively. Drug could not be detected in other tissues over a long enough time period to confirm the half-life. Figure 10 shows the accumulation of drug in the cortex, nucleus, and total lens for once-daily administration through 6 weeks of dosing. Drug concentrations in the nucleus show an increase in accumulation throughout the time period, however, accumulation in the cortex appears to reach a steady state by 3 weeks. Although dugs administered systemically nearly always show rapid distribution equilibrium between plasma and most tissues, results for ocular studies indicate that eye tissues, particularly the lens, cannot be assumed to be in rapid equilibrium with their circulating fluid (i.e., aqueous or vitreous humor).

B. ELIMINATION

Elimination of drug from the eye occurs most commonly by aqueous humor turnover, which in the rabbit eye is 1.5% of the volume of anterior chamber per minute (i.e., $t_{1/2}$ =

42.7 min). Assuming a volume of aqueous of 0.311 ml, ocular clearance by aqueous turnover is 4.67 μl/min. Whenever ocular clearance is significantly larger than 4.67 μl/min, additional pathways can be considered, e.g., metabolism and /or systemic uptake by the highly vascular tissues of the anterior uvea.

If ocular clearance is significantly below 4.67 μl/min, binding of drug to aqueous components could be suspected. However, measurements of free and not total (bound and free) drug would correct for binding and yield clearance values equal to or greater than 4.67 μl/min. On the other hand, binding to tissue components can decrease the ocular clearance and provide too little drug to invoke a pharmacological response. However, the same phenomenon, upon multiple dosing, can account for significant accumulation and a drug-enhancing effect. It is also possible for ocular clearances to be underestimated because of slow redistribution from the lens or choroid back into aqueous humor. This phenomenon can be corrected by making certain that the log-linear latter slope is truly linear and not subtly decreasing.

Metabolic pathways in the eye have only recently been acknowledged as important information leading to the development of new ophthalmic drugs. In particular, esterases have been studied most extensively because of their importance in the development of prodrugs.[32,59,83] Other enzyme systems that have been studied in the eye are catechol-*O*-methyltransferase, monoamine oxidase, steroid 6-betahydroxylase, oxidoreductase, lysosomal enzymes, peptidases, glucuronide and sulfate transferase, glutathione conjugating enzymes,[17,38] and arylamine acetyltransferase.[84] In the rabbit, the corneal epithelium and endothelium, ciliary process, and the retina are the tissues with the greatest capacity for metabolism.

REFERENCES

1. **Gibaldi, M. and Perrier, D.,** *Pharmacokinetics,* 2nd ed., Marcel Dekker, New York, 1982.
2. **Jones, R. F. and Maurice, D. M.,** New methods of measuring the rate of aqueous flow in man with fluorescein, *Exp. Eye Res.,* 5, 208, 1966.
3. **Makoid, M. C. and Robinson, J. R.,** Pharmacokinetics of topically applied pilocarpine in the albino rabbit eye, *J. Pharm. Sci.,* 68, 435, 1979.
4. **Sieg, J. W. and Robinson, J. R.,** Mechanistic studies on transcorneal permeation of pilocarpine, *J. Pharm. Sci.,* 65, 1816, 1976.
5. **Lee, V. H.-L. and Robinson, J. R.,** Mechanistic and quantitative evaluation of precorneal pilocarpine disposition in albino rabbits, *J. Pharm. Sci.,* 68, 673, 1979.
6. **Vigo, J. F., Rafart, J., Concheiro, A., Martinez, R., and Cordido, M.,** Ocular penetration and pharmacokinetics of cefotaxime: an experimental study, *Curr. Eye Res.,* 7, 1149, 1988.
7. **Chiang, C. H. and Schoenwald, R. D.,** Ocular pharmacokinetic models of clonidine-^{3}H hydrochloride, *J. Pharmacokinet. Biopharm.,* 14, 175, 1986.
8. **Gibaldi, M. and Perrier, D.,** *Pharmacokinetics,* Marcel Dekker, New York, 1975, 35.
9. **Conrad, J. M. and Robinson, J. R.,** Aqueous chamber drug distribution volume measurements in rabbits, *J. Pharm. Sci.,* 66, 219, 1977.
10. **Lee, V. H. L. and Robinson, J. R.,** Review: topical ocular drug delivery: recent developments and future challenges, *J. Ocular Pharmacol.,* 2, 67, 1986.
11. **Eller, M. G., Schoenwald, R. D., Dixson, J. A., Segarra, T., and Barfknecht, C. F.,** Topical carbonic anhydrase inhibitors IV: relationship between excised corneal permeability and pharmacokinetic factors, *J. Pharm. Sci.,* 74, 525, 1985.
12. **Schoenwald, R. D. and Chien, D. S.,** Ocular absorption and disposition of phenylephrine and phenylephrine oxazolidine, *Biopharm. Drug Disposit.* 9, 527, 1988.
13. **Rao, C. S., Schoenwald, R. D., Barfknecht, C. F., and Laban, S. L.,** Biopharmaceutical evaluation of ibufenac, ibuprofen, and their hydroxyethoxy analogs in the rabbit eyes, *J. Pharmacokinetics Biopharmaceutics,* 1992 (in press).

14. **Putnam, M. L., Schoenwald, R. D., Duffel, M. W., Barfknecht, C. F., Segarra, T. M., and Campbell, D. A.,** Ocular disposition of aminozolamide in the rabbit eye, *Invest. Ophthalmol. Vis. Sci.,* 28, 137, 1987.
15. **Eng, I. S.,** N-Methylacetazolamide; ocular disposition and enzyme kinetics, Ph.D. thesis, University of Iowa College of Pharmacy, Iowa City, 1986.
16. **Tang-Liu, D. D. S., Liu, S. S., and Weinkam, R. J.,** Ocular and systemic bioavailability of ophthalmic flurbiprofen, *J. Pharmacokinet. Biopharm.,* 12, 611, 1984.
17. **Tang-Liu, D. D. S., Liu, S., Neff, J., and Sandri, R.,** Disposition of levobunolol after an ophthalmic dose to rabbits, *J. Pharm. Sci.,* 76, 780, 1987.
18. **Ling, T. L. and Combs, D. L.,** Ocular bioavailability and tissue distribution of [^{14}C] ketorolac tromethamine in rabbits, *J. Pharm. Sci.,* 76, 289, 1987.
19. **Patton, T.,** Ophthalmic drug delivery systems, in *Ocular Drug Disposition,* Robinson, J. R., Ed., American Pharmaceutical Association, Washington, D.C., 1980, chap. 2.
20. **Himmelstein, K. J., Guvenir, I., and Patton, T. P.,** Preliminary pharmacokinetic model of pilocarpine uptake and distribution in the eye, *J. Pharm. Sci.,* 67, 603, 1978.
21. **Miller, S. C., Himmelstein, K. J., and Patton, T. F.,** A physiologically based pharmacokinetic model for the intraocular distribution of pilocarpine in rabbits, *J. Pharmacokinet. Biopharm.,* 9, 653, 1981.
22. **Mikkelson, T. J., Chrai, S. S., and Robinson, J. R.,** Altered bioavailability of dugs in the eye due to drug-protein interactions, *J. Pharm. Sci.,* 62, 1648, 1973.
23. **van Haeringen, N. J., Oosterhuis, J. A., van Delft, J. L., Glasius, E., and Noach, E. L.,** A comparison of the effects of non-steroidal compounds on the disruption of the blood-aqueous barrier, *Exp. Eye Res.,* 35, 271, 1982.
24. **Schoenwald, R. D., Folk, J. C., Kumar, V., and Piper, J. G.,** In vivo comparison of phenylephrine and phenylephrine oxazolidine instilled in the monkey eye, *J. Ocular Pharmacol.,* 3, 333, 1987.
25. **Putnam, M. L., Schoenwald, R. D., Duffel, M. W., Barfknecht, C. F., Segarra, T. M., and Campbell, D. A.,** Ocular disposition of aminozolamide in the rabbit eye, *Invest. Ophthalmol. Vis. Sci.,* 28, 1374, 1987.
26. **Auclair, E., Laude, D., Wainer, I. W., Chauouloff, F., and Elghozi, J. L.,** Comparative pharmacokinetics of D- and L- alphamethyldopa in plasma, aqueous humor, and cerebrospinal fluid in rabbits, *Fundam. Clin. Pharmacol.,* 2, 283, 1988.
27. **Ling, T. L. and Combs, D. L.,** Ocular bioavailability and tissue distribution of [^{14}C] ketorolac tromethamine in rabbits, *J. Pharm. Sci.,* 76, 291, 1987.
28. **Leibowitz, H. M., Berrospi, A. R., Kupferman, A., Restropo, G. V., Galvis, V., and Alvarez, J. A.,** Penetration of topically administered prednisolone acetate into the human aqueous humor, *Am. J. Ophthalmol.,* 83, 402, 1977.
29. **Saettone, M. F., Giannaccini, B., Teneggi, A., Savigni, P., and Tellini, N.,** Vehicle effects on ophthalmic bioavailability: the influence of different polymers on the activity of pilocarpine in rabbit and man, *J. Pharm. Pharmacol.,* 34, 464, 1982.
30. **Saettone, M. F., Giannaccini, B., Ravecca, S., La Marca, F., and Tota, G.,** Polymer effects on ocular bioavailability—the influence of different liquid vehicles on the mydriatic response of tropicamide in humans and in rabbits, *Int. J. Pharm.,* 20, 187, 1984.
31. **McDonald, T. O. and Shadduck, J. A.,** Eye irritation, in *Dermatatoxicology and Pharmacology,* Maibach, H. and Marzulli, F. N., Eds., John Wiley & Sons, New York, 1977, 139.
32. **Lee, V. H. L., Chang, S. C., Oshiro, C. M., and Smith, R. E.,** Ocular esterase composition in albino and pigmented rabbits: possible implications in ocular prodrug design and evaluation, *Curr. Eye Res.,* 4, 1117, 1985.
33. **Lee, V. H. L. and Robinson, J. R.,** Disposition of pilocarpine in the pigmented rabbit eye, *Int. J. Pharm.,* 11, 155, 1982.
34. **Chrai, S. S., Patton, T. F., Mehta, A., and Robinson, J. R.,** Lacrimal and instilled fluid dynamics in rabbit eyes, *J. Pharm. Sci.,* 62, 1112, 1973.
35. **Chrai, S. S., Makoid, M. C., Eriksen, S. P., and Robinson, J. R.,** Drop size and initial dosing frequency problems of topically applied ophthalmic drugs, *J. Pharm. Sci.,* 63, 333, 1974.
36. **Patton, T. F. and Robinson, J. R.,** Quantitative precorneal disposition of topically applied pilocarpine nitrate in rabbit eyes, *J. Pharm. Sci.,* 65, 1295, 1976.
37. **Schoenwald, R. D.,** Ocular drug delivery. Pharmacokinetic considerations, *Clin. Pharmacokinet.,* 18, 255, 1990.
38. **Plazonnet, B., Grove, J., Durr, M., Mazuel, C., Quint, M., and Rozier, A.,** Pharmacokinetics and biopharmaceutical aspects of some anti-glaucoma drugs, in *Ophthalmic Drug Delivery Biopharmaceutical Technological and Clinical Aspects* Vol. 11, Saettone, M. F., Bucci, M., and Speiser, P., Eds., Liviana Press, Springer-Verlag, Berlin, 1977, 118.

39. **Bundgaard, H., Falch, E., Larsen, C., Mosher, G. L., and Mikkelson, T.,** Pilocarpine prodrugs II. Synthesis, stability, bioconversion, and physicochemical properties of sequentially labile pilocarpine acid diesters, *J. Pharm. Sci.,* 75, 775, 1886.

40. **Burstein, N. L. and Anderson, J. A.,** Review: corneal penetration and ocular bioavailability of drugs, *J. Ocular Pharmacol.,* 3, 309, 1985.

41. **Wei, C.-P., Anderson, J. A., and Leopold, I.,** Ocular absorption and metabolism of topically applied epinephrine and a dipivalyl ester of epinephrine, *Invest. Ophthalmol. Vis. Sci.,* 17, 315, 1978.

42. **Karback, M. B., Podos, S. M., Harbin, T. S., Mandell, A., and Becker, B.,** The effects of dipivalyl epinephrine on the eye, *Am. J. Ophthalmol.,* 81, 768, 1976.

43. **Patton, T. F. and Francoeur, M.,** Ocular bioavailability and systemic loss of topically ophthalmic drugs, *Am. J. Ophthalmol.,* 86, 820, 1978.

44. **Brown, R. H., Wood, T. S., Lynch, M. G., Schoenwald, R. D., and Chien, D.-S.,** Improving the therapeutic index of topical phenylephrine by reducing drop volume, *Ophthalmology,* 94, 847, 1987.

45. **Lynch, M. G., Brown, R. H., Goode, S. M., Schoenwald, R. D., and Chien, D.-S.,** Reduction of phenylephrine drop size in infants achieves equal dilation with decreased systemic absorption, *Arch. Ophthalmol.,* 105, 1364, 1987.

46. **Hendrickson, R. O. and Hanna, C.,** Use of drugs in ointment for routine mydriasis, *Arch. Ophthalmol.,* 96, 333, 1977.

47. **Cable, M. K., Hendrickson, R. O., and Hanna, C.,** Evaluation of drugs in ointment for mydriasis and cycloplegia, *Arch. Ophthalmol.,* 96, 84, 1978.

48. **Brown, C. and Hanna, C.,** Use of dilute drug solutions for routine cycloplegia and mydriasis, *Am. J. Ophthalmol.,* 86, 820, 1978.

48a. **DeSantis, L. M. and Schoenwald, R. D.,** The lack of influence of the rabbit nictitating membrane on the miosis effect of pilocarpine, *J. Pharm. Sci.,* 67, 1189, 1978.

49. **Wang, W., Sasaki, H., Chien, D.-S., and Lee, H. L. V.,** Lipophilicity influence on conjunctival drug penetration in the pigmented rabbit: a comparison with corneal penetration, *Curr. Eye Res.,* 10, 571, 1991.

50. **Chien, D. S. and Schoenwald, R. D.,** Improving the ocular absorption of phenylephrine, *Biopharm. Drug Disposit.,* 7, 453, 1986.

51. **Schoenwald, R. D. and Huang, H. S.,** Corneal penetration behavior of beta-blocking agents I: physicochemical factors, *J. Pharm. Sci.,* 72, 1266, 1983.

52. **Huang, H. S., Schoenwald, R. D., and Lach, J. L.,** Corneal penetration behavior of beta-blocking agents II: assessment of barrier contributions, *J. Pharm. Sci.,* 72, 1272, 1983.

53. **Igarashi, H., Sato, Y., Hamada, S., and Kawasaki, T.,** Studies on rabbit corneal permeability of local anesthetics, *Jpn. J. Pharmacol.,* 34, 429, 1984.

54. **Schoenwald, R. D. and Ward, R. L.,** Relationship between steroid permeability across excised rabbit cornea and octanol-water partition coefficients, *J. Pharm. Sci.,* 67, 786, 1978.

55. **Eller, M. G., Schoenwald, R. D., Dixson, J. A., Segarra, T., and Barfknecht, C. F.,** Topical carbonic anhydrase inhibitors III: optimization model for corneal penetration of ethoxzolamide analogues, *J. Pharm. Sci.,* 74, 155, 1985.

56. **Mosher, G. L. and Mikkelson, T. J.,** Permeability of the n-alkyl p-aminobenzoate esters across the isolated corneal membrane of the rabbit, *Int. J. Pharm.,* 2, 239, 1979.

57. **Grass, G. M. and Robinson, J. R.,** Relationship of chemical structure to corneal penetration and influence of low-viscosity solution on ocular bioavailability, *J. Pharm. Sci.,* 73, 1021, 1984.

58. **Fatt, I.,** *Physiology of the Eye,* Butterworths, Boston, 1978, chap. 6.

59. **Chien, D. S., Bundgaard, H., and Lee, V. H. L.,** Influence of corneal epithelial integrity on the penetration of timolol prodrugs, *J. Ocular Pharmacol.,* 4, 137, 1988.

60. **Chang, S.-C. and Lee, V. H. L.,** Influence of chain length on the in vitro hydrolysis of model ester prodrugs by ocular esterases, *Curr. Eye Res.,* 2, 651, 1983.

61. **Lien, E. J., Alhaider, A. A., and Lee, V. H.-L.,** Phase partition: it use in the prediction of membrane permeation and drug action in the eye, *J. Paren. Sci. Technol.,* 36, 86, 1982.

62. **Schoenwald, R. D. and Stewart, P.,** Effect of particle size on the ophthalmic bioavailability of dexamethasone suspensions in rabbits, *J. Pharm. Sci.,* 69, 391, 1980.

63. **Sieg, J. W. and Robinson, J. R.,** Vehicle effects on ocular drug bioavailability I: evaluation of fluorometholone, *J. Pharm. Sci.,* 64, 931, 1975.

64. **Sieg, J. W. and Triplett, J. W.,** Precorneal retention of topically instilled micronized particles, *J. Pharm. Sci.,* 69, 863, 1980.

65. **Hansch, C. and Leo, A.,** *Log P and Parameter Database.* Comtex Scientific, New York, 1983.

66. **Chien, D. S., Homsy, J. J., Gluchowski, C., and Tang-liu, D. D. S.,** Corneal and conjunctival/scleral penetration of p-aminoclonidine, AGN 190342, and clonidine, *Curr. Eye Res.,* 9, 1051, 1990.

67. **Ahmed, I., Gokhale, R. D., Shah, M. V., and Patton, T. F.,** Physicochemical determinants of drug diffusion across the conjunctiva, sclera, and cornea, *J. Pharm. Sci.,* 76, 583, 1987.

68. **Ahmed, I. and Patton, T. F.**, Importance of the noncorneal absorption route in topical ophthalmic drug delivery, *Invest. Ophthalmol. Vis. Sci.*, 26, 584, 1985.

69. **Doane, M. G., Jensen, A. D., and Dohlman, C. H.**, Penetration routes of topically applied eye medications, *Am. J. Ophthalmol.*, 85, 383, 1978.

70. **Edelhauser, H. F. and Maren, T. H.**, Permeability of human cornea and sclera to sulfonamide carbonic anhydrase inhibitors, *Arch. Ophthalmol.*, 106, 1110, 1988.

71. **Hitoshi, S., Bundgaard, H., and Lee, V. H. L.**, Design of prodrugs to selectively reduce timolol absorption on the basis of the differential lipophilic characteristics of the cornea and the conjunctiva, *Invest. Ophthalmol. Vis. Sci.*, Suppl. 30, 25, 1989.

72. **Lee, D.-Y. and Schoenwald, R. D.**, unpublished data, 1991.

73. **Lewis, R. A., Schoenwald, R. D., Eller, M. G., Barfknecht, C. F., and Phelps, C. D.**, Ethoxzolamide analogue gel: a topical carbonic anhydrase inhibitor, *Arch. Ophthalmol.*, 102, 1821, 1984.

74. **DeSantis, L., Sallee, V., Barnes, G., Schoenwald, R., Barfknecht, C., Duffel, M., and Lewis, R.**, The effect of topically applied analogs of the carbonic anhydrase inhibitor, ethoxzolamide, on intraocular pressure in alert laser-induced ocular hypertensive cynomolgus monkeys, *Invest. Ophthalmol. Vis. Sci.*, Suppl. 27, 179, 1986.

75. **Zigman, S.**, Photobiology of lens, in *Ocular Lens,* Maisel, H. Ed., Marcel Dekker, New York, 1985, 301.

76. **Maurice, D. M.**, Structures and fluids involved in the penetration of topically applied drugs, in *Clinical Pharmacology of the Anterior Segment,* Holly, F., Ed., Little, Brown, Boston, 1980, 7.

77. **Havener, W. H.**, Autonomic drugs, in *Ocular Pharmacology,* 5th ed., V. V. Mosby, St. Louis, 1983, 269.

78. **Brazzell, R. K., Wooldridge, C. B., Hackett, R. B., and McCue, B. A.**, Pharmacokinetics of the aldose reductase inhibitor imirestat following topical ocular administration, *Pharm. Res.*, 7, 192, 1990.

79. **Maurice, D. M. and Mishima, S.**, Ocular pharmacokinetics , in *Pharmacology of the Eye,* Sears, M. L., Ed., Springer-Verlag, Berlin, 1984, 19.

80. **Maurice, D.**, Kinetics of topically applied ophthalmic drugs, in *Ophthalmic Drug Delivery: Biopharmaceutical, Technological and Clinical Aspects,* Vol. 11, (Fidia Research Series), Saettone, M. F., Bucci, M., and Speiser, P., Eds., Liviana Press, Springer-Verlag, Berlin, 1987, 19.

81. **Salvancet, A., Fisch, A., Lafaix, C., Montay, G., Dubayle, P., Forestier, F., and Haroche, G.**, Pefloxacin concentration in human aqueous humor and lens, *J. Antimicrob. Chem.*, 18, 199, 1986.

82. **Lee, V. H. L., Morimoto, K. M., and Stratford, R. E., Jr.**, Esterase distribution in the rabbit cornea and its implications in ocular drug bioavailability, *Biopharm. Drug Disposit.*, 3, 291, 1982.

83. **Lee, V. H.**, Esterase activities in adult rabbit eyes, *J. Pharm. Sci.*, 72, 239, 1983.

84. **Campbell, D. A., Schoenwald, R. D., Duffel, M. W., and Barfknecht, C. F.**, Characterization of arylamine acetyltransferase in the rabbit eye, *Invest. Ophthalmol. Vis. Sci.*, 32, 2190, 1991.

85. **Chiang, C. H., Huang, H. S., and Schoenwald, R. D.**, Corneal permeability of adrenergic agents potentially useful in glaucoma, *J. Taiwan. Pharm. Assoc.*, 38, 67, 1986.

86. **Chang, S. C., Bundgaard, H., Burr, A., and Lee, V. H. L.**, Improved corneal penetration of timolol by prodrugs as a means to reduce systemic drug load, *Invest. Ophthalmol. Vis. Sci.*, 28, 487, 1987.

87. **Schoenwald, R. D.**, The control of drug bioavailability from ophthalmic dosage forms, in *Controlled Drug Bioavailability,* Vol. 3, Smolen, V. F. and Ball, L. A., Eds., John Wiley & Sons, New York, 1985, 257.

88. **Grass, G. M. and Robinson, J. R.**, Mechanisms of corneal drug penetration I: in vivo and in vitro kinetics, 77, 3, 1988.

89. **Schoenwald, R. D. and Houseman, J. A.**, Disposition of cyclophosphamide in the rabbit and human cornea, *Biopharm. Drug Disposit.*, 3, 231, 1982.

90. **Ellingson, C. M.**, Biopharmaceutic considerations in the development of a topical ocular prodrug of ibuprofen, Ph.D. thesis, University of Iowa College of Pharmacy, Iowa City, 1991.

91. **Campbell, D. A. S. and Schoenwald, R. D.**, unpublished data, 1988.

INDEX

A

ABE copolymer, 64–65
Absorption
　into anterior chamber, see under Anterior
　　chamber
　of clonidine, 184
　corneal, 176–183
　of epinephrine, 125
　mean time of, 166
　of phenylephrine, 125
　of pilocarpine, 125
　preservatives and, 125
　prodrugs and, 125–128
　rate constants for, 169
　scleral, 183–185
　systemic, 125–128
　of vasoconstrictors, 125
Absorption, distribution, metabolism, and excretion
　(ADME), 160, 165, 166, 173
Absorption half-lives, 167, 169
Aceclidine, 30
Acetazolamide, 130
Acetylcholine, 4, 10
Acetylcholinesterase, 95
N-Acetyl-β-glucosamine, 106
Acquired immunodeficiency syndrome (AIDS), 96
Acrylic acid, 65
Acyclovir, 30, 96, 122, 135
Adenylate cyclase, 12
Adhesives, see Bioadhesives; Mucoadhesives
Adjuvants, 29–30, 33–34, see also specific types
ADME, see Absorption, distribution, metabolism,
　and excretion
Age, 44, 45
AGN 190342, 184
AIDS, see Acquired immunodeficiency syndrome
Albumin, 5
Aldehydes, 135
Alginic acid, 69
n-Alkyl p-aminobenzoate esters, 132, 176
All-trans-retinal, 16, 17
Amacrine neurons, 16
Amide prodrugs, 129
β-Aminoalcohols, 135
p-Aminoclonidine, 184
Amoxycillin, 30
Ampholytic surfactants, 30, see also specific types
Amphotericin B, 30, 96
Anatomy, 3–18
　of anterior uvea, 9–15
　bioadhesives and, 146–148
　of chamber angle, 9–15
　of chamber system, 9–15
　of choroid, 17–18
　of ciliary body, 10–12
　of conjuctiva, 5–8
　of cornea, 3–5, 44
　of extraocular orbital structures, 18
　of eyelids, 5–8
　of iris, 12–13
　of lacrimal apparatus, 7–9
　of lens, 14–15
　of optic nerve, 15–17
　of posterior segment of eye, 15–18
　of retina, 15–17
　of Schlemm's canal, 13
　of sclera, 17–18
　of trabecular meshwork, 13
　of vitreous, 17
Anesthesia, 18, 30, 45, 155, see also specific types
Anionic latices, 84
Anionic liposomes, 154
Anionic surfactants, 30, see also specific types
Antazoline, 30
Anterior chamber, 9–15, 19
　absorption into, 176–185
　　cornea, 176–183
　　sclera, 183–185
　disposition in, 185–188
Anterior hyaloid membrane, 17
Anterior segment of eye, 3, see also specific parts
Anterior uvea, 18, 22
　anatomy of, 9–15
　inflammation of, 22
　physiology of, 9–15
Antibiotics, 17, 20, 30, 96, see also specific types
Antibodies, 93
Anticholinergics, 128, see also specific types
Antidepressants, 30, see also specific types
Antiglaucoma agents, 20, 30, 82, 96, see also
　specific types
Antihistamines, 30, see also specific types
Anti-inflammatory agents, 95, 172, see also specific
　types
Antimicrobials, 128, see also specific types
Antineoplastic agents, 97, see also specific types
Antioxidants, 51, 93, see also specific types
Antiviral agents, 30, 96, see also specific types
Aphakic eyes, 20
Aqueous humor, 2, 9, 10, 13, 15, 188
　aveoscleral outflow of, 9
　clearance of, 168
　concentrations of, 88
　continuous flow of, 9
　diffusion into, 20
　distribution of drugs in, 185
　drainage of, 19–20
　dynamics of, 18
　flow of, 9, 13, 20, 21, 22
　formation of, 11
　increase in outflow of, 22
　intraocular pressure and, 13
　organic anions from, 20

production of, 11, 12
rate of flow of, 20
resistance to outflow of, 13
turnover in, 187, 188
weight of, 173
Aqueous solubility, 133–134
Aqueous veins, 13
Artificial tears, 67, 113
Arylamine acetyltransferase, 188
Ascorbic acid, 9
Atropine, 30, 94, 95
Autacoids, 3, 22, see also specific types

B

Bacitracin, 30
Back-diffusion, 172
Bactericidal preservatives, 34
BAK, see Benzalkonium chloride
Basement membrane, 44
Benzalkonium chloride (BAK), 19, 30, 35, 44,
    46–48, 49
    dry eye and, 115
    prodrugs and, 136
Benzodiazepines, 30, see also specific types
Benzofuran-sulfonamides, 136
2-Benzothiazolesulfonamide, 182, 183
β-adrenergic antagonists, 12, 19, 125, see also
    specific types
β-adrenergic receptors, 12, see also specific types
β-blockers, 12, 21, 30, 73, see also specific types
    corneal permeability of, 181
    multiple linear regression models of, 176
    prodrugs and, 130, 132
    soft drugs and, 128
6-Betahydroxylase, 188
Betaxolol, 122, 125
Bioadhesives, 111, 145–155, see also specific types
    anatomy and, 146–148
    defined, 150–152
    disposition of drugs and, 148–150
    factors affecting delivery of, 154–155
    ocular, 152–154
    viscosity and, 154
Bioavailability, 63, 66, 67, 111
    bioadhesives and, 155
    decrease in, 155
    enhancement of, 69
    hyaluronic acid and, 115, 117
    of pilocarpine, 176
Bio-Cor, 69
Bionite, 71
Blinking frequency, 7
Blood-aqueous barrier, 10, 19, 20, 21, 172
Blood flow, 13, 18
Blood-retinal barrier, 19, 20
Blood-vitreous barrier, 172
Borate solutions, 32
Bowman's membrane, 4, 5, 44
Bromhexidine, 30
Bruch's membrane, 17
Buffer capacity, 31

Butylcyanoacrylate, 82
Butyrylcholinesterase, 130
O-Butyryltimolol, 133

C

CA, see Carbonic anhydrase
Calcitonin gene-related peptide (CGRP), 12
Calcium, 154
Canal of Schlemm, 2, 9
CAP, see Cellulose acetate phthalate
Caprylic acid, 49
Carbachol, 30
Carbohydrates, 98, see also specific types
Carbomer, 35
Carbonic anhydrase (CA), 186
Carbonic anhydrase inhibitors, 130, 136, 186, see
    also specific types
Carbopol, 151
Carboxyfluorescein (CF), 97
Carboxymethylcellulose (CMC), 111, 151
Carrier-mediated transport system, 20
Carteolol, 125
Caruncle, 5
Catalase, 51
Cataracts, 15, 154, 185
Catecholamines, 12, see also specific types
Catechol-O-methyltransferase, 188
Cationic surfactants, 30, 46, 48, see also specific
    types
CDG, see Chlorhexidine digluconate
Cefotaxime, 164–165
Cellulose acetate phthalate (CAP), 67, 87
Cephalosporins, 30, see also specific types
Cetylpyridinium chloride (CPC), 44, 48
CF, see Carboxyfuorescein
CGRP, see Calcitonin gene-related peptide
Chamber angle, 9–15
Chamber system, 9–15
CHD, see Chlorhexidine digluconate
Chelating agents, 51, see also specific types
Chemical stability, 134–135
Chemotherapy, 96, see also specific types
Chitin, 69
Chloramphenicol, 30, 177
Chlorhexidine, 30, 35
Chlorhexidine digluconate (CHD), 44, 49, 50
Chlorobutanol, 44, 49, 51
Chloroquine, 19
Chlorpromazine, 19, 186
Chlortracycline, 30
Cholecystokinin, 13
Cholesterol, 93, 95
Choline acetyltransferase, 4
Choline esterases, 4, 95
Cholinergical innervation, 10
Chondroitin, 5
Chondroitin sulfate A, 5
Choriocapillaries, 18
Choriocapillary layer, 17
Choroid, 2, 17–18, 20, 188
Choroidal blood flow, 18

Ciliary body, 2, 9, 16, 17, 20
    anatomy of, 10–12
    distribution of drugs in, 185, 186
    physiology of, 10–12
    weight of, 173
Ciliary epithelium, 20
Ciliary epithelium organic anion pump system,
    19–20
Ciliary muscle, 9, 10, 18, 20
Ciliary processes, 2, 9, 10, 11, 20, 188
    vascularization of, 13
    zonules of Zinn and, 14
11-Cis-retinal, 16
Citrate buffers, 32
Cleaning of eye surface, 28
Clearance, 87, 88, 168, 170, 188
Clearance half-life, 99
Clindamycin, 30, 96
Clonidine, 125, 165, 171, 184
CMC, see Carboxymethylcellulose
Colistin, 30
Collagen, 5, 17, 68, 70, 153, 154
Colloidal carriers, 82
Colloidal silver, 30
Collyres secs gradues, 62
Collyria, 62
Compartmental modeling, 160–165
Compression technique, 66
Cones, 16
Conjunctiva, 5–8, 19, 28, 173
Conjunctival epithelium, 6
Conjunctival hyperemia, 128
Conjunctival membranes, 94
Consensual eye responses, 21
Contact lens cleaning solutions, 48
Contact lenses, 70–71, 125
Contralateral control eye, 21
Cornea, 2, 9, 13, 18, 28
    absorption in, 176–183
    anatomy of, 3–5, 44
    as barrier to drugs, 19
    as drug reservoir, 20–21
    physiology of, 3–5, 44
    thickness of, 3, 44
    weight of, 173
Corneal endothelium, 9, 188
Corneal epithelial cells, 48, 49, 50
Corneal epithelium, 45, 130, 136, 188
Corneal penetration
    paracellular pathways to, 133
    preservatives and, 136
    prodrugs and, 122–124, 132, 136
    rate of, 177
    resistance to, 176, 180
    transcellular pathways to, 133
Corneal permeability, 43–53, 181, 182
    age and, 44, 45
    coefficients of, 177, 178–179
    endothelial, 47
    epithelial, 48
    factors that influence, 177
    mechanisms of, 147, 148

pH and, 44, 45
    preservatives and, 44, 46–52
    surfactants and, 44, 46–48
Corneal stroma, 5
Corneoscleral meshwork, 13
Cortical vitreous, 17
Corticosteroids, 135, see also specific types;
    Steroids
CPC, see Cetylpyridinium chloride
Cromolyn, 177
Cryoprecipitate, 154
Cyanoacrylates, 99, 151
Cyclo-oxygenase inhibitors, 22, see also specific
    types
Cyclosporin, 97, 125, 177
Cytarabine, 96
Cytochalasin D, 96
Cytomegalovirus retinitis, 96
Cytosine arabinoside, 97
Cytostatics, 30, see also specific types
Cytotoxicity, 45

D

N-Dealkylating enzyme, 130
Denaturation, 98
Descemet's membrane, 4, 5
Desolvation, 98
Dexamethasone, 48, 49, 67, 95
Dexamethasone valerate, 48
Dextran, 21, 35
DFP, see Di-isofluorophosphate
Diclofenac, 172
Diethylenetriaminepentaacetic acid (DTPA), 87
Diffusion, 172, 186
Di-isofluorophosphate (DFP), 95
Dilator muscle, 2, 12
Dipalmitoyl phosphatidylcholine, 92
Dipivalyl epinephrine, 125, 186
Dipiverfin, 30, 174
Disodium phosphate, 32, 67
Dispersions, 82, 83, 84, 87
Disposition of drugs, 148–150
Distribution, 185–188
Distribution coefficients, 179, 180, 181
Diuretics, 30, see also specific types
Double prodrug formation (pro-prodrugs), 135
Drop size, 35, 36
Drug retention, 29–33, 68
Drug tolerance, 68
Dry eye, 6, 112, 113–115
DTPA, see Diethylenetriaminepentaacetic acid
Dyes, 97, see also specific types
Dynamic surface tension, 35

E

EC, see Ethyl cellulose
Echothiophate, 30
Edema, 5
EDTA, see Ethylenediaminetetraacetic acid
EGDMA, see Ethylene glycol dimethacrylate

Eicosanoids, 22
Electrical potential difference, 45
Elimination, 28–29, 168, 185–188
Embryologic development of eye, 2
Empty liposomes, 95
Emulsification, 82
Emulsion polymerization, 98
Emulsions, 125
Encapsulation, 96, 97
Endothelial cells, 5
Endothelial corneal permeability, 47
Endothelium, 4, 9, 19, 176, 188
Enfluran, 30
Enzymes, 95, 130–131, 188, see also specific types
Eosin, 186
Ephedrine, 30, 135
Epinephrine, 9, 12, 19, 22, 30, 73, 177
    prodrugs and, 122, 131
    systemic absorption of, 125
Episcleral veins, 13
Episcleral venous pressure, 13
Epithelial cell layers, 10
Epithelial cells, 48, 49, 50, 151
Epithelial corneal permeability, 48
Epithelial potential difference, 46
Epithelium, 4, 19, 176
    ciliary, 20
    conjunctival, 6
    corneal, 45, 130, 136, 188
    damage to, 136
    keratinization of, 6
    pigment, 16, 17, 21
    retinal, 17
Erythromycin estolate, 71
Esterases, 19, 130, 188, see also specific types
Esterification, 19
Ethoxzolamide, 182, 184, 185
Ethyl acrylate, 71
Ethyl cellulose (EC), 67
Ethylenediaminetetraacetic acid (EDTA), 44, 47,
    48, 49, 51–52
Ethylene glycol dimethacrylate (EGDMA), 70
Ethylene-vinyl acetate (EVA), 72
Ethylene-vinyl alcohol (EVA), 73
Eudragil, 66, 67
EVA, see Ethylene-vinyl acetate
EVAl, see Ethylene-vinyl alcohol
Evaporation, 96
Extraocular muscle, 18
Extraocular orbital structures, 18
Extrusion, 66
Eyelashes, 6
Eyelids, 5–8, 28

F

Factor XII, 154
Fatty acids, 87, see also specific types
Fibrin, 69, 153, 154
Fibrinogen, 154
Fibronectin, 154
Flip-flop model, 163

Fluorouracil, 30
Fluorescein, 20, 21
    corneal permeability of, 45, 47, 48, 50
    corneal uptake of, 49
    diffusion of, 186
    distribution of, 186
    hyaluronic acid and, 112
    liposome-encapsulated, 97
    pharmacokinetics of, 161
Fluorometholone, 122
5-Fluoro-orotate, 96
Fluorophotometry, 20, 21
5-Fluorouracil, 96, 97, 123
5-Fluorouridine, 97
5-Fluorouridine monophosphate, 97
Flurbiprofen, 124, 125, 169, 170, 172
Foreign matter elimination, 28–29, 168, 185–188
Fovea, 16, 18
Free enzyme, 95
Functional groups, 129–130, 151, see also specific
    types

G

Gamma scintigraphy, 87, 99, 111, 112
Ganciclovir, 135
Gelrite, 83
General anesthetics, 30, see also specific types
Gentamicin, 30, 68, 96, 97, 153
Gentamicin sulfate (GS), 117
Glands of Krause, 7
Glands of Moll, 6
Glands of Wolfring, 7
Glands of Zeis, 6, 7
Glaucoma, 17, 20, 30, 65, 82, 96, 128
Glucuronic acid, 106
Glucuronidine, 188
Glutathione conjugating enzymes, 188, see also
    specific types
Glutathione redox cycle, 51
Glycerin, 45
Glycidyl methacrylate, 71
Glycocalix, 4
Glycolix, 6
Glycoprotein D, 93
Glycoproteins, 154, see also specific types
Glycosaminoglycans, 5, 106, 117, 154, see also
    specific types
Goblet cells, 7
G-protein, 12
GS, see Gentamicin sulfate

H

Half-lives, 99, 135, 167, 169, 172
Halothan, 30
Harder's gland, 2
HEC, see Hydroxyethylcellulose
Hefilcon-A, 70
HEMA, see 2-Hydroxyethyl methacrylate
Heroin, 30
Herpes simplex virus, 93

Hibiclens, 50
Histamine, 30
Homatropine, 30
Hormones, see also specific types
  luteinizing hormone-releasing, 124
  steroid, 68, 95, 122, 128, 132, 176, 188
  thyrotropin releasing, 124
HPC, see Hydroxypropylcellulose
HPCL (low-molecular-weight
    hydroxypropylcellulose), 111
HPCM (medium-molecular-weight
    hydroxypropylcellulose), 111
Hyalocytes, 17
Hyaloid membrane, 17
Hyaluronic acid, 5, 17, 105–118
  biological properties of, 107–109
  in dry eye treatment, 113–115
  in eye surgery, 109
  in inserts, 109, 112
  molecular structure of, 107–108
  physicochemical properties of, 108
  precorneal residence time and, 109–113
  residence time and, 106, 109–113
  solutions of, 109
  source of, 107
  viscosity of, 108
Hydrocortisone, 67, 106, 125
Hydrocortisone acetate, 68
Hydrogel contact lenses, 70–71
Hydrogen bonding, 154
Hydrogen ion concentration, 31–32
Hydrogen peroxide, 44, 50–51
Hydrophilic substances, 19, 20, 73, 151, see also
    specific types
Hydroxyamphetamine, 30
6-Hydroxy-2-benzothiazolesulfonamide, 185
Hydroxyethylcellulose (HEC), 35, 88, 112
2-Hydroxyethyl methacrylate (HEMA), 70
Hydroxyl-ion-induced polymerization, 98
Hydroxypropylcellulose (HPC), 35, 65, 66, 67, 70,
    151
Hydroxypropylmethylcellulose, 35, 66
Hyperemia, 128
Hypertonic solutions, 31
Hypotonic solutions, 31

I

Idiosyncratic responses, 48
Idoxuridine, 30, 68, 71, 93, 122, 123
4-Imidazolidones, 124
Imirestat, 187
Immunoglobulins, 7
Immunoliposomes, 93
Indole-2-sulfonamides, 136
Indomethacin, 172
Inflammation, 20, 21, 22
Innervation, 6, 10, 18
Inserts, see also specific types
  advantages of, 63
  defined, 62
  history of, 62–63

hyaluronic acid in, 109, 112
insoluble, 70–73
membrane-controlled reservoir, 71–72
naturally occurring polymers in, 68–69
prodrugs in, 70
shape of, 68
size of, 68
solic polymeric, see Solid polymeric inserts
soluble, 63–70
In situ gelling systems, 81–88
Insoluble solid polymeric inserts, 70–73
Instilled volume, 29, 35–36
Insulin, 45, 47
Interfacial polymerization, 98
Intraocular pressure (IOP), 2, 12, 13–14, 21
  hyaluronic acid and, 109
  increase in, 18
  prodrugs and, 128
  reduction in, 12, 19, 22, 182, 186
Intraocular pressure (IOP)-lowering drugs, 14, see
    also specific types
Intravitreal injections, 20, 96–97
Inulin, 184
Ionization, 176
Ion-pair formation, 124
IOP, see Intraocular pressure
Iridial sphincter muscle, 18
Iris, 2, 9, 17, 19
  anatomy of, 12–13
  distribution of drugs in, 185–186
  physiology of, 12–13
  vascularization of, 13
  weight of, 173
Iritis, 19
Irritants, 34, see also specific types
Irritation, 30, 33
Isotonic solutions, 32

K

Kanamycin, 30
KCS, see Keratoconjunctivitis sicca
Keratan sulfate, 5
Keratinization, 6
Keratitis, 46, 48
Keratoconjunctivitis sicca (KCS), 112, 114, 115
Ketone reductase, 130
Ketones, 135
Ketorolac tromethamine, 167
Ketoximes, 130, see also specific types
Kinetic models, 176
Kinetics, 45, 160, see also Pharmacokinetics
Krause glands, 7

L

L-643,799, 122
Lacrimal apparatus, 7–9
Lacrimal drainage, 87
Lacrimal fluid, 30, 31–32, 173
Lacrimal glands, 7, 33
Lacrimal secretion, 8

Lacrimation, 18, 30, 45, 111, 155
Lacrisert, 66, 68
Lactoferrin, 7
Lamellae, 62
Lamina cribrosa, 15, 17
Langerhans' cells, 6
Large unilamellar vesicles (LUVs), 92
Latex, 82, 83
Latices, 125
Lecithin:cholesterol:stearylamine, 95
Lectin-mediated binding of liposomes, 93
Lectins, 153, 154, see also specific types
Lens, 2, 9, 10, 20
    anatomy of, 14–15
    distribution of drugs in, 186–187
    opacification of, 14–15
    physiology of, 14–15
    weight of, 173
Lens capsule, 14, 15, 17, 20
Lens fibers, 14
LET, see Liposome-encapsulated tobramycin
Levator palpebrae superioris muscle, 6, 7
Levobunolol, 125, 136, 167
LHRH, see Luteinizing hormone-releasing hormone
Limbus, 3, 5, 6
Linear kinetics, 160
Lipids, 92, see also specific types
Lipophilic butylcyanoacrylate, 82
Lipophilicity, 132–133
Lipophilic substances, 19, 20, 44, see also specific
        types
Liposome constituents, 92–93
Liposome-encapsulated fluorescein, 97
Liposome-encapsulated tobramycin (LET), 96
Liposome encapsulation, 96, 97
Liposomes, 92, 93–97
    adhesive, 153
    anionic, 154
    binding of, 95, 96, 153
    biphasic nature of, 93
    components of, 92–93
    defined, 153
    empty, 95
    enzyme-containing, 95
    intravitreal injection of, 96–97
    lectin-mediated binding of, 93
    nanoparticles compared to, 99
    neutral, 154
    positively charged, 99
    in tears, 94
    temperature-sensitive, 97
    topical instillation of, 93–96
Local anesthesia, 30, 45, see also specific types
Luteinizing hormone-releasing hormone, 124
LUVs, see Large unilamellar vesicles
Lysosomal enzymes, 188, see also specific types
Lysozyme, 7

M

Maleic anhydride, 64
1,4-β,D-Mannuronic (alginic) acid, 69

MAO-inhibitors, 30, see also specific types
MAT, see Mean absorption time
Maximum penetration rate (MPR), 182, 183
Mean absorption time (MAT), 166
Mean residence time (MRT), 166
Meibomian glands, 7
Melanin, 12, 19, 186
Melanocytes, 6, 12, 17
Membrane-controlled reservoir inserts, 71–72
Membranes, 151, see also specific types
    anterior hyaloid, 17
    basement, 44
    Bowman's, 4, 5, 44
    Bruch's, 17
    conjunctival, 94
    corneal permeability and, 177
    Descemet's, 4, 5
    ethylene-vinyl acetate, 72
    hyaloid, 17
    nictitating, 2
    scleral, 94
Meprobamate, 30
Mercuric compounds, 30, see also specific types
Mercuric oxide, 30
Metabolic pathways to eye, 188
Methaoxedrine, 67
Methazolamide, 184
N-Methylacetazolamide, 130
Methylacrylic polymers, 66
Methylcellulose, 45, 67, 69
1'-Methylcyclopropanolytimolol, 133
Methyl mercury, 44
Methyl methacrylate, 71
Methylparaben, 44, 49
Methylprednisolone (MP), 69, 70
MIC, see Minimal inhibitory concentration
Minimal inhibitory concentration (MIC), 97
Miosis, 12
Miotics, 30, see also specific types
MLVs, see Multilamellar vesicles
Moll glands, 6
Monoamine oxidase, 188
Monoclonal antibody, 93
Monosodium phosphate, 32
Morphine, 67
MP, see Methylprednisolone
MPR, see Maximum penetration rate
MRT, see Mean residence time
Mucin, 6, 7, 28, 69, 112, 113, 151
Mucoadhesives, 69–70, 125, 150, 151, 154–155,
        see also specific types
Müller cells, 16
Müller's muscle, 6, 7
Multilamellar vesicles (MLVs), 92–95
Multiple linear regression models, 176
Muscle, see also specific types
    ciliary, 9, 10, 18, 20
    contraction of, 10
    dilator, 2, 12
    extraocular, 18
    iridial sphincter, 18
    levator palpebrae superioris, 6, 7

Müller's, 6, 7
  orbicularis oculi, 6
  sphincter, 2, 12, 18
Mydriasis, 12
Mydriatics, 30, see also specific types
Myopia, 14

N

Nadolol, 122, 184
Nanodispersions, 84
Nanoparticles, 70, 83, 97–98, 99–100
  bioadhesives and, 152
  defined, 97
  drug release from, 99
  liposomes compared to, 99
  residence time of, 99
Naphazoline, 30
Naphthyl esters, 176
Nasal mucosa, 125
Nasolacrimal occlusion, 125
Neomycin, 30
Neostigmine, 30
Neuronal transmission phenomena, 22
Neurons, 16, see also specific types
Neuropeptides, 3, 5, 12, 22, see also specific types
Nictitating membrane, 2
Nitrous oxide, 30
Noncompartmental modeling, 165–168
Nonionic detergents, 48
Nonionic surfactants, 30, 35, see also specific types
Nonisotomic solutions, 31
Nonsteroidal anti-inflammatory drugs (NSAIDs),
    172
NSAIDs, see Nonsteroidal anti-inflammatory drugs
Nutrition,

O

Ocular pemphigoid, 6
Ocusert, 71, 174
Opacification, 14–15
Ophthalmitis, 21
Ophthalmosystemic administration, 67
Opsin, 16
Optic nerve, 15–17
Orbicularis oculi muscle, 6
Organomercurials, 30, see also specific types
Osmolality, 31
Osmotically driven monolithic devices, 73
Ouabain, 20
Overdose, 92
Oxazolidines, 123, 135, see also specific types
5-Oxazolidinones, 124, see also specific types
Oxidoreductase, 188
Oxymetazoline, 125

P

PAA, see Polyacrylic acid
Painful force, 32
Para-aminoclonidine, 22

Paracellular pathways to corneal penetration, 133
Parahydroxybenzoic acid esters, 49
Pars plana, 14, 16, 17, 19, 20
Partition coefficients, 123, 132, 171
Penbutolol, 184
Penicillins, 20, 30, 48
Peptidases, 188, see also specific types
Peptides, 12, 124, 151, see also specific types
Permeability, 183, 184
  corneal, see Corneal permeability
pH, 31–32
  bioadhesives and, 154, 155
  corneal permeability and, 44, 45
  in situ gelling systems and, 81–88
  of solutions, 125
Phagocytosis, 17
Phakic eyes, 19
Pharmacokinetics, 159–188
  of anterior chamber disposition, 185–188
  of cefotaxime, 164–165
  classical modeling of, 160–173
    compartmental, 160–165
    flip-flop, 163
    limitations of, 172–173
    noncompartmental, 165–168
    physiologic, 169–172
  of clonidine, 165, 171
  compartmental modeling of, 160–165
  of corneal absorption, 176–183
  of distribution, 185–188
  of elimination, 185–188
  flip-flop model of, 163
  of fluorescein, 161
  noncompartmental modeling of, 165–168
  physiologic modeling of, 169–172
  of pilocarpine, 161–164, 170, 172, 175
  precorneal loss and, 173–175
  of scleral absorption, 183–185
Phenylephrine, 30, 122, 123, 125, 175, 177
2-Phenylethanol, 30
Phosphatidic acid, 96
Phosphatidylcholine, 96
Phospholipids, 92, see also specific types
Photoreceptors, 16, 17
Physiological aspects of ocular drug therapy, 19–22
Physiologic modeling, 169–172
Physiology, 3–18
  of anterior uvea, 9–15
  of chamber angle, 9–15
  of chamber system, 9–15
  of choroid, 17–18
  of ciliary body, 10–12
  of conjuctiva, 5–8
  of cornea, 3–5, 44
  of extraocular orbital structures, 18
  of eyelids, 5–8
  of iris, 12–13
  of lacrimal apparatus, 7–9
  of lens, 14–15
  of optic nerve, 15–17
  of posterior segment of eye, 15–18
  of retina, 15–17

of Schlemm's canal, 13
of sclera, 17–18
of trabecular meshwork, 13
of vitreous, 17
Pigment epithelium, 16, 17, 21
Pilocarpine, 10, 30, 45, 49
   bioadhesives and, 153
   bioavailability of, 176
   degradation of, 186
   distribution of, 186
   duration of action of, 125
   half-life of, 172
   hyaluronic acid and, 115, 116
   nanoparticles and, 100
   pharmacokinetics of, 161–164, 170, 172, 175
   precorneal loss of, 175
   prodrugs and, 122, 137
   solid polymeric inserts and, 64, 65
   systemic absorption of, 125
Pilocarpine hydrochloride, 88
Pilocarpine nitrate, 175
Pilopine H.S., 174
O-Pivaloyltimolol, 133
Plica semilunaris, 5
PMMA, see Polymethylmethacrylate
Polyacrylic acid (PAA), 65, 67, 69
Polyalkylcyanoacrylates, 70, 98, 99, 153
Polyanhydrides, 64
Polybutylcyanoacrylate, 100
Polycarbophil, 69, 151, 154
Poly-hexyl-2-cyanoacrylate, 99
Polyisohexylcyanoacrylate, 99
Polymeric dispersions, 82, 83, 87
Polymeric inserts, see Solid polymeric inserts
Polymerization, 98
Polymers, 99, 151, 152, 154, see also specific types
Polymethylmethacrylate (PMMA), 82
Polymyxin B, 30, 71
Poly(ortho esters), 64
Polypeptides, 18, 68, see also specific types
Polyvinylalcohol (PVA), 35, 64, 65, 66, 67, 70
   hyaluronic acid and, 111, 112
Polyvinylpyrrolidone (PVP), 35, 66, 71, 111, 112
Posterior chamber, 10, 17, 19, 21
Posterior segment of eye, 3, see also specific parts
Precorneal loss, 173–175
Precorneal residence time, 106, 109–113
Prednisolone acetate, 68, 122, 173
Presbyopia, 14
Preservatives, 30, 34, 93, see also specific types
   corneal penetration and, 136
   corneal permeability and, 44, 46–52
   dry eye and, 113
   systemic absorption and, 125
Pressure, 13, see also specific types
   intraocular, see Intraocular pressure (IOP)
Prodrugs, 4, 121–137, see also specific types
   activation of, 130–131
   amide, 129
   applications of, 122–128
   aqueous solubility and, 133–134
   chemical stability and, 134–135

corneal penetration and, 122–124, 132, 136
design of, 131–135
development of, 188
double (pro-prodrugs), 135
duration of action and, 125
enzymes in activation of, 130–131
esterases and, 188
formulation of, 136
functional groups amenable to derivatization by,
   129–130
in inserts, 70
lipophilicity and, 132–133
physicochemical considerations in design of,
   131–135
side effects and, 122, 123, 128
systemic absorption and, 125–128
toxicity of, 136–137
Proliferative vitreoretinopathy, 96
Propranolol, 130, 184
Pro-prodrugs (double prodrug formation), 135
Propylparaben, 44, 49
Prostaglandin F, 14, 19, 122, 128, 136
Prostaglandins, 9, 14, 20, 22, 128, see also specific
   types
Proteins, 12, 14, 30, 92, 98, see also specific types
Pseudolatex, 82
Pseudolatices, 82
Pseudophakic eyes, 20
Pseudoplastic behavior, 108, 113
Pseudoplastic character of tears, 32
Punctate keratitis, 46, 48
Pupils, 9, 19
PVA, see Polyvinylalcohol
PVP, see Polyvinylpyrrolidone

R

Radioactivity, 28, 99
Rapid loading of drugs, 92
Reflection coefficient, 20
Refractive power, 3, 10, 14
Residence time, 34–36, 69, 87
   hyaluronic acid and, 106
   of nanoparticles, 99
   precorneal, 106, 109–113
Retention of drugs, 29–33, 68
Retina, 2, 15–17, 19, 21, 188
all-trans-Retinal, 16
11-cis-Retinal, 16
Retinal pigment epithelium, 17
Retinitis, 96
Retrobulbar anesthesia, 18
Retrobulbar injection, 19, 20
Reverse phase evaporation method, 96
Rhodamine B, 186
Rhodopsin, 16
Rods, 16

S

Salting-out processes, 82, 83
SCC, see Short circuit current

Schlemm's canal, 2, 9, 13
Scintigraphy, 87, 99, 111, 112
Sclera, 2, 13, 20
  absorption in, 183–185
  anatomy of, 17–18
  as barrier to drugs, 19
  physiology of, 17–18
  weight of, 173
Scleral membranes, 94
Scleral permeability, 183, 184
Scopolamine, 30
SH (sodium hyaluronic acid), see Hyaluronic acid
Short circuit current (SCC), 46, 49
Sialic acids, 153
Side effects, 92, 122, 123, 128
Silicone reservoir devices, 73
Silver compounds, 30, see also specific types
Silver nitrate, 30
Silver protein, 30
Slow release artificial tears (SRAT), 67, 68
SLS, see Sodium lauryl sulfate
Small unilamellar vesicles (SUVs), 92, 93, 94
SODIs, see Soluble ophthalmic drug inserts
Sodium, 45
Sodium bisulfite, 44, 51
Sodium dodecylsulfate, 48
Sodium fluorescein, 4
Sodium hyaluronate, 35
Sodium hyaluronic acid (SH), see Hyaluronic acid
Sodium lauryl sulfate (SLS), 35, 48
Sodium/postassium ATPase, 10
Soflens, 71
Soft contact lenses, 71, 125
Soft drugs, 128
Solid polymeric inserts, 61–74, see also specific
    types
  advantages of, 63
  defined, 62
  history of, 62–63
  insoluble, 70–73
  naturally occurring polymers in, 68–69
  prodrugs in, 70
  semisynthetic, 64–68
  soluble, 63–70
  synthetic, 64–68
Soluble ophthalmic drug inserts (SODIs), 64, 65,
    see also specific types
Soluble solid polymeric inserts, 63–70, see also
    specific types
Solutions, see also specific types
  administration of, 36
  contact lens cleaning, 48
  elimination of, 28–29
  emulsification of, 82
  formulation of, 34
  of hyaluronic acid, 109
  hypertonic, 31
  hypotonic, 31
  isotonic, 32
  nonisotonic, 31
  pH of, 125
  residence of, 34–36

viscosity of, 32–33
  viscous, 125
Sorbic acid, 44, 51
Sphincter muscle, 2, 12, 18
SRAT, see Slow release artificial tears
Stearylamine, 95
Steroids, 68, 95, 122, 128, 132, 176, 188, see also
    specific types
Streptomycin, 30
Stroma, 4, 5, 176
Subconjunctival injection, 20, 97
Substance P, 5, 12, 22
Sucrose, 184
Sulfacetamide, 177
Sulfate transferase, 188
Sulfonamides, 30, 130, 186, see also specific types
Suprachoroidal space, 9, 18
Supraciliary space, 9
Surface tension, 30, 35
Surfactants, 35, see also specific types
  ampholytic, 30
  anionic, 30
  cationic, 46, 48
  corneal permeability and, 44, 46–48
  irritation power of, 30
  nonionic, 30, 35
Suspensions, 28, 33, see also specific types
SUVs, see Small unilamellar vesicles
Swelling-controlled devices, 64
Sympathetic ophthalmitis, 21
Sympathomimetics, 7, 30, see also specific types
Systemic absorption, 125–128
Systemic administration, 19, 30, 97

T

Tableting, 66
Tarsus of eyelids, 7
Tear film, 7, 68, 112, 113
Tear fluid, 7, 9, 31
Tear fluid proteins, 92
Tears, 28
  chemical composition of, 8
  composition of, 7, 8
  flow of, 9, 87
  physical properties of, 8
  pseudoplastic character of, 32
  secretion of, 30
  slow release artificial, 68
  systemic administration and, 30
  turnover in, 92, 155
  viscosity of, 32
TEL (tobramycin and liposome-encapsulated saline
    mixture), 96–97
Temperature-sensitive liposomes, 97
Tenon's capsule, 18
Terbutaline, 122, 125
Tetrahydrocannabinol, 125
Thimerosal, 44, 48–49
Thrombin, 154
Thyrotropin-releasing hormone, 124
Timolol, 19, 70, 72, 122, 126, 132

irritant properties of, 30
  scleral penetration of, 184
Tobramycin, 30, 96, 97, 177
Tobramycin phosphate-buffered saline, 96
α-Tocopherol, 96
Tolerance, 68
Tonicity, 44, 45, 125, 155
Topical instillation of liposomes, 93–96
Toxicity of prodrugs, 136–137
Toxicology, 47
Trabecular meshwork, 9, 10, 13, 19, 20
Tranquilizers, 30, see also specific types
Transcellular pathways to corneal penetration, 133
TRH, see Thyrotropin-releasing hormone
Triamcinolone acetonide, 94
Tricyclic antidepressants, 30, see also specific types
Trisodium phosphate, 32
Tropicamide, 30, 69, 111, 117

U

Unilamellar vesicles, 92, 93, see also specific types
Uridine 5′-diphospho *N*-acetyl glucosamine, 117
Uridine 5′-diphosphoglucuronic acid, 117
Uveal meshwork, 13
Uveoscleral outflow, 9, 12, 14

V

Vascular effects, 12
Vascular endothelium in retina, 19
Vasoactive intestinal polypeptide (VIP), 18
Vasoconstrictors, 67, 125, see also specific types

Veins, 13
Verapamil, 22
Vidarabine, 122
Vinyl acetate, 71
Vinyl methyl ether, 64
VIP, see Vasoactive intestinal polypeptide
Viruses, 93, 96, see also specific types
Viscoelasticity, 33, 35, 108
Viscolyzers, 30, 33, 35, see also specific types
Viscosity, 32–33, 108, 154
Viscosity-enhancing materials, 44, 45, see also
  specific types
Viscosity-inducing agents, 93, see also specific
  types
Viscosurgery, 108
Viscous solutions, 125
Vitreoretinopathies, 20, 96
Vitreous, 2, 14, 17, 19, 20–21
Vitreous humor, 173

W

Water soluble substances, 19, 20, see also specific
  types
Wolfring glands, 7

X

Xanthan gum, 66

Z

Zeis glands, 6, 7
Zonules of Zinn, 14

Printed in the United States
by Baker & Taylor Publisher Services